Depressive Disorder

Won-Myong Bahk • Moon-Doo Kim
Young Sup Woo • Young-Eun Jung
Editors

Depressive Disorder

Bridging Clinical Practice and Evidence-Based Research

Springer

Editors
Won-Myong Bahk
Department of Psychiatry
College of Medicine,
The Catholic University of Korea
Seoul, Korea (Republic of)

Woo and Bahk Psychiatry Clinic
Seoul, Korea (Republic of)

Young Sup Woo
Woo and Bahk Psychiatry Clinic
Seoul, Korea (Republic of)

Moon-Doo Kim
Department of Psychiatry
Jeju National University Hospital,
School of Medicine,
Jeju National University
Jeju, Korea (Republic of)

Young-Eun Jung
Department of Psychiatry
Jeju National University Hospital,
School of Medicine,
Jeju National University
Jeju, Korea (Republic of)

ISBN 978-981-92-1330-6   ISBN 978-981-92-1331-3 (eBook)
https://doi.org/10.1007/978-981-92-1331-3

English translation of the 3rd original Korean edition published by KOONJA PUBLISHING INC., Paju-si, 2023

This Springer imprint is published by the registered company Springer Nature Singapore Pte Ltd.
The registered company address is: 152 Beach Road, #21-01/04 Gateway East, Singapore 189721, Singapore

Preface

Clinical Complexity and Scientific Rigor: New Evidence-Based Insights into Depressive Disorders

Bridging Clinical Complexity and Scientific Rigor in Depressive Disorders

Depressive disorders remain among the most extensively investigated yet persistently challenging conditions in contemporary psychiatry. Despite decades of accumulated research, the lived clinical reality of depression continues to exceed the explanatory power of any single theoretical framework. For many years, the monoamine hypothesis provided a coherent and productive foundation for both scientific inquiry and pharmacological innovation. It guided generations of clinicians and researchers in conceptualizing depressive symptomatology and in developing antidepressant therapies targeting serotonergic and noradrenergic systems.

Yet, as we engage daily with patients in clinical practice, it becomes increasingly evident that depressive disorders cannot be adequately reduced to disturbances in monoamine neurotransmission alone. The heterogeneity of symptom profiles, variability in treatment response, and the frequent coexistence of medical and psychiatric comorbidities compel us to adopt a broader and more integrative perspective. We are currently witnessing a paradigmatic shift—from a predominantly monoaminergic model toward multidimensional frameworks encompassing neuroanatomical circuitry, neuroinflammation, synaptic plasticity, neuroendocrine regulation, and rapidly acting therapeutic agents such as glutamatergic modulators. This evolution reflects not only advances in neuroscience but also a growing recognition of depression as a disorder of complex systems rather than isolated chemical imbalance.

Beyond Didactic Structure: Addressing the Questions That Arise in Practice

Understanding Depressive Disorder: Evidence-Based Insights for Clinicians and Researchers was conceived with a deliberate intention: to move beyond the conventional architecture of traditional textbooks. Foundational manuals remain indispensable for training and reference; however, they often emphasize diagnostic categories and standardized treatment algorithms without sufficiently addressing the ambiguities and controversies that characterize real-world practice.

In clinical settings, the questions we confront extend far beyond diagnostic criteria. We encounter patients with treatment-resistant depression who have undergone multiple pharmacological trials without sustained remission. We navigate depressive episodes accompanied by mixed features, subthreshold hypomanic symptoms, or fluctuating affective instability. We manage depression in the context of chronic pain syndromes, metabolic disorders such as obesity, neurocognitive aging, and the hormonal transitions associated with adolescence, pregnancy, postpartum states, and menopause. These scenarios demand nuanced judgment that integrates empirical evidence with individualized clinical reasoning.

In selecting the themes for this volume, we prioritized areas that are both clinically consequential and intellectually contested. Topics such as the therapeutic potential of psychedelic-assisted interventions, the role of the gut–brain axis and microbiome, neuroimmune mechanisms, and the transgenerational transmission of trauma represent domains where emerging data are reshaping conceptual boundaries. While certain discussions necessarily engage with evolving hypotheses rather than definitive consensus, we believe that responsible engagement with developing science is essential in a field characterized by rapid advancement. Our objective has been to synthesize the best available evidence while maintaining transparency regarding its current limitations.

Editorial Perspective: Integrating Clinical Intuition and Scientific Evidence

The impetus for this volume arose not from abstract academic ambition but from the reflective moments inherent in clinical practice. There is a distinct professional unease that arises when evidence-based guidelines—though indispensable—do not yield meaningful improvement for a particular patient. In such circumstances, we are reminded that randomized controlled trials provide population-level averages, whereas clinical care unfolds within the singular and multidimensional context of an individual life.

We have repeatedly observed that treatment outcomes are shaped by factors extending beyond symptom checklists: aging processes, medical comorbidities, psychosocial stressors, family psychiatric history, and cultural context. The challenge, therefore, is not to abandon evidence-based medicine, but to interpret and apply it with methodological rigor and clinical humility.

In assembling this work, we collaborated with leading experts who contribute actively to both national and international academic discourse. Many are established scholars within Korea's psychiatric community, while remaining deeply engaged in global scientific dialogue. Through this collective effort, we have sought to produce a volume that is empirically grounded, methodologically robust, and attentive to the lived experience of patients.

Concluding Reflections

This book is intended for psychiatrists, clinical researchers, trainees, and allied mental health professionals, including clinical psychologists, psychiatric nurses, and interdisciplinary clinicians, who seek a deeper and more integrative understanding of depressive disorders. Above all, it is dedicated to clinicians who persist in asking difficult questions and to patients and families whose resilience continually challenges and refines our scientific assumptions.

We hope that this volume serves not only as a reference grounded in contemporary evidence, but also as a framework for thoughtful clinical reasoning when standardized answers prove insufficient. In bridging scientific rigor with clinical complexity, we aspire to contribute meaningfully to the evolving understanding and treatment of depressive disorders.

Seoul, Republic of Korea — Won-Myong Bahk
Jeju, Republic of Korea — Moon-Doo Kim
Seoul, Republic of Korea — Young Sup Woo
Jeju, Republic of Korea — Young-Eun Jung

Contents

Part I

Concepts and Diagnosis

Unipolar Depression and Bipolar Depression

1

Sung Man Chang and Inki Sohn

1.1 History

When a patient presents with a current depressive episode, it is difficult to clearly distinguish unipolar depression from bipolar depression on cross-sectional evaluation alone, and this controversy goes back at least to the era of Kraepelin. Traditionally, mood disorders were divided into depressive states, marked by low mood, and manic states, characterized by elevated mood. Hippocrates provided systematic descriptions of mania and depression and introduced the term melancholia. Around the first century Aretaeus noted the interrelationship between depression and mania, arguing that depression might progress into mania. In the 1850s, modern conceptions of bipolar disorder emerged: Falret and Baillarger described that depression and mania may alternate in the same person—Falret termed this folie circulaire (circular insanity), and three years later Baillarger proposed la folie à double forme (dual-form insanity). Their ideas remain strikingly consistent with the contemporary concept of bipolar disorder. Kraepelin regarded depression and circular insanity as symptom expressions of a single illness—manic-depressive illness—rather than separating unipolar depression, mania, and hypomania as distinct entities. Until the mid-1950s, this broad rubric framed bipolar disorder. However, in 1957, Leonhard distinguished unipolar depression, characterized by recurrent depressive episodes only, from bipolar depression, which encompasses both depressive and manic episodes. By 1966, the notion that bipolar disorder was distinct from unipolar disorder was established by Jules Angst, Carlo Perris, and Winokur, and was subsequently codified in international diagnostic systems such as the International Classification of Diseases (ICD) and Diagnostic and Statistical Manual of Mental Disorders (DSM) in the early 1980s, where it remains so today.

Even now, ongoing research continues to refine these two concepts to better account for treatment and prognosis. Key questions include how far to broaden the diagnostic boundaries of bipolar disorder and how to further subdivide unipolar depression. Conceptual uncertainty persists, particularly in pediatric and adolescent mood disorders, which present with diverse forms and defy precise definition. Ongoing efforts aim to define bipolar spectrum states—conditions that display (hypo)manic elements yet fall short of the full diagnostic threshold for hypomania or mania—with greater clarity.

S. M. Chang (✉)
Department of Psychiatry, School of Medicine, Kyungpook National University, Daegu, Republic of Korea
e-mail: psyjang@knu.ac.kr

I. Sohn
Department of Psychiatry, Keyo Hospital, Uiwang, Republic of Korea

W.-M. Bahk et al. (eds.), *Depressive Disorder*, https://doi.org/10.1007/978-981-92-1331-3_1

1.2 Development of Diagnostic Systems and Classification

The historical distinction between unipolar and bipolar depression was formalized in modern diagnostic systems. The DSM-III (1980) was the first to formally adopt the term *bipolar disorder*, replacing the earlier category of *manic-depressive illness* and thereby underscoring its nosological separation from unipolar depression. Later, the ICD-10 (1992) further delineated this distinction, and the DSM-5 (2013) reinforced it by presenting unipolar depression (major depressive disorder) and bipolar disorder as distinct diagnostic entities with specific criteria. This evolution in classification has provided a standardized framework for clinical practice and research, linking historical observations with contemporary psychiatric nosology.

1.3 Epidemiology

Earlier studies reported the prevalence of bipolar disorder to be about 1.5% [1]. More recent work suggests that when bipolar spectrum disorders are included—defined as clinically significant mood fluctuations that do not meet full criteria for bipolar I or II—the prevalence may reach 5.5% [2]. An increase in recognized bipolar disorder inversely reduces the apparent prevalence of unipolar depression. Patients initially diagnosed with unipolar depression may be reclassified as bipolar disorder if subsequent (hypo) manic episodes are identified. Indeed, epidemiologic studies often initially register patients as depressed; in high-risk groups, further interviews frequently lead to reclassification.

In the World Health Organization (WHO) World Mental Health Survey Initiative synthesizing data from 11 countries, lifetime prevalence estimates were 0.6% for bipolar I, 0.4% for bipolar II, and 1.4% for subthreshold bipolar disorder. Taken together, the bipolar spectrum prevalence was 2.4% [3]. Although this broader conception continues to evolve—and is sometimes criticized for fostering overdiagnosis and overtreatment—bipolar depression is now recognized as more common than previously thought and frequently encountered in clinical practice.

Genetically, bipolar depression shows stronger familial aggregation and greater genetic vulnerability than unipolar depression. First-degree relatives of individuals with bipolar disorder have a five- to tenfold increased risk compared with the general population, and concordance for mood disorder among monozygotic twins of bipolar patients is 45–75 versus 15–25% in unipolar depression [4]. The sex ratio in bipolar disorder is approximately equal (1:1). Recent epidemiological work similarly reports prevalence of bipolar I at 0.8% in men versus 1.1% in women, bipolar II at 0.9 versus 1.3%, and subthreshold bipolar at 2.6 versus 2.1% [5]. By contrast, unipolar depression shows a sex ratio of roughly 1:1.7, with a higher prevalence in women [6].

1.4 Misdiagnosis of Bipolar Depression

Most individuals with bipolar disorder first present with a depressive episode, and many are initially misdiagnosed with unipolar depression. With DSM-5, bipolar disorder concepts were clarified and the diagnostic criteria for mania and hypomania were revised compared with DSM-IV [7]. Notably, the DSM-IV category of *bipolar disorder not otherwise specified* was replaced with *other specified bipolar and related disorder*. This category provides explicit criteria for cases showing bipolar features without meeting full criteria for a specific bipolar subtype—such as short-duration hypomanic episodes with major depressive episodes, hypomanic episodes with insufficient symptoms with major depressive episodes, hypomanic episodes without a history of major depression, and cyclothymia under 24 months. Although application of DSM-5 may increase recognition of bipolar depression, in clinical practice the prevailing view remains that a manic or hypomanic episode is essential for a definitive bipolar diagnosis, as in DSM-IV. Diagnostic challenges include clinicians' failure to detect prior (hypo)manic episodes and patients' denial or unawareness of them. Despite their diagnostic centrality, (hypo) manic episodes are often overlooked.

In early stages, approximately 10–40% of patients with bipolar depression are misdiagnosed as having other depressive disorders [8]. Misdiagnosis is particularly frequent early in the illness course, especially in the absence of collateral information from close contacts. Patients often do not report (hypo)manic episodes, as the associated increases in mood, energy, libido, or activity are often not perceived as pathological and may even be experienced as desirable. Collateral information from family or friends who know the patient's mood cycles, particularly during (hypo)mania, can be extremely helpful. Rigid application of (hypo)manic criteria or reliance solely on symptom checklists without collateral information can obscure bipolar depression. On average, there is a 5–10 year lag from the onset of depression to a correct bipolar diagnosis and appropriate treatment [9].

1.5 Duration of Episodes

In general, depressive episodes are shorter in bipolar disorder than in unipolar depression [10]. Although reported durations vary, meta-analyses indicate that the median duration of major depressive episodes in unipolar depression ranges from 3 to 12 months (or longer), with 10–30% showing a chronic course [11]. Variability likely reflects methodological biases—such as variable definitions of recovery, differing inclusion windows, and mixing inpatient with outpatient samples—which may overestimate chronicity. Recent studies report median durations of about 3 months [11] and 4 months (17.3 weeks) [12] for unipolar depression.

Without distinguishing polarity, Angst and colleagues estimated a mean episode duration of 3–6 months in bipolar disorder [13]. Among patients with bipolar I disorder, the median duration of depressive episodes was 13 weeks [14]. In longitudinal cohorts of recurrent depression, the longest depressive episode averaged 26 weeks in bipolar disorder versus 69 weeks in unipolar depression [15]. Naturalistic follow-up shows that 44% of major depressive episodes remit within 8 weeks and 78% recover within 1 year in bipolar disorder [16, 17].

1.6 Clinical Features

Phenomenological features of bipolar and unipolar depression have long attracted attention and have gained importance with the advent of new therapies. A wide array of depressive symptoms observed in unipolar depression can also occur during depressive phases of bipolar disorder, and distinguishing the two based on symptoms alone remains challenging. Although early views posited no differences, many subsequent studies have identified distinctions. However, limitations include samples not meeting full bipolar I criteria and inconsistent findings across investigators [10, 18].

Despite these limitations, some generalizations are possible. Unipolar depression tends to have a longer illness duration, greater severity, absence of qualitative mood change, more frequent initial insomnia, more weight loss, greater indecisiveness, and more somatic complaints than bipolar depression. By contrast, bipolar depression is more often associated with diurnal mood variation (worse in the morning), mood instability, and derealization (Table 1.1). Regarding psychomotor signs, agitation and observable anxiety-related activity are reported more often in unipolar depression, although findings vary. Psychotic symptoms, irritability, and aggression are reported more frequently in bipolar depression, although opposite findings have also been reported [10]. Such discrepancies likely reflect reliance on cross-sectional observation, which carries a risk of false-positive conclusions (Type I error) [10].

Longitudinal follow-up of patients initially diagnosed with unipolar depression provides further insight. Psychotic symptoms during the index depressive episode and multiple prior hospitalizations predict later conversion to bipolar I [19]. Prominent psychic anxiety, concentration difficulties, social withdrawal, and feelings of

Table 1.1 Research findings on phenomenological differences between bipolar and unipolar depression

Category	Clinical feature	Unipolar > Bipolar	Bipolar > Unipolar	Similar/Mixed
Episode	Duration	✓ [18, 21]		
Symptom	Severity of depression	✓ [22]		
	Unvarying depression	✓ [23]	✓ [18]	
	Suicidal thoughts/attempts	✓ [18, 23]		
	Initial insomnia	✓ [18, 23]		
	Weight loss	✓ [21]		
	Muddled thoughts	✓ [23]		
	Somatic complaints	✓ [22]	✓ [23]	✓ [24]
	Depression worse in morning		✓ [23]	
	Lability of mood		✓ [23]	
	Mania score		✓ [21]	
	Derealization		✓ [23]	
	Pathological guilt		✓ [25]	
	Psychotic features		✓ [18, 26]	✓ [27]
Mental state	Activity	✓ [28]		
	Agitation	✓ [22]	✓ [21]	
	Retardation		✓ [18]	✓ [29]
	Observed anxiety	✓ [23]		
	Anger/aggression	✓ [30]	✓ [21]	
	Arrogant attitude		✓ [23]	

Authors' synthesis based on multiple sources (see References [18, 21–30])

frustration also predict conversion to bipolar I, whereas mood instability during depressive episodes is more characteristic of conversion to bipolar II [20].

Additional Clinical Findings Suggestive of Bipolar Depression

Other findings suggestive of bipolar depression include onset in adolescence or young adulthood (before age 25), atypical depressive symptoms such as hypersomnia and weight gain, psychomotor retardation and psychotic features, and comorbid substance abuse [10]. A family history of bipolar disorder also increases the likelihood of bipolar depression. Frequent recurrence (≥3 episodes), short illness duration (≤3 months), and antidepressant-induced (hypo)mania are likewise indicative of bipolarity [31]. In bipolar depression, it is common for mixed-episode symptoms or hypomanic features to be present even during depressive episodes [32]. Loss of sustained antidepressant response after initial improvement is another clinical clue [31]. Although anxiety symptoms and anxiety disorders are common in unipolar depression, bipolar depression also frequently co-occurs with panic disorder and obsessive-compulsive disorder [33]. Such anxiety disorders may constitute prodromal features of bipolar depression [34].

The risk of postpartum mood disorders is notably high. Postpartum psychosis may represent an extreme manifestation of an underlying bipolar diathesis [35], and postpartum depression is approximately 2.5 times more likely to reflect bipolar rather than unipolar depression [36]. A history of postpartum depression therefore suggests a bipolar spectrum condition. Many women with bipolar disorder experience their first clini-

Table 1.2 Findings suggestive of bipolar disorder

	Bipolar	Unipolar
Substance abuse	+++	++
Family history of bipolar disorder	+++	++
Seasonality	++	+
Onset before age 25	+++	+
Postpartum psychiatric illness	+++	+
Psychotic symptoms before age 35	+++	±
Atypical features	++	+
Episodic course with rapid onset and remission	+++	±
Frequent recurrent major depression (≥3 episodes)	++	±
Short duration of major depressive episodes (≤3 months)	+++	±
Antidepressant-induced (hypo) mania	+++	±
Loss of antidepressant efficacy	+++	±
Mixed depression (hypomanic elements during depressive episodes):	+++	-

Scoring symbols: +++ strong; ++ moderate; + weak; ± possible; – absent.
Authors' synthesis based on multiple sources (see References [10, 31–37])

cal symptoms during the postpartum period [37], and women with prior postpartum depression should be monitored closely over follow-up for potential progression to bipolar disorder. These findings are summarized in Table 1.2.

1.7 Treatment-Resistant Depression and Risk of Bipolar Disorder

When treating a patient with depression unresponsive to antidepressants, an underlying bipolar disorder should be one of the first differential diagnoses considered. In a prospective cohort of 599 patients with antidepressant-resistant depression followed for up to 11 years, 12.5% ($n = 70$) were ultimately diagnosed with bipolar disorder [20]. Among those who failed at least two antidepressant classes, 35% were re-diagnosed as bipolar within the first year, 52% within 10 years of follow-up, and nearly 80% by study end [38]. In another study with a mean follow-up of 5.6 years, about 38% of patients with treatment-resistant depression experienced manic or hypomanic episodes [39]. These findings underscore the importance of considering bipolarity in the management of antidepressant-resistant depression. Indeed, treatment resistance itself may be an important clinical clue suggestive of bipolar depression.

Today, the bipolar concept has expanded into a bipolar spectrum. Drawing on clinical studies, various investigators have proposed broadened definitions. Ghaemi and colleagues defined bipolar spectrum disorder as a condition that does not fully meet criteria for unipolar depression or bipolar I disorder but lies along the continuum between them [31]. Bipolar spectrum disorder can be considered in patients who have experienced at least one major depressive episode but have had no spontaneous hypomanic or manic episodes. Support for this diagnosis increases when either a first-degree family history of bipolar disorder or an antidepressant-induced hypomanic/manic switch is present together with at least two additional features, or when both of these are present together with at least one additional feature. When neither a family history nor an antidepressant-induced switch is present, at least six of the following nine features are suggested: hyperthymic temperament in the euthymic state; recurrent major depressive episodes; brief depressive episodes averaging less than three months; atypical depressive symptoms (DSM-IV); psychotic depression; onset of the first major depressive episode before age 25; postpartum depression; loss of sustained antidepressant benefit over time (acute response without prophylactic effect); and nonresponse to three or more adequate antidepressant trials [31]. Accordingly, when such features are observed in patients presenting with depressive episodes, they may be considered suggestive of bipolar depression.

1.8 Neuropsychological Assessment

Neuropsychological test findings overlap substantially between unipolar and bipolar depression. Both are primarily associated with impairments in memory and executive function [40]. Nevertheless, some domains differ.

Compared with unipolar depression, bipolar depression demonstrates more severe deficits in sustained attention, immediate recall, and delayed recall [41]. Executive dysfunction occurs in both conditions, but patients with bipolar depression exhibit poorer performance in concept formation, problem-solving, and judgment [42].

In verbal fluency tasks, patients with unipolar depression exhibit both semantic and phonemic fluency deficits, whereas those with bipolar depression demonstrate selective impairment in semantic fluency alone [43]. Deficits in early information processing—such as inspection time and reaction time—are seen in both disorders [44], suggesting shared neural substrates for depressive symptom expression. These deficits are thought by some to represent trait rather than state markers, whereas overall intelligence remains largely preserved [45].

1.9 Suicide and Suicide Attempts

Misdiagnosis of bipolar depression can have grave—and even fatal—consequences, with suicide being the most devastating. Patients with bipolar disorder attempt suicide at higher rates than those with unipolar depression—lifetime attempt rates of 26–29% versus 14–16%, respectively [46]. Kessler and colleagues reported a lifetime suicide-attempt rate of 48% in bipolar I disorder [47]. Suicide in bipolar disorder occurs far more frequently during depressive than (hypo) manic episodes—approximately 30-fold more often [48]. The rate of completed suicide is likewise high in bipolar disorder, estimated at 10–19% [49]. A meta-analysis of suicide across psychiatric disorders found suicide rates more than 15-fold higher than the general population in bipolar disorder and more than 20-fold higher in major depression [50]. While patients with bipolar disorder have higher attempt rates, the overall population burden of suicide is higher in unipolar depression due to its greater prevalence.

1.10 Use of Screening Tools

In differentiating bipolar from unipolar depression, careful history taking is paramount. To uncover latent bipolarity among depressed patients, clinicians should ascertain family history of bipolar disorder; obtain collateral information from close contacts about past manic or hypomanic episodes; review not only the diagnostic criteria for a depressive episode but also the manic criteria that may co-occur; and consider standardized screening tools. The most widely used instruments include the Mood Disorder Questionnaire (MDQ), the Bipolar Spectrum Diagnostic Scale (BSDS), and the Hypomania Checklist-32 (HCL-32).

1.11 Use of Antidepressants in the Treatment of Bipolar Depression

In bipolar disorder, pharmacotherapy varies by episode type and inter-episode period, and treatment algorithms have been revised stepwise as evidence accumulates. There remains no clear consensus on antidepressant use in bipolar depression, and skepticism is common. Concerns include iatrogenic induction of (hypo) mania and promotion of rapid cycling. Accordingly, most guidelines and reviews recommend mood stabilizers such as lithium or valproate as first-line during depressive episodes, rather than antidepressants; lamotrigine and quetiapine are also recognized first-line options. If antidepressants are used, they should be considered second-line and always combined with a mood stabilizer to reduce switch risk [51].

A systematic review of randomized controlled trials examined the efficacy and safety of antidepressants in bipolar depression, including a meta-analysis of 12 randomized controlled studies that found significant improvement over 4–10 weeks [52]. Importantly, the risk of early manic switching was not higher with antidepressants than with placebo: 3.8 versus 4.7%, respectively. However, tricyclic antidepressants (TCAs) carried a higher switch rate (10%) compared with Selective Serotonin Reuptake Inhibitors (SSRIs) (3.2%). A major limitation is that approximately 75% of subjects were concurrently taking mood stabilizers or atypical antipsychotics [52].

In a large randomized trial comparing mood stabilizer monotherapy with adjunctive paroxetine or bupropion in bipolar depression, there was no advantage to adding antidepressants, as sustained recovery rates at 26 weeks did not differ [53]. Another study comparing adjunctive venlafaxine, bupropion, and sertraline found significantly higher rates of (hypo)manic switching with venlafaxine than with the other two agents, particularly in rapid-cycling patients [54]. Thus, in bipolar depression—especially in those with a history of rapid cycling—venlafaxine should be used with greater caution than bupropion or sertraline.

Maintenance therapy to prevent relapse is of major clinical importance in bipolar disorder. The efficacy of mood stabilizers and atypical antipsychotics for maintenance is well established. However, evidence supporting long-term antidepressant use for relapse prevention remains weak. A systematic review of seven randomized trials ($n = 363$) in bipolar I and II found no clear benefit to adding long-term antidepressants to lithium; antidepressant monotherapy without a mood stabilizer was likewise ineffective [55]. Moreover, prolonged antidepressant exposure may precipitate mixed episodes and mood instability. In sum, while some studies demonstrate short-term efficacy of antidepressants in bipolar depression, recent large-scale studies caution that benefits may be minimal and switch risks increased. Quetiapine, lamotrigine, and lurasidone are recommended as alternatives. If antidepressants are used, they should be combined with a mood stabilizer or atypical antipsychotic, and SSRIs or bupropion are generally preferred over TCAs or venlafaxine.

More recent international treatment guidelines have increasingly de-emphasized antidepressants in the management of bipolar depression. Contemporary guidelines—including updates from the Canadian Network for Mood and Anxiety Treatments (CANMAT)/ International Society for Bipolar Disorders (ISBD) and other expert consensus statements—recommend mood stabilizers and selected second-generation antipsychotics as first-line treatments, with antidepressants reserved for carefully selected cases and only as adjunctive therapy. In this context, agents such as lurasidone, quetiapine, and lamotrigine have emerged as evidence-based options with demonstrated efficacy for acute bipolar depression and a lower risk of mood switching.

In particular, lurasidone has been supported by multiple randomized controlled trials demonstrating efficacy both as monotherapy and as adjunctive treatment to lithium or valproate, with a favorable metabolic and tolerability profile [56]. Similarly, cariprazine, a dopamine D3-preferring partial agonist, has shown efficacy in bipolar depression at lower dose ranges, further expanding pharmacological options beyond traditional mood stabilizers and antidepressants [57]. These developments have shifted treatment paradigms toward earlier use of atypical antipsychotics with established antidepressant effects, rather than reliance on conventional antidepressants.

Accordingly, while antidepressants may still have a limited role in selected patients—particularly those without a history of antidepressant-induced switching and with predominant depressive polarity—their use should be cautious, time-limited, and always combined with a mood stabilizer or an approved atypical antipsychotic. Overall, recent guideline updates underscore a move away from antidepressant-centered strategies toward mechanism-based pharmacological approaches tailored to bipolar depression.

Key Principles for Antidepressant Use in Bipolar Depression

1. *Avoid Monotherapy*: Antidepressants must always be combined with a mood stabilizer (e.g., lithium, valproate) or an atypical antipsychotic.
2. *Not a First-Line Treatment*: Mood stabilizers or atypical antipsychotics (e.g., quetiapine, lamotrigine, lurasidone) are recommended as first-line options; antidepressants are considered second-line.

3. *Choose Cautiously*: SSRIs or bupropion are generally preferred over TCAs or venlafaxine due to their relatively lower risk of inducing mania or hypomania.
4. *Consider Short-Term Use*: Antidepressants should be used for acute depressive episodes only, with early discontinuation after recovery, as evidence for long-term maintenance efficacy is weak.

1.12 Summary

Depression is very common in clinical practice; however, distinguishing unipolar from bipolar depression based solely on phenomenology remains challenging. Although their courses and treatments differ, both can deteriorate and lead to severe psychosocial impairment if inadequately treated, making early, accurate diagnosis and appropriate treatment essential. Understanding phenomenological characteristics and differences, and conducting thorough interviews that integrate cross-sectional symptom assessment with longitudinal features of mood episodes, *are* useful for differential diagnosis. Applying this information in clinical settings can substantially improve diagnostic accuracy and guide appropriate treatment. Accordingly, when evaluating a patient with depression, clinicians should *maintain a high index of suspicion* for underlying bipolarity by integrating multifaceted information—including cross-sectional symptoms, longitudinal course, family history, and prior treatment responses.

Declarations

Competing Interests The authors have no competing interests to declare that are relevant to the content of this manuscript.

Ethics Approval The authors declare that this manuscript does not include primary research with human participants.

The authors also declare that this manuscript does not include primary studies involving animals.

References

1. Regier DA, Farmer ME, Rae DS, Locke BZ, Keith SJ, Judd LL, et al. Comorbidity of mental disorders with alcohol and other drug abuse. Results from the Epidemiologic Catchment Area (ECA) Study. JAMA. 1990;264(19):2511–8.
2. Benazzi F. Frequency of bipolar spectrum in 111 private practice depression outpatients. Eur Arch Psychiatry Clin Neurosci. 2003;253(4):203–8.
3. Merikangas KR, Jin R, He JP, Kessler RC, Lee S, Sampson NA, et al. Prevalence and correlates of bipolar spectrum disorder in the world mental health survey initiative. Arch Gen Psychiatry. 68(3):241–51.
4. Craddock N, Jones I. Molecular genetics of bipolar disorder. Br J Psychiatry Suppl. 2001;41:s128–33.
5. Merikangas KR, Akiskal HS, Angst J, Greenberg PE, Hirschfeld RM, Petukhova M, et al. Lifetime and 12-month prevalence of bipolar spectrum disorder in the National Comorbidity Survey replication. Arch Gen Psychiatry. 2007;64(5):543–52.
6. Kessler RC, Berglund P, Demler O, Jin R, Koretz D, Merikangas KR, et al. The epidemiology of major depressive disorder: results from the National Comorbidity Survey Replication (NCS-R). JAMA. 2003;289(23):3095–105.
7. Angst J. Bipolar disorders in DSM-5: strengths, problems and perspectives. Int J Bipolar Disord. 2013;1:12.
8. Benazzi F. Classifying mood disorders by age-at-onset instead of polarity. Prog Neuro-Psychopharmacol Biol Psychiatry. 2009;33(1):86–93.
9. Baldessarini RJ, Tondo L, Baethge CJ, Lepri B, Bratti IM. Effects of treatment latency on response to maintenance treatment in manic-depressive disorders. Bipolar Disord. 2007;9(4):386–93.
10. Mitchell PB, Malhi GS. Bipolar depression: phenomenological overview and clinical characteristics. Bipolar Disord. 2004;6(6):530–9.
11. Spijker J, de Graaf R, Bijl RV, Beekman AT, Ormel J, Nolen WA. Duration of major depressive episodes in the general population: results from The Netherlands Mental Health Survey and Incidence Study (NEMESIS). Br J Psychiatry. 2002;181:208–13.
12. Patten SB. A major depression prognosis calculator based on episode duration. Clin Pract Epidemiol Ment Health. 2006;2:13.
13. Angst J, Sellaro R. Historical perspectives and natural history of bipolar disorder. Biol Psychiatry. 2000;48(6):445–57.
14. Solomon DA, Leon AC, Coryell WH, Endicott J, Li C, Fiedorowicz JG, et al. Longitudinal course of bipolar I disorder: duration of mood episodes. Arch Gen Psychiatry. 67(4):339–47.

15. Forty L, Smith D, Jones L, Jones I, Caesar S, Cooper C. Clinical differences between bipolar and unipolar depression. 2008.
16. Keller MB. The course of manic-depressive illness. J Clin Psychiatry. 1988;49(Suppl):4–7.
17. Keller MB, Lavori PW, Coryell W, Andreasen NC, Endicott J, Clayton PJ, et al. Differential outcome of pure manic, mixed/cycling, and pure depressive episodes in patients with bipolar illness. JAMA. 1986;255(22):3138–42.
18. Mitchell PB, Wilhelm K, Parker G, Austin MP, Rutgers P, Malhi GS. The clinical features of bipolar depression: a comparison with matched major depressive disorder patients. J Clin Psychiatry. 2001;62(3):212–6. quiz 7
19. Coryell W, Endicott J, Maser JD, Keller MB, Leon AC, Akiskal HS. Long-term stability of polarity distinctions in the affective disorders. Am J Psychiatry. 1995;152(3):385–90.
20. Akiskal HS, Maser JD, Zeller PJ, Endicott J, Coryell W, Keller M, et al. Switching from 'unipolar' to bipolar II. An 11-year prospective study of clinical and temperamental predictors in 559 patients. Arch Gen Psychiatry. 1995;52(2):114–23.
21. Abrams R, Taylor MA. A comparison of unipolar and bipolar depressive illness. Am J Psychiatry. 1980;137(9):1084–7.
22. Katz MM, Robins E, Croughan J, Secunda S, Swann A. Behavioural measurement and drug response characteristics of unipolar and bipolar depression. Psychol Med. 1982;12(1):25–36.
23. Brockington IF, Altman E, Hillier V, Meltzer HY, Nand S. The clinical picture of bipolar affective disorder in its depressed phase. A report from London and Chicago. Br J Psychiatry. 1982;141:558–62.
24. Dunner DL, Dwyer T, Fieve RR. Depressive symptoms in patients with unipolar and bipolar affective disorder. Compr Psychiatry. 1976;17(3):447–51.
25. Parker G, Roy K, Wilhelm K, Mitchell P, Hadzi-Pavlovic D. The nature of bipolar depression: implications for the definition of melancholia. J Affect Disord. 2000;59(3):217–24.
26. Endicott J, Nee J, Andreasen N, Clayton P, Keller M, Coryell W. Bipolar II. Combine or keep separate? J Affect Disord. 1985;8(1):17–28.
27. Black DW, Nasrallah A. Hallucinations and delusions in 1,715 patients with unipolar and bipolar affective disorders. Psychopathology. 1989;22(1):28–34.
28. Kupfer DJ, Weiss BL, Foster G, Detre TP, McPartland R. Psychomotor activity in affective states. Arch Gen Psychiatry. 1974;30(6):765–8.
29. Popescu C, Ionescu R, Jipescu I, Popa S. Psychomotor functioning in unipolar and bipolar affective disorders. Rom J Neurol Psychiatry. 1991;29(1–2):17–33.
30. Beigel A, Murphy DL. Unipolar and bipolar affective illness. Differences in clinical characteristics accompanying depression. Arch Gen Psychiatry. 1971;24(3):215–20.
31. Ghaemi SN, Ko JY, Goodwin FK. The bipolar spectrum and the antidepressant view of the world. J Psychiatr Pract. 2001;7(5):287–97.
32. Benazzi F, Akiskal HS. The modified SCID Hypomania Module (SCID-Hba): a detailed systematic phenomenologic probing. J Affect Disord. 2009;117(3):131–6.
33. Zutshi A, Kamath P, Reddy YC. Bipolar and nonbipolar obsessive-compulsive disorder: a clinical exploration. Compr Psychiatry. 2007;48(3):245–51.
34. Papolos D, Mattis S, Golshan S, Molay F. Fear of harm, a possible phenotype of pediatric bipolar disorder: a dimensional approach to diagnosis for genotyping psychiatric syndromes. J Affect Disord. 2009;118(1–3):28–38.
35. Sit D, Rothschild AJ, Wisner KL. A review of postpartum psychosis. J Womens Health (Larchmt). 2006;15(4):352–68.
36. Rybakowski JK, Suwalska A, Lojko D, Rymaszewska J, Kiejna A. Types of depression more frequent in bipolar than in unipolar affective illness: results of the Polish DEP-BI study. Psychopathology. 2007;40(3):153–8.
37. Abbott R, Dunn VJ, Robling SA, Paykel ES. Long-term outcome of offspring after maternal severe puerperal disorder. Acta Psychiatr Scand. 2004;110(5):365–73.
38. Sharma V, Khan M, Smith A. A closer look at treatment resistant depression: is it due to a bipolar diathesis? J Affect Disord. 2005;84(2–3):251–7.
39. Inoue T, Nakagawa S, Kitaichi Y, Izumi T, Tanaka T, Masui T, et al. Long-term outcome of antidepressant-refractory depression: the relevance of unrecognized bipolarity. J Affect Disord. 2006;95(1–3):61–7.
40. Borkowska A, Rybakowski JK. Neuropsychological frontal lobe tests indicate that bipolar depressed patients are more impaired than unipolar. Bipolar Disord. 2001;3(2):88–94.
41. Ilsley JE, Moffoot AP, O'Carroll RE. An analysis of memory dysfunction in major depression. J Affect Disord. 1995;35(1–2):1–9.
42. Murphy FC, Sahakian BJ. Neuropsychology of bipolar disorder. Br J Psychiatry Suppl. 2001;41:s120–7.
43. Calev A, Nigal D, Chazan S. Retrieval from semantic memory using meaningful and meaningless constructs by depressed, stable bipolar and manic patients. Br J Clin Psychol. 1989;28(Pt 1):67–73.
44. Tsourtos G, Thompson JC, Stough C. Evidence of an early information processing speed deficit in unipolar major depression. Psychol Med. 2002;32(2):259–65.

45. Ferrier IN, Stanton BR, Kelly TP, Scott J. Neuropsychological function in euthymic patients with bipolar disorder. Br J Psychiatry. 1999;175:246–51.
46. Jamison KR. Suicide and bipolar disorder. J Clin Psychiatry. 2000;61(Suppl 9):47–51.
47. Kessler RC, Rubinow DR, Holmes C, Abelson JM, Zhao S. The epidemiology of DSM-III-R bipolar I disorder in a general population survey. Psychol Med. 1997;27(5):1079–89.
48. Compton MT, Nemeroff CB. The treatment of bipolar depression. J Clin Psychiatry. 2000;61(Suppl 9):57–67.
49. Goodwin FK, Jamison KR. Manic-depressive illness. New York: Oxford University Press; 1990. xxi, 938 p.
50. Harris EC, Barraclough B. Suicide as an outcome for mental disorders. A meta-analysis. Br J Psychiatry. 1997;170:205–28.
51. Fountoulakis KN, Grunze H, Panagiotidis P, Kaprinis G. Treatment of bipolar depression: an update. J Affect Disord. 2008;109(1–2):21–34.
52. Gijsman HJ, Geddes JR, Rendell JM, Nolen WA, Goodwin GM. Antidepressants for bipolar depression: a systematic review of randomized, controlled trials. Am J Psychiatry. 2004;161(9):1537–47.
53. Sachs GS, Nierenberg AA, Calabrese JR, Marangell LB, Wisniewski SR, Gyulai L, et al. Effectiveness of adjunctive antidepressant treatment for bipolar depression. N Engl J Med. 2007;356(17):1711–22.
54. Post RM, Altshuler LL, Leverich GS, Frye MA, Nolen WA, Kupka RW, et al. Mood switch in bipolar depression: comparison of adjunctive venlafaxine, bupropion and sertraline. Br J Psychiatry. 2006;189:124–31.
55. Ghaemi SN, Lenox MS, Baldessarini RJ. Effectiveness and safety of long-term antidepressant treatment in bipolar disorder. J Clin Psychiatry. 2001;62(7):565–9.
56. Loebel A, Cucchiaro J, Silva R, et al. Effectiveness and safety of lurasidone in the treatment of bipolar I depression. Am J Psychiatry. 2014;171(2):160–8.
57. Durgam S, Earley W, Guo H, et al. Effectiveness and safety of cariprazine in the treatment of bipolar I depression. Am J Psychiatry. 2016;173(3):271–81.

A Multidimensional Perspective of Treatment-Resistant Depression: The Staging Model

2

Kang Soo Lee and Jonghun Lee

Treatment-resistant depression (TRD) is relatively common in clinical practice; however, the lack of a consistent definition and characterization has posed a major challenge [1]. Despite increasing clinical and academic attention, no universally accepted operational definition of TRD currently exists [2]. Definitions vary across studies and clinical guidelines, resulting in inconsistencies in diagnoses, treatment strategies, and outcome measurements. Furthermore, none of these classifications has been systematically examined, verified for reliability, or validated for prognosis. Guideline definitions of TRD vary; there is no consensus on what constitutes adequate prior treatment, and recommended next-step interventions often differ [3–6]. Various clinical guidelines and studies propose definitions of TRD, yet numerous conceptual and practical challenges remain. A key limitation is that the existing definitions do not adequately reflect the diversity of therapeutic strategies used in clinical practice. Within the scope of pharmacotherapy, TRD definitions often overlook the widespread use of non-antidepressant agents such as atypical antipsychotics. The Canadian Network for Mood and Anxiety Treatments (CANMAT) [5], The National Institute for Health and Care Excellence (NICE) [6], as well as multiple clinical trials fail to reflect the real-world use of these medications as common first- or second-line treatments. Another concern is the lack of consensus regarding the adequacy of the antidepressant dose and duration, clarifying treatment failure, and determining whether TRD requires prior use of different pharmacological classes of antidepressants. Other effective treatment factors, such as electroconvulsive therapy, neurostimulation, and psychotherapy, also influence the therapeutic outcomes of TRD, further complicating its classification. Because of these complexities, many international guidelines refrain from explicitly defining TRD or specifying corresponding treatment protocols. For instance, the NICE guideline presents a stepped-care model without direct reference to TRD [6]. The American Psychological Association's 2019 guideline similarly focuses on treatment response without establishing a formal TRD definition [3]. Only the Department of Veterans Affairs and Department of Defense (VA/DoD) and Nationale Versorgungs Leitlinie (NVL) guidelines define TRD as a lack of response to at least two ade-

K. S. Lee
Department of Psychiatry, CHA Bundang Medical Center, CHA University, Seongnam, Republic of Korea

J. Lee (✉)
Department of Psychiatry, School of Medicine, Catholic University of Daegu, Daegu, Republic of Korea
e-mail: rheejh@cu.ac.kr

W.-M. Bahk et al. (eds.), *Depressive Disorder*, https://doi.org/10.1007/978-981-92-1331-3_2

quately dosed and timed pharmacological trials and offer next-step recommendations [4, 7].

Another debate is whether TRD should be treated as a categorical diagnosis or as a spectrum of responsiveness to treatment. Although TRD has been historically defined as a dichotomous concept, this definition has been criticized for not reflecting clinical reality, as demonstrated by findings from antidepressant treatment switch trials, including STAR*D [8, 9]. Nevertheless, the dichotomous definition aids in identifying and differentiating responders from those with less severe forms of treatment resistance [10–12]. The continuous approach utilizes a staging model, proposed as a more refined transitional diagnostic approach, with the potential to improve the logic and timing of intervention [13]. Staging depression in a way similar to that of medical diseases, such as cancer, may provide the opportunity to systematically guide treatment selection based on clinical presentation and the progression of the disorder. Presently, the conceptualization and operationalization of TRD in both research and clinical practice are consensus-driven rather than data-driven [14]. This is largely due to the limited understanding of TRD and the challenges in empirically testing its definitions, which are limited by heterogeneous research methodologies and inconsistent findings [15]. This has delayed the translation of research findings into clinical practice and impeded the development of new treatment strategies aimed at improving the outcomes of TRD. The classification of TRD into stages has been recently proposed, where the greater the degree of treatment resistance, the lower the probability of response to any new treatment.

Thase and Rush first proposed a five-level staging model of treatment resistance, based on the number and classes of antidepressants that failed to elicit a response. Stage I is described as failure of at least one adequate trial of one antidepressant. Stage II is described as failure of at least two adequate trials of two or more distinctly different classes of antidepressants. Stage III is described as stage II resistance plus failure of an adequate trial of a tricyclic antidepressant. Stage IV is described as stage III resistance plus failure of an adequate trial of a monoamine oxidase inhibitor. Stage V is described as stage IV resistance plus a course of bilateral electroconvulsive therapy. This hierarchical model implies that medications used at higher stages of resistance are presumed to have superior efficacy [16]. Major drawbacks of this model include its hierarchical assumptions and limited flexibility to accommodate the potentially numerous medications that may be deployed to treat a resistance episode, as well as the lack of defined criteria for trial intensity in terms of dosing and duration [17–20]. Although the model has been extensively criticized in the last decade, it is easy to use and implicitly provides a strategy for clinicians to treat patients with TRD [21].

The European Staging Method proposes a distinction between nonresponse, TRD, and chronic resistant depression [22]. This model includes the duration of treatment for a depressive episode and does not suggest an implicit hierarchy of the efficacy of antidepressants. Non-responder is defined as nonresponse to one adequate trial of Tricyclic Antidepressant (TCA), Selective Serotonin Reuptake Inhibitor (SSRI), Monoamine Oxidase Inhibitor (MAOI), Serotonin-norepinephrine Reuptake Inhibitor (SNRI), Electroconvulsive Therapy (ECT), or other antidepressants for 6–8 weeks. TRD is defined as resistance to two or more adequate antidepressant trials of different classes. According to the duration of trial, TRD1 is defined as 12–16 weeks of trial while TRD2 for 18–24 weeks, TRD3 for 24–32 weeks, TRD4 for 30–40 weeks, and TRD5 for 36 weeks to 1 year. Chronic resistant depression is defined as resistant to several antidepressant trials, including augmentation strategy with at least 12 months. The main features of this model are characterized with the establishment of a required minimum number of failed antidepressant medications for TRD and the consideration given to the chronic nature of TRD. Limitation of this model is that symptom severity or medication augmentation strategies are not addressed.

A group from the Massachusetts General Hospital proposed a slightly different approach that considers both the number of failed trials and the intensity or optimization of each trial, but without classes [19]. Points are assigned based on whether a trial was adequate (correct dose and duration) or inadequate and extra weight is given if the trial was optimized (dose adjustments, augmentation strategies). The more the adequate trials failed, the higher the score, and undergoing ECT adds to the score, reflecting advanced treatment resistance. This method generates continuous scores reflecting the level of resistance in depression, which might better discriminate between low and high levels of TRD and has the flexibility to incorporate as many factors as possible. However, with the large number of treatment options currently available, these systems may be less efficient and discriminatory [16, 18].

The Maudsley staging method summarizes the TRD stage into a single score ranging from 3 to 15 (Table 2.1) [23]. This model includes the number of treatment failures, augmentation strategies, and ECT treatments. Unlike other models, this model includes additional clinical information on the duration and severity of illness to add to the level of TRD. This model is the only one with validity assessed using prospective data and higher scores associated with failure to achieve remission: it correctly predicts treatment resistance in more than 85% of cases [24]. However, the authors suggested that the model should include the level of functional impairment and psychosocial stressors as additional dimensions [23].

Table 2.1 Maudsley staging model

Domain		Clinical implications
Number of treatment failures	Level 1 → 1–2 medications failed Level 2 → 3–4 medications failed Level 3 → 5–6 medications failed Level 4 → 7–10 medications failed Level 5 > 10 medications failed	More failures higher points 1–5
Augmentation	Not used 0 Used 1	
ECT	Not used 0 Used 1	
Duration	Acute (≤12 months) Sub-acute (13–24 months) Chronic (>24 months)	Longer duration → higher points 1–3 points
Symptom severity (at baseline)	Subsyndromal Syndromal Mild Moderate Severe without psychosis Severe with psychosis	1–5 points
Scoring	Maudsley staging model (MSM) total = Treatment (1–7) + Duration (1–3) + Severity (1–5) = 3–15	Mild TRD: 3–6 Moderate TRD: 7–10 Severe TRD: 11–15

TRD is a significant concept in both clinical practice and research. However, the lack of consistency in the definition and assessment of TRD is a major barrier to progress in clinical research and the treatment of resistant depression [25]. An operational definition for TRD would guide clinicians to better select treatment options and may ultimately help prevent prolonged depressive illness. Future empirical studies should address the inconsistencies between the current evidence- and expert-based guidelines for TRD. Biological markers may help integrate the overlapping areas of treatment resistance, chronicity, duration of illness, and illness progression.

Declarations

Competing Interests The authors have no competing interests to declare that are relevant to the content of this manuscript.

Ethics Approval The authors declare that this manuscript does not include primary research with human participants.

The authors also declare that this manuscript does not include primary studies involving animals.

References

1. Souery D, Lipp O, Massat I, Mendlewicz J. The characterization and definition of treatment-resistant mood disorders. In: Amsterdam JD, Hornig M, Nierenberg AA, editors. Treatment-resistant mood disorders. New York (NY): Cambridge University Press; 2001. p. 3–29.

2. Trevino K, McClintock SM, McDonald Fischer N, Vora A, Husain MM. Defining treatment-resistant depression: a comprehensive review of the literature. Ann Clin Psychiatr. 2014;26(3):222–32.
3. American Psychological Association. Clinical practice guideline for the treatment of depression across three age cohorts. Washington, DC: APA; 2019.
4. Department of Veterans Affairs, Department of Defense. VA/DoD clinical practice guideline for the management of major depressive disorder. Washington, DC: Department of Veterans Affairs and Department of Defense; 2016.
5. Lam RW, Kennedy SH, Grigoriadis S, McIntyre RS, Milev R, Ramasubbu R, et al. Canadian Network for Mood and Anxiety Treatments (CANMAT) Clinical guidelines for the management of major depressive disorder in adults. J Affect Disord. 2009;117(Suppl 1):S26–43.
6. National Institute for Health and Clinical Excellence (NICE) Depression. The treatment and management of depression in adults (updated edition). Leicester, UK: British Psychological Society; 2018.
7. Härter M, Schorr S, Schneider F, editors. S3-Leitlinie: nationale versorgungsleitlinie unipolare depression langfassung. 2nd ed. Berlin: Springer; 2015.
8. Rush AJ, Kraemer HC, Sackeim HA, Fava M, Trivedi MH, Frank E, et al. Report by the ACNP task force on response and remission in major depressive disorder. Neuropsychopharmacology. 2006;31(9):1841–53.
9. Rush AJ, Trivedi MH, Wisniewski SR, Nierenberg AA, Stewart JW, Warden D, et al. Acute and longer-term outcomes in depressed outpatients requiring one or several treatment steps: a STAR*D report. Am J Psychiatry. 2006;163(11):1905–17.
10. Malhi GS, Byrow Y. Is treatment-resistant depression a useful concept? Evid Based Ment Health. 2016;19(1):1–3.
11. Murphy JA, Sarris J, Byrne GJ. A review of the conceptualisation and risk factors associated with treatment-resistant depression. Depress Res Treat. 2017;2017:4176825.
12. Pérez-Wehbe AI, Perestelo-Pérez L, Bethencourt-Pérez JM, Cuéllar-Pompa L, Peñate-Castro W. Treatment-resistant depression: a systematic review of systematic reviews. Int J Clin Health Psychol. 2014;14(2):145–53.
13. McGorry PD, Hickie IB, editors. Clinical staging in psychiatry: making diagnosis work for research and treatment. Cambridge University Press; 2019.
14. Berlim MT, Turecki G. What is the meaning of treatment resistant/refractory major depression (TRD)? A systematic review of current randomized trials. Eur Neuropsychopharmacol. 2007;17(11):696–707.
15. Malhi GS, Parker GB, Crawford J, Wilhelm K, Mitchell PB. Treatment-resistant depression: resistant to definition? Acta Psychiatr Scand. 2005;112(4):302–9.
16. Thase ME, Rush AJ. When at first you don't succeed: sequential strategies for antidepressant nonresponders. J Clin Psychiatry. 1997;58(Suppl 13):23–9.
17. Ruhé HG, van Rooijen G, Spijker J, Peeters FP, Schene AHJ. Staging methods for treatment resistant depression. A systematic review. Affect Disord. 2012;137(1–3):35–45.
18. Berlim MT, Turecki G. Definition, assessment, and staging of treatment-resistant refractory major depression: a review of current concepts and methods. Can J Psychiatr. 2007;52(1):46–54.
19. Fava M. Diagnosis and definition of treatment-resistant depression. Biol Psychiatry. 2003;53:649–59.
20. Souery D, Papakostas GI, Trivedi MH. Treatment-resistant depression. J Clin Psychiatry. 2006;67(Suppl 6):16–22.
21. Souery D, Van der Auwera K. The multiple facets of treatment resistant depression. CNS Spectr. 2004;9(11):803–7.
22. Souery D, Amsterdam J, de Montigny C, Lecrubier Y, Montgomery S, Lipp O, et al. Treatment resistant depression: methodological overview and operational criteria. Eur Neuropsychopharmacol. 1999;9:83–91.
23. Fekadu A, Wooderson S, Donaldson C, Markopoulou K, Masterson B, Poon L, et al. A multidimensional tool to quantify treatment resistance in depression: the Maudsley staging method. J Clin Psychiatry. 2009;70(2):177–84.
24. Fekadu A, Wooderson SC, Markopoulou K, Cleare AJ. The Maudsley staging method for treatment-resistant depression: prediction of longer-term outcome and persistence of symptoms. J Clin Psychiatry. 2009;70(7):952–7.
25. Rybak YE, Lai KSP, Ramasubbu R, Vila-Rodriguez F, Blumberger DM, Chan P, et al. Treatment-resistant major depressive disorder: Canadian expert consensus on definition and assessment. Depress Anxiety. 2021;38(4):456–67.

3 Mixed Specifier

In Hee Shim, Won-Myong Bahk, and Won Kim

3.1 Concept and Evolution of Mixed Features

Historical Concepts and Early Theories

Heinroth [1] was the first psychiatrist to describe mixed states, classifying mental disorders into states of excitation, depression, and mixed conditions. Wilhelm Griesinger [2] later described mixed states as "melancholia accompanied by destructive impulses" or "melancholia characterized by persistent fluctuations in volition over a prolonged period."

Subsequently, Emil Kraepelin [3] systematized the concept of mixed states and became the most representative figure in its theoretical development. He coined the term "manic-depressive insanity" for mood disorders and noted that most clinical manifestations appear in mixed forms. Based on three elements—mood, thought, and volition—he categorized mixed states into several subtypes, including depression with flight of ideas, excited depression, depressive-anxious mania, unproductive mania with poverty of thought, inhibited mania, and manic stupor. His colleague and disciple, Weygandt, introduced the concept of agitated depression in relation to mixed states.

However, these early conceptualizations have several limitations. First, they relied solely on clinical observation without incorporating neurobiological or other relevant clinical factors. Second, objective tools for evaluating depressive or manic states, as well as the dichotomous classification between major depressive disorder (MDD) and bipolar disorder (BD), had not yet been developed. Third, the classification was excessively subdivided, limiting its applicability in clinical practice.

Changes in Diagnostic Classification

In both the first and second editions of the *Diagnostic and Statistical Manual of Mental Disorders* (DSM)-I and DSM-II, mixed states were described under categories such as "other

I. H. Shim
Department of Psychiatry, Dongnam Institute of Radiological & Medical Sciences, Busan, Republic of Korea

W.-M. Bahk (✉)
Department of Psychiatry, College of Medicine, The Catholic University of Korea, Seoul, Republic of Korea

Woo and Bahk Psychiatry Clinic, Seoul, Republic of Korea
e-mail: wmbahk@catholic.ac.kr

W. Kim
Department of Psychiatry, Sanggye Paik Hospital, College of Medicine, Inje University, Seoul, Republic of Korea

W.-M. Bahk et al. (eds.), *Depressive Disorder*, https://doi.org/10.1007/978-981-92-1331-3_3

manic-depressive reactions" and "mixed manic-depressive illness; manic and depressive symptoms occurring almost simultaneously" [4, 5]. With the publication of the DSM-III, mood disorders were dichotomized into MDD and BD, marking a departure from Kraepelin's broad unitary concept of "manic-depressive insanity" [6]. This shift created a greater need for clarity regarding states in which both mood poles are simultaneously present.

However, DSM-III, DSM-IV, and the *International Classification of Diseases* (ICD)-10 primarily emphasized manic episodes accompanied by prominent depressive symptoms, considering them rare presentations linked to BD. Until DSM-IV-TR (*Diagnostic and Statistical Manual of Mental Disorders*, fourth Edition, Text Revision), the classification applied a strict categorical criterion that recognized only "mixed episodes" as full syndromes meeting the diagnostic criteria for both manic and depressive episodes concurrently—and only within the context of BD. This classification applied solely to cases involving manic episodes, thus excluding the more commonly observed "mixed depression" from consideration. In clinical reality, fully syndromal mixed episodes that meet both sets of criteria are rare. Instead, presentations in which manic and depressive symptoms coexist, with either manic or depressive predominance, are more frequently encountered. This led to criticism that the DSM framework limited diagnostic flexibility and underestimated the clinical relevance of mixed features.

In response to these limitations, the DSM-5, published in 2013, replaced the term "mixed episode" with the specifier "with mixed features," allowing its application not only in BD but also in MDD. The specifier can now be applied to various mood episodes, including depressive, hypomanic, and manic episodes. Mixed depression under DSM-5 refers to a major depressive episode accompanied by at least three of the seven manic symptoms. However, nonspecific and overlapping symptoms—such as psychomotor agitation, irritability, and distractibility—were excluded due to their potential to appear in both manic and depressive states. Nevertheless, several studies have argued that these overlapping symptoms may represent core features of mixed states [7, 8]. As a result, their exclusion has been criticized for lacking empirical support and for potentially omitting a large proportion of clinically relevant mixed presentations.

Anxiety and restlessness also overlap with depression and mania and can act as confounding factors in identifying mixed states. Nonetheless, these symptoms are considered highly relevant for assessing mixed states and are more closely linked to pathophysiology than typical mood symptoms. The Systematic Treatment Enhancement Program–Bipolar Disorder Study (STEP-BD, $N = 1380$) identified distractibility, racing thoughts, and restlessness as the most common manic symptoms in mixed depression [9]. Similarly, studies conducted in Asia reported elevated self-esteem and psychomotor agitation as the most frequent symptoms [10].

Specifically, anxiety is associated with hyperarousal and predominantly appears in depressive episodes. It is also linked to mixed mania but rarely observed in pure manic episodes without comorbidity [11]. Anxiety correlates with the severity of depressive symptoms in manic episodes and the severity of manic symptoms in depressive episodes, thus being associated with mixed states across all episode types. Restlessness occurs in both depressive and manic episodes but presents differently: in mania, goal-directed activity increases, whereas in depression, non-goal-directed activity increases due to internal tension—both patterns manifesting as mixed states. Studies have also shown that agitated depression and mixed depression are highly similar, and restlessness is closely associated with severe outcomes such as weight loss and suicidal thoughts [12]. However, whether agitated depression without hypomania or mania qualifies as mixed depression remains controversial, and DSM-5 suggests it could be classified as non-mixed [13]. Additionally, comparisons of mixed manic patients and patients with agitated depression (without manic symptoms) revealed similar clinical features, including anxiety, restlessness, irritability, and cognitive dysfunction [14].

As a result, Koukopoulos et al. [15] raised concerns about the DSM-5 definition, stating that "overlapping symptoms are the most important aspect of mixed states." When attempting to understand the pathophysiology and treatment of mixed states, these overlapping symptoms form the basis of the condition, and excluding them could lead to underdiagnosis, so caution is necessary. Considering the exclusionary criteria in DSM-5, the prevalence of mixed depression remains relatively low under strict definitions. However, when overlapping symptoms and broader diagnostic criteria are permitted, the prevalence increases substantially, highlighting the clinical relevance of more inclusive definitions of mixed depression [7, 8, 16]. This suggests that despite being a case of mixed depression, the limitations of diagnostic criteria may result in patients either not being properly diagnosed or receiving inappropriate treatment. Consequently, the ongoing controversy regarding exclusion criteria for mixed depression diagnosis calls for more thoughtful revisions in future editions to reflect the academic feedback and improve diagnostic accuracy.

In contrast, the Research-Based Diagnostic Criteria (RBDC) for mixed depression define it similarly—as a depressive episode with three or more manic/hypomanic symptoms—but notably include overlapping symptoms. Using this definition, the prevalence of mixed depression is estimated to be as high as one-third of all depressive episodes. Furthermore, mixed depression defined by RBDC has shown stronger associations with clinical variables such as illness course and family history than the DSM-5 criteria [17].

In the most recent edition of the ICD-11, mixed episodes are defined exclusively within the context of BD as "a manic or depressive episode in which prominent symptoms of the opposite polarity—manic or depressive—are also present, either simultaneously or alternating very rapidly" [18]. Although the term "mixed episode" remains the same as in the DSM-IV-TR, the ICD-11 differs in that it allows for the inclusion of mixed depression. In this respect, its approach more closely resembles the "mixed features specifier" introduced in DSM-5 [19]. Notably, while DSM-5 excludes nonspecific overlapping symptoms from its criteria, ICD-11 includes symptoms commonly observed in mixed depression—such as irritability and psychomotor agitation—as manic features, thus marking a key distinction between the two systems.

Malhi and colleagues [20] have argued that the reliance on exclusionary diagnostic criteria has led to clinical failures in accurately identifying mixed depression. To address this, they proposed the ACE model, which conceptualizes mixed states as arising from asynchronous changes across three domains: Activity, Cognition, and Emotion. According to this model, various patterns of mixed states can result depending on how these components fluctuate independently. The ACE model can be seen as a refined continuation of the earlier conceptualizations of Kraepelin and Weygandt, emphasizing the heterogeneity in both etiology and clinical presentation of mixed states.

The evolution of the concept and diagnostic definitions of mixed features across different systems and authors is summarized in Table 3.1 [10, 13, 15, 17, 18, 20, 22–27].

From a diagnostic standpoint, categorical definitions—such as those distinguishing between depressive and manic episodes—can aid in classification and treatment selection by reflecting distinct syndromal entities. In contrast, dimensional approaches define mixed states along a continuum, allowing operational flexibility in how these presentations are identified and understood. Empirical studies grounded in symptomatology and observable behavior have increasingly lent support to such dimensional models of mixed states [21].

Table 3.1 Evolution of the concept of mixed features [10, 13, 15, 17, 18, 20, 22–27]

Author/source	Definition	Key features
Kraepelin	Described various mixed states arising from asynchronous changes in mood, cognition, and behavior	Subtypes: Overly subdivided; lacked practical applicability
WHO: ICD-10	Co-occurrence or rapid cycling of manic and depressive symptoms lasting ≥2 weeks	Allowed rapid alternation or combination; still restricted to bipolar disorder
APA: DSM-III, IV	Full manic and depressive episodes simultaneously present for ≥1 week, nearly every day	Abandoned Kraepelin's unitary concept; narrow, categorical definition (excluded mixed depression)
Benazzi (DMX2/ DMX3)	Depressive episode + ≥2 or 3 hypomanic symptoms (including overlapping symptoms)	Captures broader spectrum of mixed depression; higher clinical prevalence than DSM-5
Perugi et al. (RBDC)	Depressive episode + ≥3 hypomanic symptoms (including overlapping symptoms)	Higher prevalence (~1/3 of depressive episodes); stronger family history association; broadly, may risk overdiagnosis
Koukopoulos	Considered agitated depression as a core mixed state (even without hypomania)	Emphasized psychomotor agitation, inner tension, suicidality as central; not recognized by DSM-IV/5 (risk of underdiagnosis)
APA: DSM-5	Manic, hypomanic, or depressive episode + ≥3 opposite-polarity symptoms (excluding overlapping ones), present nearly every day for a substantial portion of the episode	Excludes overlapping symptoms (e.g., irritability, psychomotor agitation, distractibility)
WHO: ICD-11	Manic or depressive episode + prominent opposite-polarity symptoms co-occurring or rapidly alternating (including overlapping symptoms)	Includes irritability, psychomotor agitation as manic features; differs from DSM-5 by including mixed depression
Malhi (ACE model)	Proposed the ACE (activity, cognition, emotion) model to describe diverse mixed states from asynchronous changes in the three components	Explains heterogeneity and complexity; lacks operational diagnostic thresholds

APA American Psychiatric Association, *DMX* Depressive Mixed State, *DSM* Diagnostic and Statistical Manual of Mental Disorders, *ICD* International Statistical Classification of Diseases and Related Health Problems, *RBDC* Research Based Diagnostic Criteria, *WHO* World Health Organization

3.2 Epidemiology

The prevalence of mixed states varies depending on the diagnostic criteria. Weygandt [28] suggested that more than 60% of patients with mood disorders exhibit mixed states. When mixed states were defined as depressive episode + ≥2 or 3 hypomanic symptoms, the prevalence in patients with BD II, depressive episodes ranged from 46.3% to 73.1%, and in MDD it ranged from 7.8% to 42.1% [29, 30]. According to these statistics, mixed depression is frequently reported in MDD, and some patients diagnosed with MDD are actually part of the bipolar spectrum disorder. Notably, Zimmermann [31] reported that the proportion of bipolar spectrum disorder within MDD was 41.4%, which showed distinct clinical differences compared to pure major depressive episodes, such as a higher family history of mania, co-occurring substance use disorders and anxiety disorders, and a higher tendency toward criminal behavior.

In BD, mixed states were observed in approximately 30% of patients [32]. A 24-month prospective observational study of patients with BD and mixed episodes showed that 66% had pure manic episodes and 34% had mixed episodes [33]. However, according to DSM-III criteria, it was estimated that only about 10% of patients with BD fall into mixed states [34]. Additionally, in the STEP-BD study, the prevalence of mixed states was relatively low, about 14.8%, according to the strict DSM-IV-TR diagnostic criteria [9].

According to an Asian study, when mixed depression was defined as depressive episode + ≥3 hypomanic symptoms based on Benazzi's criteria, approximately 17.5% of patients with BD, depressive episodes were diagnosed with mixed depression [10]. Additionally, when mixed mania was defined as manic episode + ≥3 depressive symptoms based on Cincinnati's criteria, the prevalence among patients with manic episodes was 14.6% [24]. In contrast, when mixed episodes were diagnosed according to the strict DSM-IV-TR criteria, the prevalence was very low, at around 6% [35].

3.3 Neurobiological Pathophysiology

Early explanations of pathophysiology were based on biological descriptions derived from observations but were not experimentally validated. However, in the late nineteenth and early twentieth centuries, with the development of systematic medical observation, neurophysiology, and pharmacology, the classical models of mood states evolved into models based on the pathophysiology of brain and systemic diseases [36]. Although many aspects of the pathophysiology of mixed states remain unclear, studies are being conducted on neurotransmitters such as biogenic amines, inflammatory cytokines, cortisol, thyroid hormones, and other endocrine hormones.

First, in mixed states, there is an increase in urinary norepinephrine and its metabolites. While catecholamine activity in both peripheral and central systems tends to increase in pure mania, it has been found to rise by more than 50% in mixed mania [37].

Second, serum levels of inflammatory cytokines, such as tumor necrosis factor (TNF)-α and interleukin (IL)-6, were significantly higher than in the control group, and serum IL-6 levels showed a significant positive correlation with the Young Mania Rating Scale (YMRS) score in mixed states [38]. Another research has also suggested that depression with severe anxiety is associated with increased immune system activity, such as C-reactive protein (CRP) and monocyte elevation [39]. Since 2020, mixed features have increasingly been conceptualized as a distinct neuroinflammatory subtype of mood disorders. Emerging evidence suggests that elevated pro-inflammatory cytokines—particularly IL-1β, IL-6, TNF-α, and CRP—are correlated with structural and functional alterations within fronto-limbic circuits (e.g., orbitofrontal cortex, anterior cingulate), which may underlie atypical neurocircuitry and treatment resistance in mixed episodes [40]. Neuroimaging studies have linked peripheral inflammation levels with fronto-limbic gray matter reductions and connectivity disruptions, supporting a neuroimmune hypothesis. These findings raise the potential for biomarker-guided diagnosis and development of inflammation-targeted therapeutics for patients with mixed features [41].

Third, mixed states may be related to increased cortisol secretion. In mixed mania, the function of the Hypothalamic–Pituitary–Adrenal axis is increased, similar to the degree of depressive symptoms, and cerebrospinal fluid cortisol levels correlated with depressive indices [37]. However, some pure manic episodes also showed a non-suppressive pattern in the dexamethasone suppression test, so further research is still required [37, 42]. Fourth, while some studies have reported an association between thyroid dysfunction and mixed episodes, other research has not demonstrated a significant correlation [43–45].

3.4 Clinical Correlates and Temperament

There have been studies suggesting that mixed states are related to underlying emotional temperaments. In mixed episodes centered on mania, emotional elevation and irritability were found to be associated, while anxiety and depressive temperaments were frequently observed in mixed depression [46]. Mixed mania has a higher lifetime prevalence of depressive episodes, dysthymia, anxiety disorders, substance use disorders, and personality disorders compared to pure mania, and is associated with persistent and severe disease courses [47]. Additionally, early onset, female gender, increased suicide rates, a family history of depression, non-suppression in the dexamethasone suppression test, low responsiveness to lithium, and the cycling of manic and depressive states are also linked [24, 25, 48]. Resistance to lithium treatment was observed when manic symptoms co-occurred with two or more depressive symptoms [49].

As the manic symptoms increase during depressive episodes, early onset, frequent recurrence, high comorbidity rates, increased suicide attempts, and a family history of BD were significantly higher. Individuals experiencing a major depressive episode with mixed features—characterized by the presence of at least three manic symptoms—face a significantly heightened risk of suicide attempts, even in the absence of recent suicidal thoughts [50]. In bipolar depression, those with mixed features showed more elevated self-esteem and psychomotor agitation compared to pure depressive episodes, and the time to remission was significantly longer [10]. During this period, the combination of depressive symptoms and impulsivity was associated with increased substance use disorders, head trauma, and suicide attempts [51, 52].

Compared to major depressive episodes, bipolar depressive episodes showed differences in clinical factors such as early onset, frequent episode recurrence, atypical features, and a higher family history of BD. However, in MDD with mixed features, there were no significant differences in clinical factors such as age of onset, atypical features, and family history of BD compared to bipolar II depression [29]. This is an important finding regarding the relationship between BD and MDD, indicating that mixed features may serve as a link or continuum between these two disorders. Some scholars suggest that mixed features in MDD could be associated with bipolar spectrum disorders. Manic symptoms during depressive episodes were found to be more prevalent in BD, and these individuals are likely to eventually experience independent manic or hypomanic episodes. Early onset BD, especially depression onset before age 21, high recurrence (more than four depressive episodes), and frequent hospitalizations—particularly frequent mixed depression episodes—and a family history of BD are indicators suggesting bipolarity, including BD II [53, 54]. Additionally, the number of past depressive episodes and the number of manic symptoms during depressive episodes were significantly correlated [55]. Particularly in patients whose diagnosis changed from MDD to BD II, there was a higher self-report of mood fluctuations, energy activation, and daydreaming, and the early onset, high rates of substance use disorders were related [56].

In BD patients, those whose initial episode was mixed showed differences in long-term disease course compared to those whose episodes started with other types. These patients were more likely to exhibit suicide attempts and chronic courses, though the relationship with rapid cycling was inconsistent across studies [57]. They experienced a longer duration of mixed states throughout their disease course, with a relatively higher prevalence of mixed or depressive episodes and dysthymia. In contrast, patients who experienced mania as the first episode showed a higher prevalence of manic, hypomanic, and psychotic features [58]. Mixed states have diagnostic stability across episodes, and patients who experienced a mixed state during the first episode were more likely to re-experience mixed states in subsequent episodes. This was also consistent with the DSM-IV-TR criteria for mixed episodes and the criteria for mixed depression with depressive episodes as the primary polarity [59, 60].

In conclusion, regardless of the type of initial episode, patients showing one or more opposing polarity symptoms (e.g., manic and depressive features) are associated with increased anxiety, more frequent relapses, and a higher history of suicide attempts, all contributing to a more severe disease course. Furthermore, the concept and characteristics of mixed states, independent of diagnostic criteria and assessment methods, are meaningful due to their stability across episodes [23, 61].

3.5 Treatment Approaches

Pharmacological Management

The pharmacological treatment of mixed depression must not only show antidepressant effects but also demonstrate efficacy in treating manic symptoms, while simultaneously preventing the transition of mood episodes induced by medication. However, historically, mixed episodes were defined predominantly by manic symptoms, and pharmacological research has been focused on mixed mania rather than mixed depression. Therefore, evidence for pharmacological treatment strategies for mixed depression is relatively sparse compared to mixed mania. Up until recently, there have been only three randomized controlled trials on this topic, while subsequent post-hoc analyses on atypical antipsychotics have primarily focused on bipolar depression, with only a limited number specifically addressing MDD with mixed features. Thus, there is a lack of sufficient research to conclusively discuss treatment for mixed depression, making it difficult to reach a clear conclusion.

Let us first examine the three randomized, placebo-controlled studies. The first study investigated the effect of ziprasidone monotherapy in patients with DSM-IV criteria for major depressive episode with two to three manic symptoms in BD II or MDD [62]. This six-week study included 73 participants, randomly assigned to either the ziprasidone monotherapy group or the placebo group. The allowable dose of ziprasidone was 40–160 mg/day, with an average dose of 129.7 ± 45.3 mg/day. The change in Montgomery–Åsberg Depression Rating Scale (MADRS) total score at week 3 was significantly greater in the ziprasidone group compared to the placebo group, and this effect persisted through week 6. The antidepressant effect was more pronounced in BD II than in MDD. However, there was no significant difference in the change in the Mania Rating Scale total score between the two groups. Ziprasidone also showed favorable tolerability, with no significant weight gain or extrapyramidal symptoms. Post-hoc analysis of this study identified the three most common symptoms of mixed depression—flight of ideas (60%), distractibility (58%), and irritability (55%)—and raised questions about the diagnostic exclusion criteria [57]. Additionally, it was reported that the treatment response to mixed depression did not support a dichotomous classification between MDD and BD based on DSM criteria [63].

Second, a randomized, double-blind, placebo-controlled study evaluated the efficacy and safety of lurasidone in patients with MDD presenting with mixed features, defined as two or three subthreshold manic symptoms [64]. A total of 209 patients meeting DSM-IV-TR criteria for MDD were randomized to 6 weeks of lurasidone (20–60 mg/day; n = 109) or placebo (n = 100). Lurasidone significantly improved depressive symptoms and overall illness severity compared to placebo, with least squares mean changes at week 6 in the MADRS (−20.5 vs −13.0; effect size = 0.80) and Clinical Global Impressions-Severity scale (CGI-S: −1.8 vs −1.2; effect size = 0.60). Additional improvements in manic symptoms, as measured by the YMRS, were also observed. Lurasidone was well tolerated, with low rates of adverse event-related discontinuation; the most common side effects were mild nausea and somnolence. These findings support lurasidone as an effective and well-tolerated treatment option for MDD with mixed features. In post-hoc analyses related to this study, it was reported that the most common symptoms of mixed depression (in MDD) were distractibility (59.2%) and irritability (57.3%), emphasizing the importance of nonspecific exclusion symptoms [65].

In the third study, 185 patients with MDD with mixed features and 200 patients with bipolar depression with mixed features were randomized 1:1 to receive either lumateperone 42 mg (n = 193) or placebo (n = 195) for 6 weeks [66]. Significant improvements in the MADRS total score and CGI-S score were observed in the lumateperone group compared to the placebo group. These results were maintained when the MDD and BD groups were analyzed individually. Therefore, lumateperone is expected to be effective in the treatment of mixed depression.

Post-hoc analyses of randomized, placebo-controlled trials of atypical antipsychotics have included olanzapine, olanzapine/fluoxetine combination (OFC), lurasidone, cariprazine, asenapine, and lumateperone.

First, two randomized, placebo-controlled studies were conducted on 1214 patients (olanzapine group: $n = 690$, placebo group: $n = 524$) to evaluate the effect of olanzapine monotherapy in BD I with mixed depression [67]. Mixed depression was redefined as patients with YMRS ≥1 item in 0, 1, or 2, and ≥3 items at baseline. After 6 weeks, the olanzapine group showed significantly better treatment response rates and remission rates in terms of changes in MADRS scores compared to the placebo group.

Second, an 8-week randomized placebo-controlled trial was conducted to assess the effects of olanzapine and OFC in BD I with mixed depression (DSM-IV, major depressive episode with ≥2 items of YMRS) [68]. A total of 788 patients were randomized to receive olanzapine (5–20 mg/day; $n = 351$), OFC (6/25, 6/50, 12/50 mg/day; $n = 82$), or placebo ($n = 355$). After 8 weeks, both olanzapine and OFC showed significant improvements in depressive symptoms compared to placebo. However, OFC did not show superior efficacy compared to olanzapine. When comparing manic switch rates, neither olanzapine nor OFC showed significant differences compared to placebo.

Third, post-hoc analyses of randomized, placebo-controlled 6-week trials have demonstrated lurasidone's efficacy in mixed features across both MDD and bipolar depression. In MDD with mixed features accompanied by anxiety, patients meeting DSM-IV-TR criteria for MDD with ≥2 manic symptoms ($n = 209$) were randomized to lurasidone 20–60 mg/day or placebo; lurasidone significantly improved depressive symptoms measured by MADRS and reduced anxiety severity on Hamilton Anxiety Rating Scale across both mild and moderate-to-severe anxiety groups [69]. Similarly, in MDD with irritability, defined by YMRS irritability and disruptive-aggressive subscale scores ≥2, lurasidone treatment (20–60 mg/day; $n = 209$) produced significant reductions in both depressive and irritability symptoms compared to placebo [70]. In bipolar I depression with subsyndromal hypomanic features, patients with MADRS ≥20 and YMRS ≤12 were randomized to lurasidone 20–60 mg, 80–120 mg, or placebo ($N = 485$); mixed features were defined as YMRS ≥4 at baseline [71]. Lurasidone significantly reduced MADRS scores in both mixed-feature and non-mixed subgroups without increasing treatment-emergent mania or hypomania. Collectively, these studies show that lurasidone effectively improves depressive symptoms while targeting key mixed features such as anxiety, irritability, and subthreshold hypomania, with a favorable safety profile.

Fourth, a pooled post-hoc analysis of three randomized, double-blind, placebo-controlled trials evaluated the efficacy of cariprazine in bipolar I depression with and without concurrent manic symptoms [72]. Among 1383 patients with a current major depressive episode, 58.4% exhibited mixed features defined by a baseline YMRS score ≥4. At week 6, patients with manic symptoms showed significantly greater reductions in MADRS scores with cariprazine 1.5 mg/day and 3 mg/day versus placebo. In patients without manic symptoms, cariprazine 1.5 mg/day significantly reduced MADRS scores, while 3 mg/day showed a nonsignificant trend. These findings suggest cariprazine is effective for bipolar depression both with and without mixed features, with higher doses offering potential benefit in patients with concurrent manic symptoms.

Fifth, randomized controlled trial was conducted to evaluate the effectiveness of lumateperone 42 mg monotherapy for both BD I and II, depressive episode patients, and a post-hoc analysis was performed to assess its effects on mixed depression [73]. A total of 376 patients were classified as having mixed depression (41.5%), if their initial YMRS score was between 4 and 12. The remaining patients, with an initial YMRS score below 4, were classified as having non-mixed depression (51.5%). On day 43, both the mixed depression and non-mixed depression groups showed significant improvement in MADRS and CGI-Bipolar Version total scores, and treatment-related side effects were rare.

A systematic review of drug studies on mixed depression also mentions post-hoc analyses of asenapine. However, caution is needed in interpreting these studies, as the definition of mixed depression in these studies may differ from the revised DSM-5 criteria. Berk et al [74]. defined moderate-to-severe mixed depression in BD I according to DSM-IV-TR as patients meeting both MADRS ≥20 and YMRS ≥20. However, these patients may present with symptoms that would likely be classified as mixed mania under DSM-5.

Treatment Guidelines

We will review the latest trends in the pharmacological management of mixed depression in BD, as outlined in recently published treatment guidelines. Specifically, the pharmacological strategies for managing mixed depression are addressed in several major guidelines, including the Canadian Network for Mood and Anxiety Treatments–International Society for Bipolar Disorders (CANMAT–ISBD) recommendations [75], the World Federation of Societies of Biological Psychiatry (WFSBP) guidelines [76], the Stahl Group's guidelines [77], and Korean Medication Algorithm Project for Bipolar Disorder (KMAP-BP) guidelines [78]. In comparison to other pharmacological treatment guidelines, the KMAP-BP Guidelines provide more clinically useful information as they offer detailed treatment strategies for BD with mixed depression based on expert consensus.

Other guidelines, such as those from the British Association for Psychopharmacology (BAP) [79], International College of Neuro-Psychopharmacology (CINP) [80], and Royal Australian and New Zealand College of Psychiatrists (RANZCP) [20], mention mixed episodes or mixed states in BD, but they do not provide specific treatment strategies for mixed depression. Thus, they offer general insights rather than detailed recommendations.

One of the prominent features observed when summarizing the overall guidelines is the increasing concern about antidepressant monotherapy. In patients with a high likelihood of mixed depression or those who have been diagnosed with it, the use of antidepressants is not recommended, and antidepressants have been excluded from the first- and second-line treatment strategies. When applied to BD, the effectiveness of antidepressants is relatively low and may even trigger activated depression [81]. Additionally, they can increase the risk of suicidal behavior [12]. Studies suggest that when hypomanic symptoms are also present in MDD, the treatment response is similar to that in BD. These patients are especially sensitive to activation by antidepressants and tend to respond better to mood stabilizers [30, 82]. Therefore, if antidepressants must be used, it is recommended to avoid monotherapy and combine them with atypical antipsychotics or mood stabilizers.

The second notable trend is the rise of atypical antipsychotics. A variety of atypical antipsychotics, such as lurasidone, ziprasidone, olanzapine, and quetiapine, are now being recommended as monotherapy or in combination as first- and second-line treatment strategies. This shift is due to the fact that atypical antipsychotics are no longer limited to treating psychotic symptoms but are now recognized for their antidepressant and antimanic effects, highlighting their role as mood stabilizers. Since most treatments have been primarily developed to treat acute episodes of depression or mania, it is not surprising that mixed states are more difficult to treat and require more complex treatment strategies. Therefore, in order to develop effective treatments for mixed states, further research into the neurophysiology and pathophysiology of these conditions will be necessary.

According to the recently published Korean Medication Algorithm Project for Depressive Disorder (KMAP-DD) [83], the pharmacological management of MDD with mixed features recommends combining an antidepressant with either an atypical antipsychotic or a mood stabilizer as a first-line option. Second-line strategies include monotherapy with an atypical antipsychotic or a mood stabilizer, antidepressant monotherapy, combining two antidepressants, or augmenting an antidepressant with a typical antipsychotic. Notably, experts frequently selected various antidepressants as first-line treatments, and in acute-phase management, there was a stronger preference for atypical antipsychotics over mood stabilizers.

Non-pharmacological Management

Electroconvulsive therapy (ECT) is known to be effective in the treatment of mixed mania and mixed depression in bipolar disorder as a non-pharmacological treatment. In this context, the severity of depressive symptoms in mixed depression may be related to the treatment response to ECT [84]. Since mixed states are often complex and associated with a high risk of suicide, making treatment difficult, ECT could be a good treatment strategy, particularly when the response to pharmacological treatment is weak or there is a high risk of suicide. Additionally, various psychotherapeutic approaches can also serve as effective treatment methods.

3.6 Remaining Challenges and Future Directions

The classical description of mood disorders depicted them as chronic systemic conditions in which depressive and manic episodes were not systematically distinguished. Following Kraepelin's work, advancements in neuroscience and the serendipitous discovery of episodic-based treatments necessitated a more analytical approach to mood episodes. This led to the development of categorical and mutually exclusive diagnostic criteria for depression and mania, with a focus on the differences between depressive and manic episodes when distinguishing BD from MDD. Furthermore, the approach shifted from a systemic mechanism to a brain-centered perspective on mood disorders, emphasizing the characteristics of episodes over the overall disease course. As a result, mixed states have gradually been regarded as exceptional.

However, as it was discovered that mixed states have a lower response to treatment and a more severe disease course, efforts to define them became necessary. Various diagnostic criteria have been proposed, ranging from a state where depressive and manic episodes are fully mixed as a syndrome, to cases where a depressive or manic episode appears with some symptoms of the opposite polarity. While a unified criterion has not yet been presented, it is generally defined as a case where three or more symptoms of the opposite polarity accompany a major mood episode. However, mixed states cannot simply be understood as a condition where some symptoms of mania and depression overlap. The DSM-5 criteria require at least three symptoms of the opposite episode type to be present alongside a depressive or manic episode, excluding symptoms like anxiety and restlessness, which are considered "overlapping." This is an improvement over the previous criteria, which referred to a complete syndrome including both depressive and manic episodes. However, there is still controversy over whether exclusion diagnoses should be required, whether it is appropriate to partially adopt diagnostic criteria for the opposite polarity episode based on major mood episodes, or whether new diagnostic criteria need to be developed.

In summary, there are still several unresolved issues regarding mixed states. First, there is a need for the establishment of appropriate clinical diagnostic criteria. This will help avoid underdiagnosis due to the ongoing debate surrounding diagnostic criteria. Second, the role of mixed states in the binary classification of bipolar disorder versus major depressive disorder needs to be clarified. Third, efforts are required to develop effective treatments or treatment strategies. Fourth, caution is needed regarding the worsening of disease course due to the priority use of antidepressants. However, further research is needed to determine whether this also applies to mixed states in MDD. To address these issues, ongoing research on pathophysiology and disease classification, as well as continuous discussion, will be necessary.

Declarations

Competing Interests The authors have no competing interests to declare that are relevant to the content of this manuscript.

Ethics Approval The authors declare that this manuscript does not include primary research with human participants.

The authors also declare that this manuscript does not include primary studies involving animals.

References

1. Heinroth JCA. Lehrbuch der Störungen des Seelenlebens oder der Seelenstörungen und ihrer Behandlung – aus rationaler Sicht. Leipzig: Vogel; 1818.
2. Griesinger W. Die Pathologie und Therapie der psychischen Krankheiten für Ärzte und Studierende. Stuttgart: Verlag von Adolph Krabbe; 1861.
3. Kraepelin E. Manic-depressive illness and paranoia. Robertson GM, editor. Edinburgh: E & S Livingstone; 1921.
4. American Psychiatric Association. Diagnostic and statistical manual of mental disorders: DSM-I. 1st ed. Washington, DC: American Psychiatric Association; 1952.
5. American Psychiatric Association. Diagnostic and statistical manual of mental disorders: DSM-II. 2nd ed. Washington, DC: American Psychiatric Association; 1975.
6. American Psychiatric Association. Diagnostic and statistical manual of mental disorders: DSM-III. 3rd ed. Washington, DC: American Psychiatric Association; 1980.
7. Kim W, Kim H, Citrome L, Akiskal HS, Goffin KC, Miller S, Holtzman JN, Hooshmand F, Wang PW, Hill SJ, Ketter TA. More inclusive bipolar mixed depression definitions by requiring fewer non-overlapping mood elevation symptoms. Acta Psychiatr Scand. 2016;134(3):189–98. https://doi.org/10.1111/acps.12598.
8. Kim H, Kim W, Citrome L, Akiskal HS, Goffin KC, Miller S, Holtzman JN, Hooshmand F, Wang PW, Hill SJ, Ketter TA. More inclusive bipolar mixed depression definition by permitting overlapping and non-overlapping mood elevation symptoms. Acta Psychiatr Scand. 2016;134(3):199–206. https://doi.org/10.1111/acps.12599.
9. Goldberg JF, Perlis RH, Bowden CL, Thase ME, Miklowitz DJ, Marangell LB, et al. Manic symptoms during depressive episodes in 1,380 patients with bipolar disorder: findings from the STEP-BD. Am J Psychiatry. 2009;166(2):173–81. https://doi.org/10.1176/appi.ajp.2008.08030343.
10. Shim IH, Woo YS, Jun TY, Bahk WM. Mixed-state bipolar I and II depression: time to remission and clinical characteristics. J Affect Disord. 2014;152–154:340–6. https://doi.org/10.1016/j.jad.2013.09.031.
11. Swann AC, Steinberg JL, Lijffijt M, Moeller GF. Continuum of depressive and manic mixed states in patients with bipolar disorder: quantitative measurement and clinical features. World Psychiatry. 2009;8(3):166. https://doi.org/10.1002/j.2051-5545.2009.tb00246.x.
12. Akiskal HS, Benazzi F, Perugi G, Rihmer Z. Agitated "unipolar" depression reconceptualized as a depressive mixed state: implications for the antidepressant–suicide controversy. J Affect Disord. 2005;85(3):245–58. https://doi.org/10.1016/j.jad.2004.10.004.
13. Koukopoulos A, Sani G, Koukopoulos AE, Manfredi G, Pacchiarotti I, Girardi P. Melancholia agitata and mixed depression. Acta Psychiatr Scand Suppl. 2007;433:50–7. https://doi.org/10.1111/j.1600-0447.2007.01059.x.
14. Swann AC, Secunda SK, Katz MM, Croughan J, Bowden CL, Koslow SH, et al. Specificity of mixed affective states: clinical comparison of dysphoric mania and agitated depression. J Affect Disord. 1993;28(2):81–9. https://doi.org/10.1016/0165-0327(93)90079-c.
15. Koukopoulos A, Sani G. DSM-5 criteria for depression with mixed features: a farewell to mixed depression. Acta Psychiatr Scand. 2014;129(1):4–16. https://doi.org/10.1111/acps.12140.
16. Miller S, Suppes T, Mintz J, Hellemann G, Frye MA, McElroy SL, et al. Mixed depression in bipolar disorder: prevalence rate and clinical correlates during naturalistic follow-up in the Stanley bipolar network. Am J Psychiatry. 2016;173(10):1015–23. https://doi.org/10.1176/appi.ajp.2016.15091133.
17. Perugi G, Angst J, Azorin JM, Bowden CL, Mosolov S, Reis J, et al. Mixed features in patients with a major depressive episode: the BRIDGE-II-MIX study. J Clin Psychiatry. 2015;76(3):e351–8. https://doi.org/10.4088/JCP.14m09030.
18. World Health Organization. International statistical classification of diseases and related health problems. 11th ed. Geneva: WHO; 2019.
19. Perugi G. ICD-11 mixed episode: nothing new despite the evidence. Bipolar Disord. 2019;21(4):376–7. https://doi.org/10.1111/bdi.12785.
20. Malhi GS, Bell E, Bassett D, Boyce P, Bryant R, Hazell P, et al. The 2020 Royal Australian and New Zealand College of Psychiatrists clinical practice guidelines for mood disorders. Aust N Z J Psychiatry. 2021;55(1):7–117. https://doi.org/10.1177/0004867420979353.
21. Benazzi F. Mixed states in bipolar II disorder: should full hypomania always be required? Psychiatry Res. 2004;127(3):247–57. https://doi.org/10.1016/j.psychres.2004.04.007.
22. Benazzi F, Akiskal HS. Psychometric delineation of the most discriminant symptoms of depressive mixed

states. Psychiatry Res. 2006;141(1):81–8. https://doi.org/10.1016/j.psychres.2005.06.008.
23. Swann AC, Lafer B, Perugi G, Frye MA, Bauer M, Bahk WM, et al. Bipolar mixed states: an International Society for Bipolar Disorders task force report of symptom structure, course of illness, and diagnosis. Am J Psychiatry. 2013;170(1):31–42. https://doi.org/10.1176/appi.ajp.2012.12030301.
24. Shim IH, Woo YS, Jun TY, Bahk WM. A reevaluation of the possibility and characteristics in bipolar mania with mixed features: a retrospective chart review. Psychiatry Res. 2014;215(2):335–40. https://doi.org/10.1016/j.psychres.2013.11.013.
25. McElroy SL, Keck PE Jr, Pope HG Jr, Hudson JI, Faedda GL, Swann AC. Clinical and research implications of the diagnosis of dysphoric or mixed mania or hypomania. Am J Psychiatry. 1992;149(12):1633–44. https://doi.org/10.1176/ajp.149.12.1633.
26. Berner P, Katschnig H, Keiffer W, Koehler K, Lenz G, Simhandl C. Diagnostic criteria for schizophrenia and affective psychoses (World Psychiatric Association). Washington, DC: American Psychiatric Association; 1983.
27. American Psychiatric Association. Diagnostic and statistical manual of mental disorders. 4th ed, text revision (DSM-IV-TR). Washington, DC: American Psychiatric Association; 2000.
28. Weygandt W. Über die Mischzustände des manisch-depressiven Irreseins. Munich: Verlag von JF Lehmann; 1899.
29. Akiskal HS, Benazzi F. Family history validation of the bipolar nature of depressive mixed states. J Affect Disord. 2003;73(1–2):113–22. https://doi.org/10.1016/s0165-0327(02)00352-5.
30. Benazzi F, Akiskal HS. Delineating bipolar II mixed states in the Ravenna-San Diego collaborative study: the relative prevalence and diagnostic significance of hypomanic features during major depressive episodes. J Affect Disord. 2001;67(1–3):115–22. https://doi.org/10.1016/S0165-0327(01)00443-8.
31. Zimmermann P, Brückl T, Nocon A, Pfister H, Lieb R, Wittchen HU, et al. Heterogeneity of DSM-IV major depressive disorder as a consequence of subthreshold bipolarity. Arch Gen Psychiatry. 2009;66(12):1341–52. https://doi.org/10.1001/archgenpsychiatry.2009.158.
32. Himmelhoch JM, Mulla D, Neil JF, Detre TP, Kupfer DJ. Incidence and significance of mixed affective states in a bipolar population. Arch Gen Psychiatry. 1976;33(9):1062–6. https://doi.org/10.1001/archpsyc.1976.01770090032002.
33. Azorin JM, Aubrun E, Bertsch J, Reed C, Gerard S, Lukasiewicz M. Mixed states vs pure mania in the French sample of the EMBLEM study: results at baseline and 24 months—European mania in bipolar longitudinal evaluation of medication. BMC Psychiatry. 2009;9:33. https://doi.org/10.1186/1471-244X-9-33.
34. Goodwin FK, Jamison K. Manic-depressive illness. New York: Oxford University Press; 1990.
35. Shim IH, Woo YS, Bahk WM. Prevalence rates and clinical implications of bipolar disorder "with mixed features" as defined by DSM-5. J Affect Disord. 2015;173:120–5. https://doi.org/10.1016/j.jad.2014.10.066.
36. Berk M, Kapczinski F, Andreazza AC, Dean OM, Giorlando F, Maes M, et al. Pathways underlying neuroprogression in bipolar disorder: focus on inflammation, oxidative stress and neurotrophic factors. Neurosci Biobehav Rev. 2011;35(3):804–17. https://doi.org/10.1016/j.neubiorev.2010.10.001.
37. Swann AC, Stokes PE, Secunda SK, Maas JW, Bowden CL, Berman N, et al. Depressive mania versus agitated depression: biogenic amine and hypothalamic-pituitary-adrenocortical function. Biol Psychiatry. 1994;35(10):803–13. https://doi.org/10.1016/0006-3223(94)91139-4.
38. Luo Y, He H, Zhang M, Huang X, Fan N. Altered serum levels of TNF-α, IL-6 and IL-18 in manic, depressive, and mixed states of bipolar disorder patients. Psychiatry Res. 2016;244:19–23. https://doi.org/10.1016/j.psychres.2016.07.033.
39. Shim IH, Woo YS, Bahk WM. Associations between immune activation and the current severity of the "with anxious distress" specifier in patients with depressive disorders. Gen Hosp Psychiatry. 2016;42:27–31. https://doi.org/10.1016/j.genhosppsych.2016.06.001.
40. Benedetti F, Poletti S, Hoogenboezem TA, Locatelli C, Colombo C, de Wit H, et al. Inflammation and bipolar disorder: new evidence of a neuroinflammatory subtype. Front Psych. 2020;11:71. https://doi.org/10.3389/fpsyt.2020.00071.
41. Altamura M, Leccisotti I, Mollica A, Maddalena S, Altamura C, Moretti M, Bellomo A. Inflammatory biomarkers, cognitive functioning, and brain imaging abnormalities in bipolar disorder: a systematic review. Clin Neuropsychiatry. 2024;21(1):32–62. https://doi.org/10.36131/cnfioritieditore20240103.
42. Swann AC, Stokes PE, Casper R, Secunda SK, Bowden CL, Berman N, et al. Hypothalamic-pituitary-adrenocortical function in mixed and pure mania. Acta Psychiatr Scand. 1992;85(4):270–4. https://doi.org/10.1111/j.1600-0447.1992.tb01471.x.
43. Shim IH, Woo YS, Bae DS, Bahk WM. Thyroid functioning in patients with bipolar disorder with mixed features. Psychiatry Res. 2015;225(1–2):212–4. https://doi.org/10.1016/j.psychres.2014.11.040.
44. Cassidy F, Ahearn E, Carroll B. Thyroid function in mixed and pure manic episodes. Bipolar Disord. 2002;4(6):393–7. https://doi.org/10.1034/j.1399-5618.2002.01213.x.
45. Chang KD, Keck PE, Stanton SP, McElroy SL, Strakowski SM, Geracioti TD. Differences in thyroid function between bipolar manic and mixed states. Biol Psychiatry. 1998;43(10):730–3. https://doi.org/10.1016/s0006-3223(97)00443-3.
46. Iasevoli F, Valchera A, Di Giovambattista E, Marconi M, Rapagnani MP, De Berardis D, et al. Affective temperaments are associated with specific clusters

of symptoms and psychopathology: a cross-sectional study on bipolar disorder inpatients in acute manic, mixed, or depressive relapse. J Affect Disord. 2013;151(2):540–50. https://doi.org/10.1016/j.jad.2013.06.054.
47. Agosti V, Stewart JW. Hypomania with and without dysphoria: comparison of comorbidity and clinical characteristics of respondents from a national community sample. J Affect Disord. 2008;108(1):177–82. https://doi.org/10.1016/j.jad.2007.10.020.
48. Suppes T, Mintz J, McElroy SL, Altshuler LL, Kupka RW, Frye MA, et al. Mixed hypomania in 908 patients with bipolar disorder evaluated prospectively in the Stanley Foundation bipolar treatment network: a sex-specific phenomenon. Arch Gen Psychiatry. 2005;62(10):1089–96. https://doi.org/10.1001/archpsyc.62.10.1089.
49. Swann AC, Bowden CL, Morris D, Calabrese JR, Petty F, Small J, et al. Depression during mania: treatment response to lithium or divalproex. Arch Gen Psychiatry. 1997;54(1):37–42. https://doi.org/10.1001/archpsyc.1997.01830130041008.
50. Peyre H, Hoertel N, Pignon B, Amad A, Roelandt JL, Benradia I, et al. Mixed features and nonfatal suicide attempt among individuals with major depressive episode: insights from the French MHGP survey. J Clin Psychiatry. 2024;85(4):24m15445. https://doi.org/10.4088/JCP.24m15445.
51. Swann AC, Moeller FG, Steinberg JL, Schneider L, Barratt ES, Dougherty DM. Manic symptoms and impulsivity during bipolar depressive episodes. Bipolar Disord. 2007;9(3):206–12. https://doi.org/10.1111/j.1399-5618.2007.00420.x.
52. Balazs J, Benazzi F, Rihmer Z, Rihmer A, Akiskal KK, Akiskal HS. The close link between suicide attempts and mixed (bipolar) depression: implications for suicide prevention. J Affect Disord. 2006;91(2–3):133–8. https://doi.org/10.1016/j.jad.2005.12.049.
53. Benazzi F, Akiskal HS. How best to identify a bipolar-related subtype among major depressive patients without spontaneous hypomania: superiority of age at onset criterion over recurrence and polarity? J Affect Disord. 2008;107(1–3):77–88. https://doi.org/10.1016/j.jad.2007.07.021.
54. Winokur G, Wesner R. From unipolar depression to bipolar illness: 29 who changed. Acta Psychiatr Scand. 1987;76(1):59–63. https://doi.org/10.1111/j.1600-0447.1987.tb02864.x.
55. Benazzi F. Challenging the unipolar-bipolar division: does mixed depression bridge the gap? Prog Neuro-Psychopharmacol Biol Psychiatry. 2007;31(1):97–103. https://doi.org/10.1016/j.pnpbp.2006.07.008.
56. Akiskal HS, Maser JD, Zeller PJ, Endicott J, Coryell W, Keller M, et al. Switching from 'unipolar' to bipolar II. An 11-year prospective study of clinical and temperamental predictors in 559 patients. Arch Gen Psychiatry. 1995;52(2):114–23. https://doi.org/10.1001/archpsyc.1995.03950140024004.
57. Perugi G, Micheli C, Akiskal HS, Madaro D, Socci C, Quilici C, et al. Polarity of the first episode, clinical characteristics, and course of manic depressive illness: a systematic retrospective investigation of 320 bipolar I patients. Compr Psychiatry. 2000;41(1):13–8. https://doi.org/10.1016/S0010-440X(00)90125-6.
58. Baldessarini RJ, Salvatore P, Khalsa HM, Tohen M. Dissimilar morbidity following initial mania versus mixed states in type-I bipolar disorder. J Affect Disord. 2010;126(1–2):299–302. https://doi.org/10.1016/j.jad.2010.03.017.
59. Cassidy F, Ahearn E, Carroll BJ. A prospective study of inter-episode consistency of manic and mixed subtypes of bipolar disorder. J Affect Disord. 2001;67(1–3):181–5. https://doi.org/10.1016/S0165-0327(01)00435-9.
60. Sato T, Bottlender R, Sievers M, Schröter A, Kleindienst N, Möller HJ. Evaluating the interepisode stability of depressive mixed states. J Affect Disord. 2004;81(2):103–13. https://doi.org/10.1016/S0165-0327(03)00156-3.
61. Perugi G, Medda P, Swann AC, Reis J, Rizzato S, Mauri M. Phenomenological subtypes of severe bipolar mixed states: a factor analytic study. Compr Psychiatry. 2014;55(4):799–806. https://doi.org/10.1016/j.comppsych.2013.12.004.
62. Patkar A, Gilmer W, Pae CU, Vohringer PA, Ziffra M, Pirok E, et al. A 6-week randomized double-blind placebo-controlled trial of ziprasidone for the acute depressive mixed state. PLoS One. 2012;7(4):e34757. https://doi.org/10.1371/journal.pone.0034757.
63. Pae CU, Vohringer PA, Holtzman NS, Thommi SB, Patkar A, Gilmer W, et al. Mixed depression: a study of its phenomenology and relation to treatment response. J Affect Disord. 2012;136(3):1059–61. https://doi.org/10.1016/j.jad.2011.06.049.
64. Suppes T, Silva R, Cucchiaro J, Mao Y, Targum S, Streicher C, et al. Lurasidone for the treatment of major depressive disorder with mixed features: a randomized, double-blind, placebo-controlled study. Am J Psychiatry. 2016;173(4):400–7. https://doi.org/10.1176/appi.ajp.2015.15060770.
65. Targum SD, Suppes T, Pendergrass JC, Lee S, Silva R, Cucchiaro J, et al. Major depressive disorder with subthreshold hypomania (mixed features): clinical characteristics of patients entered in a multiregional, placebo-controlled study. Prog Neuro-Psychopharmacol Biol Psychiatry. 2016;68:9–14. https://doi.org/10.1016/j.pnpbp.2016.03.002.
66. Durgam S, Kozauer SG, Earley WR, Chen C, Huo J, Lakkis H, et al. Lumateperone for the treatment of major depressive disorder with mixed features or bipolar depression with mixed features: a randomized placebo-controlled trial. J Clin Psychopharmacol. 2025;45(2):67–75. https://doi.org/10.1097/JCP.0000000000001964.
67. Tohen M, Kanba S, McIntyre RS, Fujikoshi S, Katagiri H. Efficacy of olanzapine monotherapy in the treatment of bipolar depression with mixed

features. J Affect Disord. 2014;164:57–62. https://doi.org/10.1016/j.jad.2014.04.033.
68. Benazzi F, Berk M, Frye MA, Wang W, Barraco A, Tohen M. Olanzapine/fluoxetine combination for the treatment of mixed depression in bipolar I disorder: a post hoc analysis. J Clin Psychiatry. 2009;70(10):1424–31. https://doi.org/10.4088/JCP.08m04590.
69. Tsai J, Thase ME, Mao Y, Ng-Mak D, Pikalov A, Loebel A. Lurasidone for major depressive disorder with mixed features and anxiety: a post-hoc analysis of a randomized, placebo-controlled study. CNS Spectr. 2017;22(2):236–45. https://doi.org/10.1017/S109285291600046X.
70. Swann AC, Fava M, Tsai J, Mao Y, Pikalov A, Loebel A. Lurasidone for major depressive disorder with mixed features and irritability: a post-hoc analysis. CNS Spectr. 2017;22(2):228–35. https://doi.org/10.1017/S1092852916000458.
71. McIntyre RS, Cucchiaro J, Pikalov A, Kroger H, Loebel A. Lurasidone in the treatment of bipolar depression with mixed (subsyndromal hypomanic) features: post hoc analysis of a randomized placebo-controlled trial. J Clin Psychiatry. 2015;76(4):398–405. https://doi.org/10.4088/JCP.14m09168.
72. McIntyre RS, Suppes T, Earley W, Patel M, Stahl SM. Cariprazine efficacy in bipolar I depression with and without concurrent manic symptoms: post hoc analysis of 3 randomized, placebo-controlled studies. CNS Spectr. 2020;25(4):502–10. https://doi.org/10.1017/S1092852919001444.
73. McIntyre RS, Durgam S, Huo J, Kozauer SG, Stahl SM. The efficacy of lumateperone in patients with bipolar depression with mixed features. J Clin Psychiatry. 2023;84(3):22m14739. https://doi.org/10.4088/JCP.22m14739.
74. Berk M, Tiller JW, Zhao J, Yatham LN, Malhi GS, Weiller E. Effects of asenapine in bipolar I patients meeting proxy criteria for moderate-to-severe mixed major depressive episodes: a post hoc analysis. J Clin Psychiatry. 2015;76(6):728–34. https://doi.org/10.4088/JCP.14m09618.
75. Yatham LN, Chakrabarty T, Bond DJ, Schaffer A, Beaulieu S, Parikh SV, et al. Canadian network for mood and anxiety treatments (CANMAT) and International Society for Bipolar Disorders (ISBD) recommendations for the management of patients with bipolar disorder with mixed presentations. Bipolar Disord. 2021;23(8):767–88. https://doi.org/10.1111/bdi.13110.
76. Grunze H, Vieta E, Goodwin GM, Bowden C, Licht RW, Azorin JM, et al. The World Federation of Societies of Biological Psychiatry (WFSBP) guidelines for the biological treatment of bipolar disorders: acute and long-term treatment of mixed states in bipolar disorder. World J Biol Psychiatry. 2018;19(1):2–58. https://doi.org/10.1080/15622975.2017.1384850.
77. Stahl SM, Morrissette DA, Faedda G, Fava M, Goldberg JF, Keck PE, et al. Guidelines for the recognition and management of mixed depression. CNS Spectr. 2017;22(2):203–19. https://doi.org/10.1017/S109285291700002X.
78. Kim W, Bahk WM, Woo YS, Jeong JH, Seo JS, Choo IH, et al. Korean medication algorithm project for bipolar disorder 2022: mixed features. J Korean Neuropsychiatr Assoc. 2022;61(2):133–42. https://doi.org/10.4306/jknpa.2022.61.2.133.
79. Goodwin GM, Haddad PM, Ferrier IN, Aronson JK, Barnes T, Cipriani A, et al. Evidence-based guidelines for treating bipolar disorder: revised third edition recommendations from the British Association for Psychopharmacology. J Psychopharmacol. 2016;30(6):495–553. https://doi.org/10.1177/0269881116636545.
80. Fountoulakis KN, Grunze H, Vieta E, Young A, Yatham L, Blier P, et al. The International College of Neuro-Psychopharmacology (CINP) treatment guidelines for bipolar disorder in adults (CINP-BD-2017), part 3: the clinical guidelines. Int J Neuropsychopharmacol. 2016;20(2):180–95. https://doi.org/10.1093/ijnp/pyw109.
81. Sani G, Napoletano F, Vohringer PA, Sullivan M, Simonetti A, Koukopoulos A, et al. Mixed depression: clinical features and predictors of its onset associated with antidepressant use. Psychother Psychosom. 2014;83(4):213–21. https://doi.org/10.1159/000360771.
82. Goldberg JF, Perlis RH, Ghaemi SN, Calabrese JR, Bowden CL, Wisniewski S, et al. Adjunctive antidepressant use and symptomatic recovery among bipolar depressed patients with concomitant manic symptoms: findings from the STEP-BD. Am J Psychiatry. 2007;164(9):1348–55. https://doi.org/10.1176/appi.ajp.2007.06091486.
83. Park YM, Seo JS, Woo YS, Bahk WM, Kim W, Jeong JS, et al. Korean medication algorithm project for depressive disorder 2021 (II): the subtypes of depression. J Korean Neuropsychiatr Assoc. 2021;60(3):186–92. https://doi.org/10.4306/jknpa.2021.60.3.186.
84. Small JG, Klapper MH, Kellams JJ, Miller MJ, Milstein V, Sharpley PH, et al. Electroconvulsive treatment compared with lithium in the management of manic states. Arch Gen Psychiatry. 1988;45(8):727–32. https://doi.org/10.1001/archpsyc.1988.01800320061009.

Part II

Depressive Disorder in Diverse Populations and Clinical Contexts

Reproductive Life Cycle and Depression in Women

4

Kyung-Min Kim and Young-Eun Jung

4.1 Introduction

Depression is one of the most common psychiatric disorders worldwide and is about twice as frequent in women as in men [1]. This difference is not a mere statistical observation but is understood as the result of an interplay between biological factors, psychosocial environments, and cognitive characteristics. Among these, reproductive transitions throughout a woman's life—puberty, menstrual cycling, perinatal period, and menopause—are directly linked to rapid hormonal fluctuations, and each stage has been noted as a period of increased risk for depressive episodes [1, 2].

Sex hormones such as estrogen and progesterone regulate neurotransmitters like serotonin, dopamine, and norepinephrine, and promote neuroplasticity, thereby playing a key role in mood stabilization. However, during times of abrupt hormonal change, these protective effects can weaken or become unstable, leaving some women more vulnerable to mood disorders [1, 3]. In addition, women are more frequently exposed to influential environmental risk factors such as childhood sexual abuse and intimate partner violence, while social gender roles and structural inequality further amplify these risks [1, 4]. Ultimately, the relationship between reproductive life cycle and depression in women should not be understood merely as an issue of hormonal fluctuation but as the outcome of interactions among biological sensitivity, psychosocial stress, and cognitive traits. Considering this context, the connection between reproductive stages and mental health is not simply an academic subject but has direct implications for clinical interventions and preventive strategies.

This chapter examines the relationship between the female reproductive life cycle and depression, focusing in particular on premenstrual dysphoric disorder (PMDD), perinatal depression, and menopausal depression. Figure 4.1 provides a visual overview of the main hormonal changes and depression risk across the female life cycle, serving as a foundation for understanding the detailed discussion that follows.

K.-M. Kim
Department of Psychiatry, Naju National Hospital, Naju, Republic of Korea

Y.-E. Jung (✉)
Department of Psychiatry, Jeju National University Hospital, School of Medicine, Jeju National University, Jeju, Republic of Korea
e-mail: jyejye@jejunu.ac.kr

W.-M. Bahk et al. (eds.), *Depressive Disorder*, https://doi.org/10.1007/978-981-92-1331-3_4

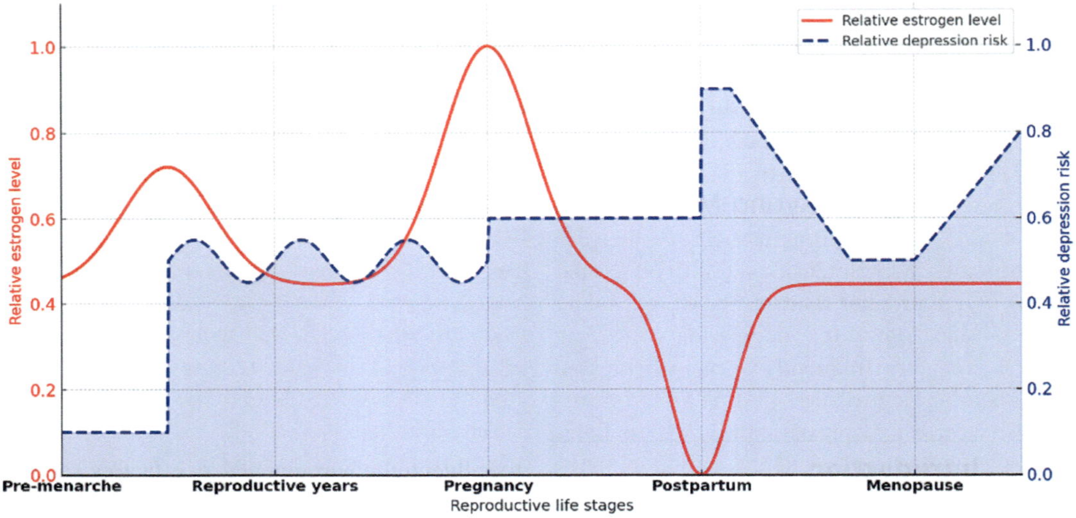

Fig. 4.1 Conceptual illustration: Estrogen fluctuation and depression risk across female reproductive stages. This schematic figure depicts the relative changes in estrogen levels (red line, left axis) and the relative risk of depression (blue dashed line with shaded area, right axis) across major female reproductive stages. Estrogen remains low before menarche, increases with cyclic fluctuations during the reproductive years, peaks during pregnancy, and drops sharply after childbirth (postpartum period). Depression risk is minimal before menarche, moderate during the reproductive years, slightly elevated in pregnancy, and reaches its highest point immediately postpartum before declining to baseline levels. The risk increases again during the menopausal transition, when estrogen levels gradually decline. The figure is intended as a conceptual representation and does not reflect quantitative data. Risk curve reflects not only prevalence but also clinical severity/acuity

4.2 Pregnancy and Depression

During the peripartum period, a variety of psychiatric problems may arise, with depressive episodes being the most common psychiatric complication. The *Diagnostic and Statistical Manual of Mental Disorders, fifth Edition* (DSM-5) replaced the older term "postpartum onset" with "peripartum onset," reflecting the fact that depressive episodes often occur not only after childbirth but also during pregnancy. In fact, more than half of perinatal depression cases are reported to have begun during pregnancy [5]. Pregnancy itself causes changes in sleep, appetite, and energy levels, making it easy to confuse these physiological shifts with depressive symptoms. Therefore, careful attention to emotional core symptoms—such as worthlessness, guilt, hopelessness, and suicidal ideation—is important for diagnosis.

Postpartum blues occur in 40–80% of women immediately after delivery and usually improve within 2 weeks [6]. However, if symptoms persist beyond this period and are accompanied by functional impairment, the diagnosis of perinatal depression should be considered.

Risk factors for perinatal depression include a personal or family history of depression, childhood trauma, personality disorders, lack of social support, intimate partner violence, low spousal support, and medical complications such as anemia, gestational diabetes, or thyroid disease [7, 8]. Perinatal depression not only causes suffering for the mother but also increases obstetric risks such as preterm birth and low birth weight, and in the long term is associated with attachment disturbances and delays in children's cognitive and emotional development [8, 9]. For these reasons, repeated depression screening is recommended throughout pregnancy and the perinatal period. The Edinburgh Postnatal Depression Scale (EPDS) is the most widely used self-report tool and serves as the standard instrument in both clinical and research settings [10]. It consists of 10 items scored from 0 to 3 (total score range, 0–30), and higher scores indicate greater depressive symptom severity. In general, scores of 13 or higher suggest clinically significant depressive symptoms, while endorsement of self-harm ideation warrants immediate clinical evaluation.

4.3 Treatment of Perinatal Depression

Perinatal depression has profound effects not only on the mother's quality of life but also on the family and the infant's development, making early intervention essential. For mild symptoms, psychotherapy is recommended as the first-line approach. Cognitive-behavioral therapy (CBT) and interpersonal therapy (IPT) have demonstrated both efficacy and safety, contributing to symptom relief as well as relapse prevention. Recently, digital interventions—such as Internet-based CBT, mobile applications, and peer-support programs—have improved accessibility and shown therapeutic benefits, leading to broader use [11–13]. Lifestyle-based interventions are also important adjunct strategies. Regular physical activity, sleep hygiene, and stress management not only help prevent perinatal depression but also support symptom reduction, and they are strongly recommended in clinical practice [14].

For moderate to severe cases, pharmacological treatment is necessary. Multiple guidelines emphasize that pharmacotherapy should not be delayed when symptoms are severe, relapse risk is high, or suicidal ideation or psychotic symptoms are present [15–17].

The most widely used antidepressants during pregnancy are selective serotonin reuptake inhibitors (SSRIs), with sertraline, escitalopram, and citalopram being most commonly recommended. Sertraline is typically used at 50–200 mg/day, escitalopram at 10–20 mg/day, and citalopram at 20–40 mg/day (with caution above 40 mg due to QT prolongation). Paroxetine may be used at 10–40 mg/day, but it has been associated with a 1.5–2-fold increased risk of congenital cardiac malformations when taken in early pregnancy and is therefore generally avoided [18, 19].

Quantitatively, a Cochrane meta-analysis of postpartum depression trials [20] demonstrated that SSRIs significantly increased remission and response rates compared with placebo (pooled odds ratio = 2.13; 95% confidence interval [CI] = 1.36–3.32), albeit with moderate heterogeneity. Although most available data are derived from postpartum samples, these findings reinforce the role of SSRIs as the first-line pharmacotherapy across the perinatal period.

If SSRIs are ineffective or poorly tolerated, serotonin-norepinephrine reuptake inhibitors (SNRIs) such as venlafaxine or duloxetine may be considered. Meta-analytic data in major depressive disorder (MDD) indicate that venlafaxine shows a small but statistically significant advantage over SSRIs (standardized mean difference = −0.14; 95% CI = −0.22 to −0.07), corresponding to a number needed to treat of approximately 17 for response improvement [18]. Although direct comparative data in perinatal depression are limited, this evidence supports the clinical rationale for considering SNRIs as an alternative option when SSRI efficacy or tolerability is suboptimal.

While these agents are not strongly linked to teratogenic risk, some studies have reported associations with gestational hypertension and preterm birth, requiring close monitoring during pregnancy [21]. Tricyclic antidepressants (TCAs) have a long history of use but are now considered adjunctive options due to anticholinergic side effects and cardiac conduction issues. Mirtazapine can be useful in women with severe nausea or insomnia, while bupropion may sometimes be prescribed, though rare cases of infant seizures have been reported [22].

Antidepressants can affect the fetus and newborn. While most SSRIs do not significantly increase the risk of major congenital malformations, paroxetine has been consistently linked to cardiac malformations. Late-pregnancy SSRI exposure may lead to neonatal adaptation syndrome (NAS) in 20–30% of infants, presenting with symptoms such as respiratory distress, hypertonia, feeding difficulties, tremors, and irritability. These symptoms are usually mild and self-limited within 2 weeks, though some cases may require intensive care [23]. In rare cases, persistent pulmonary hypertension of the newborn (PPHN) has been reported, with an incidence of 0.2–0.3%, corresponding to a relative risk increase of about 1.5–2 compared to unexposed infants [24]. Some studies report an association with preterm birth and low birth weight, but maternal depression itself is also an independent risk factor. Long-term follow-up studies generally do not support significant negative developmental effects, and untreated maternal depression appears to be more harmful for child development than pharmacological treatment [25].

Even when pharmacotherapy is necessary, breastfeeding is not automatically contraindicated. In fact, many guidelines emphasize that maintaining maternal mental health and supporting mother–infant bonding are important, and breastfeeding should be continued when possible [15–17]. Because exposure through breast milk is unavoidable, minimizing infant risk and ensuring safety are priorities. Here, the relative infant dose (RID)—the infant's weight-adjusted dose received via breast milk compared to the mother's dose—is a useful reference. An RID below 10% is generally considered safe, though immature liver and kidney function in neonates requires careful clinical monitoring even with low RID exposure.

Based on RID data, sertraline (0.5–2%), paroxetine (1–3%), and escitalopram (3–6%) are regarded as the safest SSRIs for breastfeeding. Citalopram (4–8%) is relatively safe but should be avoided in high doses. Fluoxetine has a higher RID (5–15%) and a long half-life, which can lead to elevated infant plasma concentrations and increased risks of irritability, poor feeding, and growth delay. Venlafaxine (6–9%) has been associated with irritability and sleep disturbances in infants, while bupropion (2–10%) has rare reports of infant seizures. Mirtazapine (RID <10%) is considered generally safe, though data are limited [22]. When pharmacotherapy is necessary and the mother strongly wishes to continue breastfeeding, it is recommended to choose drugs with a low RID and established clinical safety, while carefully monitoring the infant for feeding difficulties, irritability, or growth problems.

Beyond traditional antidepressants, neurosteroid-based agents such as brexanolone and zuranolone have recently emerged as new treatment options for postpartum depression, showing rapid antidepressant effects. In phase 3 trials, brexanolone produced mean additional hamilton depression rating scale (HAM-D) score reductions of 3–5.5 points versus placebo within 60 h [26], and zuranolone achieved a −4.2-point greater reduction at day 15, with odds ratios for response and remission of 2.6 and 2.5, respectively [27]. The estimated number needed to treat for response is approximately 4–5. These rapid-acting neurosteroids represent the first mechanistically novel agents approved specifically for postpartum depression. Brexanolone is administered intravenously, while zuranolone has the advantage of being oral. Both, however, are limited by high cost and insufficient data on safety during lactation [25, 27].

International guidelines emphasize several shared principles for perinatal pharmacotherapy. The lowest effective dose should be used, and unnecessary dose reduction or abrupt discontinuation should be avoided, as this can raise relapse rates by up to 50–70%. Monotherapy is preferred whenever possible, and it is generally safer to continue a medication that has previously been effective for the mother rather than switching to a new drug. In all cases, clinicians should ensure informed, shared decision-making with the mother and her family [15–17]. Table 4.1 summarizes the safety profiles of antidepressants commonly used during pregnancy and lactation. This overview allows clinicians to weigh fetal and infant risks against maternal benefits and provides a practical guide for selecting appropriate medications in the perinatal period.

Table 4.1 Safety of antidepressants during pregnancy and lactation

Drug class/Agent	Pregnancy safety	Neonatal/infant risks	Breastfeeding (RID[a])	Clinical recommendation
SSRI (sertraline, escitalopram, citalopram)	No consistent ↑ risk of major malformations; paroxetine associated with ↑ cardiac defects (Relative Risk (RR) 1.5–2.0)	Neonatal adaptation syndrome (20–30%); rare PPHN (0.2–0.3%)	RID usually <10% (lowest: Sertraline)	First-line
SNRI (venlafaxine, duloxetine)	No clear ↑ in malformations; possible ↑ risk of hypertension, preterm birth	Neonatal withdrawal symptoms; irritability	RID <10%	Consider if SSRI not tolerated
TCA	Long clinical experience; low teratogenic risk	Anticholinergic side effects; neonatal sedation	Generally safe	Adjunctive/ second-line
Mirtazapine	Limited but reassuring data; low risk of malformations	Possible sedation; feeding difficulties	Limited evidence	Useful in cases with insomnia, nausea
Bupropion	Limited data; not clearly teratogenic	Rare infant seizures reported	Detectable in breast milk	Use cautiously; avoid in epilepsy risk
Neurosteroids (brexanolone, zuranolone)	Limited pregnancy data	Unknown lactation safety; maternal side effects (sedation, dizziness)	Not recommended	Consider only in refractory postpartum depression (FDA-approved indication)

FDA Food and Drug Administration
[a]RID = relative infant dose; <10% is generally considered safe
[↑] denotes an increased risk or increased frequency

4.4 Premenstrual Dysphoric Disorder (PMDD)

PMDD is distinct from premenstrual syndrome (PMS) in that it involves severe emotional and physical symptoms that are closely tied to the menstrual cycle and cause marked impairment in social and occupational functioning. Symptoms typically begin in the late luteal phase after ovulation, improve within a few days after the onset of menstruation, and are minimal or absent until the next cycle. This cyclical pattern is a defining feature. According to DSM-5, PMDD is diagnosed when at least five emotional and physical symptoms are present and cause significant disruption to daily functioning [5].

Clinically, common emotional and cognitive symptoms include depressed mood, anxiety, anger and irritability, difficulty with impulse control, poor concentration, and loss of interest. Physical symptoms such as breast tenderness, headaches, abdominal bloating, and musculoskeletal pain are also frequent. These lead to recurrent interpersonal conflicts and reduced occupational performance, substantially lowering quality of life. Epidemiological studies estimate that PMDD affects about 2–5% of women of reproductive age, with only a small proportion of those experiencing PMS meeting criteria for clinically significant functional impairment [3, 28, 29].

Although the exact pathophysiology is not fully understood, rapid fluctuations of estrogen and progesterone in the late luteal phase are thought to trigger symptoms. Recent findings suggest that the rate of change, rather than the absolute hormone levels, may be more critical [30]. Allopregnanolone, a metabolite of progesterone, is a neurosteroid acting on Gamma-Aminobutyric Acid Type A (GABA-A) receptors. Under normal conditions, it reduces anxiety, but in women with PMDD, abnormal sensitivity of GABA-A receptors may paradoxically induce anxiety and mood instability [30, 31]. Serotonin dysfunction is also strongly implicated, explaining why SSRIs are highly effective; their benefits are thought to come not only from serotonin reuptake inhibition but also from promoting allopregnanolone synthesis and thereby indirectly modulating GABA activity [31]. Other factors such as elevated High-Sensitivity C-Reactive Protein (hs-CRP), cytokine imbalances, and reduced Hypothalamic–Pituitary–Adrenal (HPA) axis reactivity have been reported [32]. Twin studies suggest heritability over 40%, pointing to genetic vulnerability to hormonal fluctuations [33].

Diagnosis is based on clinical interviews and DSM-5 criteria, but objective confirmation of cyclicity is essential. For this, daily symptom diaries such as the Daily Record of Severity of Problems (DRSP) are widely used. The DRSP helps clinicians determine whether emotional and physical symptoms consistently worsen during the luteal phase and improve after menstruation, making it valuable for distinguishing PMS from PMDD and for tracking treatment response [5, 34]. Table 4.2 summarizes the DRSP domains and interpretation, providing an objective framework that enhances diagnostic reliability and supports ongoing evaluation of treatment effects.

Treatment should combine pharmacological and non-pharmacological approaches. Pharmacological treatment consists broadly of two categories: antidepressants and hormonal therapy. Among antidepressants, SSRIs are considered first-line, with fluoxetine, sertraline, paroxetine, and escitalopram all showing efficacy. They can be taken either continuously or only during the luteal phase, with response rates of 60–90% compared to placebo [30, 31, 35]. Fluoxetine is widely used because it is effective even at low doses (10–20 mg) and generally well tolerated. Sertraline is also effective, though relapse rates may be somewhat higher. Paroxetine works quickly and strongly but is limited by anticholinergic side effects and weight gain [30]. Escitalopram and citalopram have shown promising results, though the evidence is less robust. When SSRIs are not effective or tolerated, SNRIs such as venlafaxine or duloxetine may be alternatives, particularly for anger and irritability, though supporting evidence is limited [36]. By contrast, bupropion, mirtazapine, and tricyclic antidepressants are not recommended due to inconsistent or insufficient evidence [28].

Hormonal therapy may also be considered when physical symptoms dominate or when SSRIs are inadequate. Combined oral contraceptives containing drospirenone and ethinylestradiol are Food and Drug Administration (FDA)-approved for PMDD and have demonstrated significant benefits, particularly for somatic symptoms such as breast tenderness, bloating, and headaches, while also improving mood [37]. GnRH agonists suppress ovulation and relieve symptoms but carry side effects such as hot flashes, vaginal dryness, and bone density loss, limiting their long-term use. Recently, neurosteroid antagonists such as sepranolone and

Table 4.2 Daily record of severity of problems (DRSP) summary

Domain	Example item (summary)	Clinical meaning
Depressed mood	Felt sad or tearful	Depression
Anxiety/tension	Felt anxious, nervous, or on edge	Anxiety
Anger/irritability	Irritable or had difficulty controlling anger	Impulse control/interpersonal
Loss of interest	Lost interest in usual activities	Anhedonia; low motivation
Concentration	Trouble concentrating or distractible	Cognitive impairment
Low energy	Felt easily fatigued	Functional impairment
Appetite changes	Overate or appetite change	Physical symptom
Sleep disturbance	Trouble sleeping or oversleeping	Insomnia/hypersomnia
Physical symptoms	Headache; bloating; breast tenderness; muscle pain	PMS/PMDD-related symptoms
Functional impairment	Difficulty at work/school or social activities	Functional impairment

Source: Endicott et al. [34]

Interpretation: Each item rated 1–6. PMDD diagnosis is supported if symptoms worsen in the late luteal phase and improve after menstruation across ≥2 cycles. No absolute cut-off, but persistent high functional impairment scores indicate clinical high-risk isoallopregnanolone have shown significant benefits in randomized controlled trials [36, 38], suggesting potential new options for treatment-resistant patients. Alongside these pharmacological strategies, non-drug interventions play an important adjunctive role.

Cognitive-behavioral therapy (CBT) helps correct negative thought patterns and teaches coping strategies, and when delivered as couple-based therapy, it can also reduce interpersonal conflict and strengthen support systems [39]. Regular aerobic exercise and yoga improve both mood and physical symptoms through endorphin release and autonomic regulation, with some studies suggesting yoga may even be superior to aerobic exercise [40]. Nutritional supplements such as calcium, vitamin B_6, vitamin D, zinc, and magnesium have also been reported to reduce symptoms [30, 41], while maintaining a balanced diet, limiting caffeine and alcohol, and avoiding smoking are all important lifestyle measures.

PMDD is therefore best understood as a disorder arising from the complex interaction of hormonal fluctuations, serotonin dysfunction, and altered neurosteroid regulation, which sets it apart from PMS due to its severe functional impairment. SSRIs and drospirenone-containing oral contraceptives remain the most established treatments, while neurosteroid modulators represent a promising next-generation option. Non-pharmacological interventions, including CBT, exercise, and nutritional support, are most effective when combined with pharmacological or hormonal treatment. Ultimately, management of PMDD requires individualized, integrative approaches that consider symptom profile, patient preference, and comorbidities.

4.5 Menopausal Depression

Menopause is defined as the permanent cessation of menstruation for at least 12 consecutive months, caused by the gradual loss of ovarian function and the end of ovulation. The average age of onset is around 50 years. The period surrounding this transition, called perimenopause, is defined as the 4–8 years preceding menopause plus the first year after the final menstrual period. During this time, estrogen and progesterone secretion become irregular, accompanied by diverse physical and emotional changes. Menopause is not merely the end of reproductive ability but a significant life transition characterized by hormonal instability, psychosocial adjustments, and increased vulnerability to menopausal depression. This transition represents a critical window during which new depressive symptoms may emerge or pre-existing depression may worsen, underscoring the importance of proactive screening and early intervention [42, 43].

Menopausal depression is not a distinct diagnostic entity, but rather diagnosed according to DSM-5 criteria for major depressive disorder (MDD). Clinically, however, even women who do not meet full criteria often experience overlapping physical and emotional symptoms that substantially impair quality of life. Alongside typical depressive symptoms such as low mood, worthlessness, and loss of interest, women often report insomnia, cognitive difficulties, and chronic pain. These can cause significant functional decline and may correspond to subthreshold depression as described in DSM-5. Therefore, even if the full criteria for a major depressive episode (MDE) are not met, these presentations should be regarded as clinically meaningful and warrant early intervention.

The Menopausal Depression Scale (Meno-D) is a useful assessment tool in such cases, as it broadly covers areas particularly vulnerable during menopause, including vitality, self-esteem, anxiety, irritability, sleep, somatic symptoms, sexual interest, and cognitive functioning. A total score of 15 or more suggests clinical relevance, and higher scores in domains such as energy, self-esteem, and anxiety indicate elevated risk of developing a full depressive episode [44]. Table 4.3 outlines the Meno-D domains and their clinical implications, allowing clinicians to identify subthreshold but clinically important symptoms and intervene before they progress to an MDE.

Treatment of menopausal depression follows the evidence-based principles for MDD. First-line pharmacological options are SSRIs and

Table 4.3 Menopausal depression scale (Meno-D) domains

Domain	Clinical meaning
Energy	Fatigue, low vitality
Irritability	Anger, easily annoyed
Anxiety	Nervousness, tension
Self-esteem	Worthlessness, self-blame
Isolation	Social withdrawal
Paranoid thinking	Suspiciousness, ideas of reference
Sleep disturbance	Insomnia, night awakening
Somatic symptoms	Pain, discomfort
Weight change	Involuntary weight change
Sexual interest	Loss of libido
Memory/ concentration	Cognitive impairment

Source: Kulkarni et al. [44]
Interpretation: Total score 0–48; ≥*15* suggests clinically relevant depressive symptoms and a need for intervention; high scores in energy, self-esteem, and anxiety domains indicate an increased risk of a depressive episode

SNRIs. Standard dosages include sertraline 50–200 mg/day, escitalopram 10–20 mg/day, fluoxetine 20–40 mg/day, and paroxetine 20–40 mg/day. Escitalopram is particularly useful for insomnia and anxiety symptoms, while fluoxetine and paroxetine have shown benefits for vasomotor symptoms in some studies [45]. Venlafaxine XR 75–225 mg/day is effective for hot flashes and night sweats, while duloxetine 60–120 mg/day is especially helpful when chronic pain is present [45, 46].

Hormone replacement therapy (HRT) is not considered a first-line treatment for depression itself, but it may be used adjunctively in women with prominent vasomotor symptoms and insomnia who have no contraindications. Common regimens include oral estradiol 0.5–1 mg/day or transdermal patches (50–100 μg), typically combined with progesterone. Some randomized controlled trials have demonstrated that both low-dose estradiol and venlafaxine can effectively relieve hot flashes and have a positive impact on mood [46]. However, HRT carries long-term risks such as breast cancer, thromboembolism, and cardiovascular disease. Therefore, the 2022 position statement of the North American Menopause Society (NAMS) recommends using the lowest effective dose for the shortest duration with regular reevaluation [47].

Recently, fezolinetant, an NK3 receptor antagonist (45 mg/day), has been approved as a nonhormonal therapy for menopause-related vasomotor symptoms. It has been shown to reduce hot flashes and night sweats, as well as improve sleep quality and overall quality of life. Although not an antidepressant per se, fezolinetant may indirectly support mood stability by alleviating vasomotor and sleep-related disturbances. Rare cases of liver toxicity have been reported, so liver function monitoring is required before and during treatment [48].

First-line pharmacological options for mood symptoms during menopause include SSRIs and SNRIs. Meta-analytic data indicate that these agents yield comparable antidepressant efficacy in midlife depression, although SNRIs such as venlafaxine provide additional benefits for vasomotor symptoms [46], while escitalopram significantly reduces the frequency and severity of hot flashes [45]. Accordingly, antidepressant selection in menopausal women should be guided by both mood and vasomotor symptom profiles, as well as by individual tolerability and comorbidities.

When managing menopausal depression, individualized and integrative approaches are essential, taking into account the overall symptom profile, comorbidities, and patient preferences. Antidepressants remain the therapeutic foundation for mood symptoms, while adjunctive use of SNRIs, hormone replacement therapy (HRT), or non-hormonal agents such as fezolinetant may be appropriate for women with prominent vasomotor symptoms.

Non-pharmacological interventions—including cognitive-behavioral therapy, regular exercise, and sleep hygiene—should also be integrated to optimize symptom control and prevent relapse. Throughout treatment, clinicians should engage in shared decision-making with patients, balancing risks and benefits, and adhering to the principles of minimal effective dosing and regular reevaluation. Ultimately, while menopausal depression is diagnosed as an MDD, it can only be fully understood and managed by considering the unique context of the menopausal transition.

Table 4.4 Clinical features of depression across the female reproductive life cycle

Stage	Prevalence/risk	Core symptoms	Risk factors	Screening tools
Premenstrual (PMDD)	2–5% of reproductive-age women (DSM-defined PMDD)	Depressed mood, anxiety, irritability	Serotonin dysregulation, estrogen fluctuation	DRSP, DSM-5
Pregnancy	~10–12% (point prevalence of MDE during pregnancy)	Low energy, hopelessness, suicidal ideation	History of depression, obstetric complications	EPDS, PHQ-9
Postpartum	~7–19% (point prevalence of MDE within 6 months)	Anxiety, excessive worry about infant health	Postpartum blues, low social support	EPDS, clinical interview
Menopause (perimenopause)	Risk ≈2× higher than premenopausal women; ≈4× higher than men	Depressed mood, mood lability, anxiety, insomnia	VMS, sleep disturbance, past PMDD/Postpartum Depression (PPD)	Meno-D

Note: Prevalence figures for pregnancy and postpartum represent the point prevalence of MDE; PMDD prevalence reflects a distinct cyclical disorder. For menopause, risk is best expressed as relative risk (≈2× higher than premenopausal women, ≈4× higher than men), since absolute prevalence varies widely by study design. Clinically, postpartum carries the most significant acute risk, while menopausal depression is often more chronic with a quality-of-life impact
Abbreviations: *DRSP* Daily Record of Severity of Problems, *DSM-5* Diagnostic and Statistical Manual of Mental Disorders, fifth Edition, *EPDS* Edinburgh Postnatal Depression Scale, *Meno-D* Menopausal Depression Scale, *PHQ-9* Patient Health Questionnaire-9, *PMDD* premenstrual dysphoric disorder, *VMS* vasomotor symptoms

4.6 Summary of Depression Across the Female Reproductive Life Cycle

Depression in women is closely tied to reproductive stage, with each transition marked by characteristic prevalence, symptom patterns, and risk factors. Table 4.4 provides an overview of these key features across the female reproductive life cycle, highlighting the most commonly used screening tools for each stage. This table serves as a concise reference to guide clinicians in assessment and management.

4.7 Conclusion

Depression in women presents with different clinical features and risk factors depending on reproductive life cycle transitions, and these differences cannot be explained by hormonal fluctuations alone. In reality, biological vulnerability, psychosocial stress, and cognitive factors interact to produce distinct forms of depression at each stage. Therefore, clinicians must always consider the patient's reproductive stage when tailoring assessment and intervention.

Perinatal depression requires early screening and intervention, as it affects both the mother and the infant. PMDD is characterized by cyclicity and functional impairment, and daily symptom tracking is valuable for both diagnosis and monitoring treatment response. Menopausal depression often presents with clinically significant symptoms even if full DSM-5 criteria for MDD are not met, and subthreshold symptoms should also be actively evaluated and treated.

Pharmacological treatment is generally centered around SSRIs and SNRIs, but approaches differ by reproductive stage. During the perinatal period, drug safety is the highest priority. In PMDD, intermittent dosing strategies are possible. In menopause, the presence of vasomotor symptoms may guide the choice of SNRIs or HRT, while newer agents such as neurosteroid-based therapies or fezolinetant may be alternatives in treatment-resistant cases. At the same time, non-pharmacological interventions such as cognitive-behavioral therapy, interpersonal therapy, exercise, and lifestyle management complement medication and reduce relapse.

Ultimately, an integrated understanding of the female life cycle and mental health, along with individualized treatment strategies, is essential not only for preserving the quality of life of women but also for promoting the health of families and society at large.

Declarations

Competing Interests The authors have no competing interests to declare that are relevant to the content of this manuscript.

Ethics Approval The authors declare that this manuscript does not include primary research with human participants.

The authors also declare that this manuscript does not include primary studies involving animals.

References

1. Kuehner C. Why is depression more common among women than among men? Lancet Psychiatry. 2017;4(2):146–58.
2. Bromet E, Andrade LH, Hwang I, Sampson NA, Alonso J, De Girolamo G, et al. Cross-national epidemiology of DSM-IV major depressive episode. BMC Med. 2011;9(1):90.
3. Hantsoo L, Epperson CN. Premenstrual dysphoric disorder: epidemiology and treatment. Curr Psychiatry Rep. 2015;17(11):87.
4. Stoltenborgh M, Bakermans-Kranenburg MJ, Alink LR, van IJzendoorn MH. The prevalence of child maltreatment across the globe: review of a series of meta-analyses. Child Abuse Rev. 2015;24(1):37–50.
5. American Psychiatric A. Diagnostic and statistical manual of mental disorders. 5th ed. Arlington: American Psychiatric Association; 2013.
6. Pitt B. Maternity blues. Br J Psychiatry. 1973;122:431–3.
7. Austin MP, Priest SR. Clinical issues in perinatal mental health: new developments in the detection and treatment of perinatal mood and anxiety disorders. Acta Psychiatr Scand. 2005;112:97–104.
8. Halbreich U. Prevalence of mood symptoms and depression during pregnancy: implications for clinical practice and research. CNS Spectr. 2004;9:177–84.
9. Reck C, Hunt A, Fuchs T, Weiss R, Noon A, Moehler E. Interactive regulation of affect in postpartum depressed mothers and their infants: an overview. Psychopathology. 2004;37:272–80.
10. Cox JL, Holden JM, Sagovsky R. Detection of postnatal depression. Br J Psychiatry. 1987;150:782–6.
11. Sockol LE. A systematic review of the efficacy of cognitive behavioral therapy for treating and preventing perinatal depression. J Affect Disord. 2015;177:7–21.
12. Sockol LE. A systematic review and meta-analysis of interpersonal psychotherapy for perinatal women. J Affect Disord. 2018;232:316–28.
13. Ashford MT, Olander EK, Ayers S. Computer- or web-based interventions for perinatal mental health: a systematic review. J Affect Disord. 2016;197:134–46.
14. Daley AJ, Foster L, Long G. The effectiveness of exercise for the prevention and treatment of antenatal depression: systematic review with meta-analysis. BJOG. 2015;122(1):57–62.
15. American College of O, Gynecologists. ACOG clinical practice guideline no. 5: treatment and management of mental health conditions during pregnancy and postpartum. Obstet Gynecol. 2023;141(6):1262–91.
16. National Institute for H, Care E. Antenatal and postnatal mental health: clinical management and service guidance [CG192]. 2020.
17. Vigod SN, Frey BN, Clark CT, Grigoriadis S, Barker LC, Brown HK, et al. Canadian network for mood and anxiety treatments 2024 clinical practice guideline for the Management of Perinatal Mood, anxiety, and related disorders: guide de pratique 2024 du Canadian network for mood and anxiety treatments pour le traitement des troubles de l'humeur, des troubles anxieux et des troubles connexes perinatals. Can J Psychiatry. 2025;70(6):429–89.
18. Cipriani A, Furukawa TA, Salanti G, et al. Comparative efficacy and acceptability of 21 antidepressant drugs: a systematic review and network meta-analysis. Lancet. 2018;391(10128):1357–66.
19. Källén B, Olausson PO. Antidepressant drugs during pregnancy and infant congenital heart defect. Reprod Toxicol. 2006;21(3):221–2.
20. Brown J, Pearlstein T, Lurie S, Mulcahy R, Saunders KE, Parry BL, et al. Selective serotonin reuptake inhibitors for postpartum depression. Cochrane Database Syst Rev. 2021;2(2):CD013638.
21. Grigoriadis S, VonderPorten EH, Mamisashvili L, et al. Antidepressant exposure during pregnancy and adverse perinatal outcomes: overview of systematic reviews. CMAJ. 2013;185(7):545–53.
22. Hale TW. Medications and mothers' milk. Amarillo: Hale Publishing; 2012.
23. Sanz EJ, De-las-Cuevas C, Kiuru A, Bate A, Edwards R. Selective serotonin reuptake inhibitors in pregnant women and neonatal withdrawal syndrome: a database analysis. Lancet. 2005;365(9458):482–7.
24. Ng QX, Venkatanarayanan N, Ho CYX, et al. Selective serotonin reuptake inhibitors and persistent pulmonary hypertension of the newborn: an updated meta-analysis. J Women's Health. 2019;28(3):331–8.
25. Rommel AS, Bergink V, Liu X, et al. Long-term effects of antenatal exposure to antidepressants on child development: a systematic review. Eur Child Adolesc Psychiatry. 2020;29(2):147–56.
26. Meltzer-Brody S, Colquhoun H, Riesenberg R, et al. Brexanolone injection in post-partum depression: two multicentre, double-blind, randomised, placebo-controlled, phase 3 trials. Lancet. 2018;392(10152):1058–70.

27. Deligiannidis KM, Meltzer-Brody S, Gunduz-Bruce H, et al. Effect of zuranolone vs placebo in postpartum depression: a randomized clinical trial. JAMA Psychiatry. 2021;78(9):951–9.
28. Pearlstein TB, Halbreich U, Batzar ED, Brown CS, Endicott J, Frank E, et al. Psychosocial functioning in women with premenstrual dysphoric disorder before and after treatment with sertraline or placebo. J Clin Psychiatry. 2000;61(2):101–9.
29. Halbreich U. The etiology, biology, and evolving pathology of premenstrual syndromes. Psychoneuroendocrinology. 2004;28(Suppl 3):55–99.
30. Modzelewski S, Oracz A, Żukow X, Iłendo K, Śledzikowka Z, Waszkiewicz N. Premenstrual syndrome: new insights into etiology and review of treatment methods. Front Psych. 2024;15:1363875.
31. Rapkin AJ. A review of treatment of premenstrual syndrome and premenstrual dysphoric disorder. Psychoneuroendocrinology. 2003;28(Suppl 3):39–53.
32. Gold EB, Wells C, Rasor MO. The association of inflammation with premenstrual symptoms. J Women's Health (Larchmt). 2016;25(9):865–74.
33. Jahanfar S, Lye MS, Krishnarajah IS. The heritability of premenstrual syndrome. Twin Res Hum Genet. 2011;14(5):433–6.
34. Endicott J, Nee J, Harrison W. Daily record of severity of problems (DRSP): reliability and validity. Arch Womens Ment Health. 2006;9(1):41–9.
35. Dimmock PW, Wyatt KM, Jones PW, O'Brien PM. Efficacy of SSRIs in PMS: a systematic review. Lancet. 2000;356(9236):1131–6.
36. Bixo M, Ekberg K, Poromaa IS, Hirschberg AL, Jonasson AF, Andréen L, et al. Treatment of premenstrual dysphoric disorder with the GABAA receptor modulating steroid antagonist sepranolone: a randomized controlled trial. Psychoneuroendocrinology. 2017;80:46–55.
37. Pearlstein TB, Bachmann GA, Zacur HA, Yonkers KA. Treatment of PMDD with a new drospirenone-containing oral contraceptive formulation. Contraception. 2005;72(6):414–21.
38. Bäckström T, Bixo M, Johansson M, Nyberg S, Ossewaarde L, Ragagnin G. Allopregnanolone and mood disorders. Prog Neurobiol. 2014;113:88–94.
39. Ussher JM, Perz J. Evaluation of the relative efficacy of a couple cognitive-behaviour therapy (CBT) for premenstrual disorders, in comparison to one-to-one CBT and a wait list control: a randomized controlled trial. PLoS One. 2017;12(4):e0175068.
40. Chang HC, Cheng YC, Yang CH, Tzeng YL, Chen CH. Effects of yoga for coping with premenstrual symptoms in Taiwan: a cluster randomized study. Healthcare (Basel). 2023;11(8):1183.
41. Jafari F, Amani R, Tarrahi MJ. Effect of zinc supplementation on physical and psychological symptoms, biomarkers of inflammation, oxidative stress, and brain-derived neurotrophic factor in young women with premenstrual syndrome: a randomized, double-blind, placebo-controlled trial. Biol Trace Elem Res. 2020;194(1):89–95.
42. Cohen LS, Soares CN, Vitonis AF, Otto MW, Harlow BL. Risk for new onset of depression during the menopausal transition: the Harvard study of moods and cycles. Arch Gen Psychiatry. 2006;63(4):385–90.
43. Freeman EW. Depression in the menopause transition: risks in the changing hormone milieu as observed in the general population. Women's Midlife Health. 2015;1:2.
44. Kulkarni J, Gavrilidis E, Hudaib AR, Bleeker C, Worsley R, Gurvich C. Development and validation of a new rating scale for perimenopausal depression—the Meno-D. Transl Psychiatry. 2018;8(1):123.
45. Freeman EW, Guthrie KA, Caan B, Sternfeld B, Cohen LS, Joffe H. Efficacy of escitalopram for hot flashes in healthy menopausal women: a randomized controlled trial. JAMA. 2011;305(3):267–74.
46. Joffe H, Guthrie KA, LaCroix AZ, Reed SD, Ensrud KE, Manson JE. Low-dose estradiol and the serotonin–norepinephrine reuptake inhibitor venlafaxine for vasomotor symptoms: a randomized clinical trial. JAMA Intern Med. 2014;174(7):1058–66.
47. The 2022 hormone therapy position statement of The North American Menopause Society. Menopause. 2022;29(7):767–94.
48. Fraser GL, Lederman S, Waldbaum A, Kroll R, Santoro N, Lee M. Efficacy of fezolinetant in moderate-to-severe vasomotor symptoms associated with menopause: a randomized clinical trial. Obstet Gynecol. 2023;141(6):1262–73.

5 Childhood and Adolescent Depression

MoonSoo Lee and Se Hoon Shim

5.1 Introduction

Depressive disorders occur in children and adolescents as well as adults. Since the 1980s, increasing evidence has shown that major depressive disorder (MDD) can present even in young children, and cases of preschool-onset depression have been documented [1]. Diagnostic criteria have been adjusted for developmental context: beginning with *Diagnostic and Statistical Manual of Mental Disorders* (DSM)-III-R, chronic irritable mood was added as an allowable symptom in place of depressed mood for diagnosing MDD in children and adolescents. This modification has been retained through DSM-IV, DSM-5, and DSM-5-TR [1, 2]. Childhood-onset depression can have profound acute and long-term effects. If inadequately treated, depression in youth can lead to severe impairment in social, academic, and other vital functioning; it often persists into adult life, contributing to chronic depression, substance abuse, and increased suicide risk [3]. Unfortunately, families and even physicians may be reluctant to diagnose a young person with a psychiatric disorder due to stigma, sometimes dismissing depressive symptoms as a mere phase of development [4]. However, given the substantial personal and societal costs of untreated depression, there is a growing emphasis on preventive interventions and early treatment. Those preventive interventions and early treatment are essential for youth with known biological, psychological, or social risk factors for mental illness, or those showing subthreshold early symptoms. Notably, the majority of adult psychiatric disorders have their onset in childhood or adolescence; thus, early intervention in youth can be crucial in preventing or mitigating adult psychopathology. Early-onset depression is associated with a worse prognosis, so intervening with at-risk youth or those in the earliest stages of depression may prevent or delay the full onset of the disorder, and even delaying onset is a meaningful goal. A Cochrane review reported that psychological and educational interventions can effectively reduce the incidence of depression in children and adolescents [5]. In summary, recognition of depression in young people and prompt implementation of preventive or therapeutic strategies are essential to reduce long-term morbidity.

5.2 Epidemiology

Epidemiological studies show that the prevalence of depressive disorders increases from childhood to adolescence. A meta-analysis of community studies (birth cohorts from 1965 to 1996) that

M. Lee (✉)
Department of Psychiatry, Korea University, College of Medicine, Seoul, Republic of Korea
e-mail: npboard@korea.ac.kr

S. H. Shim
Department of Psychiatry, Soonchunhyang University, College of Medicine, Cheonan, Republic of Korea

W.-M. Bahk et al. (eds.), *Depressive Disorder*, https://doi.org/10.1007/978-981-92-1331-3_5

used structured diagnostic interviews reported an overall prevalence of depressive disorders of about 2.8% in children (under ~13 years old) and 5.6% in adolescents (13–18 years old) [6]. In that analysis, the 13–18-year-old females had a prevalence of ~5.9% compared to ~4.6% in males, reflecting the well-known emergence of higher depression rates in girls during mid-adolescence. Across most studies, depressive disorders are considerably more common after the onset of puberty than in prepubertal children [7].

Sex differences in prevalence vary with age. Prior to puberty, boys and girls have similar or even slightly higher rates of depression. By mid-adolescence, however, females predominate with roughly a 2:1 female-to-male ratio, a pattern that continues into adulthood. A recent nationwide study in South Korea (2002–2013) illustrated this developmental shift: among youth under 15 years old, boys had a higher diagnosed depression prevalence than girls, but with increasing age, the prevalence of depression rose in both sexes and eventually became higher in females than males in older adolescent age groups [7]. Globally, by late adolescence, a substantial minority of youths have experienced a depressive episode; some estimates suggest that by age 18, roughly 11–20% of adolescents may have had an episode of MDD (including subclinical cases) [8]. The rising incidence in adolescence is thought to relate to biological changes of puberty, increased psychosocial stressors, and greater cognitive–emotional complexity during the teen years. Notably, depression in adolescents is far more common than pediatric bipolar disorder or other severe psychiatric illnesses of youth [26], making it a significant public health concern.

5.3 Risk Factors

Depression in children and adolescents arises from a complex interplay of biological, psychological, and environmental factors. Known risk factors span genetic and neurobiological influences, gender and hormonal factors, as well as adverse life experiences and family environment. Key risk domains are summarized below.

Gender and Pubertal Factors

The incidence of depression increases for both sexes during puberty, but the rise is steeper in females [3]. By mid-adolescence, females have roughly twice the rate of depression as males, a disparity thought to result from a combination of biological differences (e.g., hormonal fluctuations) and psychosocial factors (e.g., higher exposure or sensitivity to interpersonal stress). The sharp increase in depression risk in girls appears more closely tied to pubertal status and hormone levels than chronological age. Depression prevalence in females peaks during periods of hormonal change—notably, it rises at puberty and again around menopause—supporting a role for gonadal steroid hormones in modulating depression risk. Aside from biology, certain psychosocial traits confer vulnerability during adolescence: insecure attachment to parents, an anxious or inhibited temperament (characterized by shyness, discomfort, or fearfulness in novel situations), and poor coping skills for stress have all been associated with a higher risk of developing depression during the pubertal transition [1].

Environmental Risk Factors

A variety of environmental and psychosocial factors influence depression risk in youth. Perinatal factors such as premature birth or low birth weight have been linked to elevated risk of childhood depression or depressive symptoms later in development. There has also been concern that in utero exposure to maternal antidepressants (particularly selective serotonin reuptake inhibitors [SSRIs]) could predispose offspring to depression or anxiety disorders in the long term. Earlier studies raised this possibility, but more recent analyses controlling for confounding variables have found no significant increase in risk of depression in children whose mothers took SSRIs during pregnancy [9]. These findings must be interpreted cautiously, but they suggest that needed antidepressant treatment in pregnancy should not be categorically avoided due to fear of causing childhood depression.

Childhood adversity is a well-established environmental risk factor. Adverse events occurring in childhood have a stronger association with the onset of psychiatric disorders during childhood than with the onset in adulthood. For example, the death of a parent, serious childhood physical illnesses, or significant economic hardship can precipitate childhood-onset mental disorders, whereas the connection to adult-onset disorders is weaker [10]. Childhood abuse and trauma are among the most potent environmental risk factors for depression. Exposure to physical, sexual, or severe emotional abuse in childhood substantially increases the likelihood of developing MDD and of experiencing a more chronic and refractory course. A meta-analysis found that a history of childhood maltreatment is associated with earlier onset, more recurrent or persistent depression, and poorer response to treatment [11]. Prospective studies have confirmed that childhood abuse and neglect are major causal contributors to subsequent depression [12]. One biological consequence linked to early trauma is reduced hippocampal volume in depressed patients with abuse histories, suggesting enduring neurobiological effects of maltreatment (e.g., via prolonged stress hormone exposure) [13].

Other environmental factors in childhood that can elevate depression risk include chronic medical illness (in the child), which, as in adults, is associated with greater emotional distress and higher rates of MDD. Specific family-related stressors, such as moving residences frequently, parental illness or hospitalization, and especially parental death, have been linked to increased risk of early-onset major depression; parental death also elevates the risk of depression persisting or recurring into adulthood. Socioeconomic disadvantage (poverty) alone appears to have a more limited direct effect on pediatric depression risk, though the evidence is not entirely consistent [14]. Disruption of the family structure—for example, divorce or prolonged parental absence—has been reported by some studies to increase depressive symptoms in adolescents (particularly females). However, findings have been mixed [15].

By contrast, certain protective factors can buffer against depression, though this area is less researched. Having close, supportive friendships in childhood is associated with a lower risk of developing depressive symptoms, and strong social support networks appear to reduce the likelihood of major depression [1]. These observations underscore the importance of psychosocial interventions (such as strengthening support and coping skills) in preventive efforts.

Biological and Neurobiological Factors

Neurobiological abnormalities observed in adult depression are often also found in depressed youths, indicating some continuity in underlying brain circuit dysfunction [16]. Pediatric depression has been frequently linked to dysregulation in corticolimbic circuits that govern emotional processing and stress response. Key brain regions implicated include: (1) the hypothalamus (and related Hypothalamic-Pituitary-Adrenal axis HPA-axis structures) and pituitary; (2) the prefrontal cortex (predominantly ventral and dorsolateral sectors); and (3) the amygdala [17]. Neuroimaging studies of depressed adolescents have shown patterns resembling adults with MDD. For instance, in adolescent depression, there is often hyperactivation of the amygdala in response to negative emotional stimuli, coupled with reduced activation to positive stimuli [18]. In addition, depressed youth have demonstrated smaller hippocampal volumes compared to healthy peers [19], a finding paralleling adult depression and thought to reflect the impact of chronic stress or genetic vulnerability on the developing brain.

Sleep disturbances provide another biological indicator. Subjective sleep complaints (such as insomnia or hypersomnia) are very prominent in early-onset depression. Polysomnographic studies in depressed youth have identified some objective changes; the most consistent sleep Electroencephalography (EEG) finding in youth depression is a prolongation of sleep latency (difficulty falling asleep), although other classical adult findings (like reduced Rapid Eye Movement (REM) latency) may be less robust in pediatric samples. A meta-analysis of early-onset depression sleep studies confirmed significantly increased sleep latency as a hallmark feature [20].

Genetic Factors

Major depression is known to aggregate in families, and having a family history of depression is a significant risk factor for depression in children. Offspring of depressed parents have a markedly elevated risk of developing MDD, often at an earlier age than their parents did. Familial (genetic) risk also contributes to the recurrence of depression: children with a depressed first-degree relative are not only more likely to experience subthreshold depressive symptoms, but also more likely to have recurrent depressive episodes over time. A positive family history of MDD increases the chance that a child's subclinical depressive symptoms will progress to a full-blown depressive episode. Additionally, the burden of depression in the mother (for example, a greater number of maternal depressive episodes) has been associated with a higher likelihood that the child's subthreshold depressive state will become protracted or develop into an MDD episode in adolescence [21]. These findings underscore an inherited vulnerability to depression. Neuroimaging research on youth at familial risk supports this: even before illness onset, high-risk children (with depressed parents) show brain structure and connectivity alterations (e.g., in limbic and cortical regions) similar to those seen in depressed patients, indicating a brain-based endophenotype reflecting genetic risk [22].

In terms of specific genes, depression is polygenic, and no single gene is determinative. However, several polymorphisms have been studied for their potential influence on depression risk, especially in interaction with environmental factors. Notable candidates include the serotonin transporter gene promoter polymorphism Serotonin transporter-linked polymorphic region (5-Serotonin Transporter-Linked Polymorphic Region [HTTLPR]), the brain-derived neurotrophic factor (BDNF) gene Val66Met polymorphism, and the catechol-O-methyltransferase (COMT) gene Val158Met polymorphism [23]. Each of these has been hypothesized to affect mood regulation and stress reactivity. While none of these variants causes depression on their own, they have been focal points for examining how genetic makeup modulates an individual's susceptibility to developing depression under adverse conditions.

Gene–Environment Interactions

Genetic predispositions for depression often manifest only in the presence of specific environmental triggers, an area of study known as gene–environment (G × E) interaction. Systematic reviews of G × E in child and adolescent depression have found that, despite heterogeneity in methods and some inconsistent results, the preponderance of evidence supports the existence of significant gene–environment interactions in pediatric depression [24]. In other words, the impact of environmental risk factors (like stress or trauma) on depression can depend on the child's genotype.

One widely cited example involves the serotonin transporter promoter polymorphism (5-HTTLPR). In adolescent girls, the short ("s") allele of 5-HTTLPR has been associated with increased depression risk *only* in the context of stressful life events—illustrating a classic G × E effect where genetic sensitivity to stress influences depression onset. In children, more complex interactions have been observed: one study reported that only those children who carried risk variants in both the 5-HTTLPR and the BDNF gene, *and* who were exposed to childhood maltreatment, showed elevated depression symptom scores—a gene–gene–environment interaction [25]. Furthermore, the effect of these genetic variants and abuse was moderated by social support in a four-way interaction (gene–gene–environment–environment): high social support appeared to buffer the impact of having both genetic risk variants in maltreated children [26]. Specifically, two landmark studies by Kaufman et al. demonstrated that maltreated children with the high-risk

5-HTTLPR genotype were less likely to develop depression if they had sufficient social support, and that BDNF Val66Met could interact with 5-HTTLPR and childhood abuse in predicting depression, with social support further modifying outcomes [25, 26]. These findings highlight the intricate interplay between genes and environment: genetic factors may heighten vulnerability to depression, but supportive environmental factors can, to some extent, offset genetic risk.

5.4 Clinical Presentation and Diagnosis

Clinical Features of Depression in Youth

The core symptoms of major depression (low mood, loss of interest or pleasure, and associated cognitive and neurovegetative changes) are fundamentally similar in children, adolescents, and adults. However, the clinical presentation in youth has some distinctive nuances owing to developmental factors. Irritable mood is a prevalent symptom of pediatric depression; epidemiologic data indicate that irritability accompanies depression in a large proportion of depressed youth. Purely irritable depression (without any subjective sadness) is relatively uncommon, but irritability as a prominent feature occurs in most cases of child and adolescent depression. Notably, one population-based study found that depression in youth rarely occurred in the absence of depressed mood; virtually all depressed children who were irritable were also subjectively sad or depressed. Moreover, that study reported that children with both depressed and irritable mood were clinically indistinguishable (in developmental level and depression severity) from those with depression characterized by depressed mood alone. In other words, irritability tends to co-occur with depressed mood rather than replace it, and its presence does not necessarily signal a more severe depression—it is simply a typical manifestation of depression in youth [27].

In both preschool and school-age children, the most frequent depressive affective symptoms are *irritable mood* and *sad/depressed mood*. The overall symptom profile of MDD is remarkably similar in children and adolescents; however, specific symptoms are more prevalent in adolescents. Compared to depressed children, depressed adolescents report higher rates of hopelessness, fatigue, hypersomnia (excessive sleep), and suicidal ideation or behavior. For example, while young children with depression may have more overt anxious distress (such as separation anxiety) or somatic complaints, adolescents more often endorse pessimistic feelings about the future, low energy, excessive sleeping, and frank thoughts of death or self-harm [28, 29].

One symptom that appears predictive of a more protracted course is guilt: the presence of inappropriate or excessive guilt in a depressed youth has been associated with longer depressive episodes [30].

Depressive symptoms in young people can manifest in a variety of age-dependent ways. Common presentations include not only sadness and crying but also angry outbursts, irritability, and low frustration tolerance. In younger children, depression may present with separation anxiety, frequent temper tantrums, a range of physical (somatic) complaints (headaches, stomachaches), or psychomotor agitation. Some depressed children become withdrawn and inactive without explicitly verbalizing feeling sad—for instance, a young child might stop engaging in play or fail to enjoy interactions with family, which can be subtle signs of depression if the child cannot articulate sadness. School-aged children often show a sudden decline in academic performance due to impaired concentration and motivation; younger depressed children are also more prone to hypersomnia (excessive sleep) and hyperphagia (over-eating), whereas older adolescents more commonly experience insomnia and appetite loss. Early-onset depression (e.g., prepubertal) tends to have a higher familial (genetic) loading. It has been linked to a greater likelihood of personality disorders emerging in adulthood, suggesting a more severe developmental subtype in some cases.

It is important to note that children and adolescents might not spontaneously report "feeling depressed." Often, their irritable or demoralized mood is observed by others rather than self-reported. Parents may notice their child has become "very touchy or short-tempered" and find the behavior challenging, without recognizing it as a sign of depression. Indeed, many youths with depression present to clinical attention due to secondary problems rather than a chief complaint of low mood. Common precipitating issues that lead families to seek help include deteriorating school grades, substance abuse, excessive Internet or screen use (as maladaptive coping or anhedonia), social withdrawal, oppositional or risk-taking behavior, or even suicide attempts, with the underlying depression only identified upon evaluation. Clinicians must maintain a high index of suspicion for depression in any youth with such changes in behavior or functioning.

Developmental considerations also apply to specific DSM criteria. For example, increased appetite and weight gain, which are included among depressive symptoms (alongside weight loss or decreased appetite), may be less valid indicators of pathological depression in children and adolescents. Weight gain and heightened appetite can be part of normal growth and puberty; thus, unlike weight loss or failure to gain weight, which are red flags, a moderate increase in weight or appetite is not particularly specific to depression in this age group [28]. Consistent with this, DSM-5/5-TR specifies that *failure to make expected weight gains* can be a sign of depression in children, rather than weight loss per se. Another developmental distinction is in persistent depressive disorder (dysthymia): in youth, dysthymia is defined by only one year of chronically depressed (or irritable) mood (as opposed to two years required in adults).

Diagnosis and Assessment

When evaluating a child or adolescent for depression, the same core diagnostic criteria used in adults apply, with the developmental modifications noted above. According to DSM-5-TR, major depressive disorder is diagnosed when at least five of nine symptoms (depressed/irritable mood, loss of interest, weight/appetite change, sleep disturbance, psychomotor changes, fatigue, feelings of worthlessness or guilt, impaired concentration, recurrent thoughts of death) are present for at least 2 weeks, representing a change from prior functioning. In youth, at least one of the symptoms must be either depressed (or irritable) mood or loss of interest/pleasure, the same as in adults. The key developmental notes are: (a) the mood may be irritable rather than sad; and (b) weight loss may manifest as failure to meet expected weight gains in children. Aside from these, the phenomenology of MDD is judged by the same criteria and causes significant distress or impairment.

To improve diagnostic validity and reliability, clinicians are encouraged to use structured or semi-structured diagnostic interviews in the assessment of child and adolescent depression. One widely used instrument is the *Kiddie Schedule for Affective Disorders and Schizophrenia—Present and Lifetime Version (K-SADS-PL)*, a semi-structured interview designed for ages 6–18 [31]. The K-SADS-PL is administered by a trained person who interviews both the parent and the child about current and past episodes, thus capturing longitudinal information. In addition to interviews, rating scales can quantify symptom severity. For clinician-rated assessment, the Children's Depression Rating Scale—Revised (CDRS-R) is commonly used for ages 6–12. The CDRS-R consists of 17 items (14 are rated based on parent/child reports, and 3 are based on clinician observation during the interview) and provides a numeric severity score [32]. For self-report or parent-report, the Children's Depression Inventory (CDI) is frequently employed in youths aged ~8 to 13. The CDI has 27 items (each 0–2 points) with higher total scores indicating more severe depression [33]. These scales, alongside global functioning assessments, help in establishing baseline severity and tracking response to treatment. They can also screen for depressive symptoms in school or primary care settings.

It is crucial during the diagnostic process to assess suicide risk in any child or adolescent with suspected depression. Youth may not volunteer suicidal thoughts, so direct but sensitive inquiry is needed. Collateral information from parents or teachers about any alarming behaviors (e.g., writing suicide notes, giving away belongings, self-harm) is also important. Any indications of psychotic symptoms (such as hallucinations or delusional guilt) should be carefully evaluated, as psychotic depression requires more intensive treatment (often including antipsychotic medication or electroconvulsive therapy [ECT] in severe cases).

5.5 Differential Diagnosis and Comorbidities

Comorbidity is more the rule than the exception in pediatric depression. In the large British Child and Adolescent Mental Health Survey, 66% of children and adolescents with depression had at least one comorbid psychiatric disorder [34]. The most common co-occurring diagnoses with youth depression are anxiety disorders (such as generalized anxiety or separation anxiety), oppositional defiant disorder (ODD), and conduct disorder. Comorbid anxiety is associated with a more severe depressive symptomatology in youth and a higher likelihood of a chronic course. The presence of *any* comorbid mental disorder in a depressed child/adolescent tends to predict more frequent depressive relapses over time. Comorbid disruptive behavior disorders (ODD or conduct disorder) can worsen the overall course by exacerbating functional impairment and creating additional challenges in management. The high co-occurrence of depression with anxiety likely reflects shared etiological factors: twin studies and genetic analyses suggest that depression and anxiety have overlapping genetic vulnerabilities and temperamental bases (e.g., a tendency toward negative affectivity) more so than purely shared environmental causes. This is supported by evidence that depression–anxiety comorbidity is partly explained by genetic pleiotropy and shared personality traits (such as neuroticism) [35].

A wide range of other conditions can either co-occur with depression or mimic depressive symptoms, necessitating careful differential diagnosis. Medical conditions that can present with depressive-like symptoms include: hypothyroidism, anemia, chronic infectious or inflammatory illnesses, autoimmune diseases, certain vitamin deficiencies, and neurological disorders (e.g., epilepsy, brain tumors). A basic medical workup (physical exam, laboratory tests for thyroid function, anemia, etc.) is often indicated to rule out underlying medical causes of depressive symptoms. On the psychiatric side, one must differentiate adjustment disorder with depressed mood (where depressive symptoms are in response to a clear psychosocial stressor and do not meet full MDD criteria) from MDD itself. Other psychiatric disorders that may resemble or mask depression in youth include anxiety disorders (which can present primarily with irritability or somatic complaints), persistent depressive disorder (dysthymia; a chronic, milder depression—though note it can co-occur with MDD in a "double depression" pattern), attention-deficit/hyperactivity disorder (ADHD; which can cause demoralization or mood lability secondary to chronic frustration), oppositional defiant disorder (where irritability and anger are present but without the neurovegetative and subjective sadness of depression), autism spectrum disorder (social withdrawal and flat affect can be mistaken for depression, though in autism these are rooted in social communication deficits), and even early-onset schizophrenia (if negative symptoms present as apathy or if psychotic depression is misidentified). A thorough clinical evaluation, including a detailed psychosocial history and standardized interviews, as noted, is essential to tease apart these diagnoses. Often, collateral information from parents and teachers is invaluable in understanding the context and chronicity of symptoms.

A significant differential is between unipolar depression and bipolar depression in a youth presenting a depressive episode. The first lifetime mood episode in pediatric bipolar disorder is often depression, and distinguishing this from a unipolar depressive disorder can be challenging at the initial presentation. Certain clinical clues may raise suspicion for bipolar depression in a youth: bipolar depression tends to have more severe psychomotor slowing or anhedonia, more profound hopelessness, and more psychotic features or suicidal ideation compared to unipolar depression [36]. Adolescents with bipolar disorder often have a history of brief hyperenergized episodes or distinct periods of mood elevation/irritability that might have been overlooked. In general, studies have found that bipolar depression in teens is associated with an earlier age of onset of mood symptoms, more frequent depressive episodes, more comorbid conditions, more psychiatric hospitalizations, and greater functional impairment compared to unipolar depression in teens. Moreover, youth who experience a major depressive episode are at higher risk of eventually developing a manic or hypomanic episode than are adults with an initial depression. One longitudinal study reported that roughly 20–30% of children and adolescents initially diagnosed with MDD later were diagnosed with bipolar disorder [36]. The risk is particularly heightened if there is a family history of bipolar disorder, or if symptoms like psychomotor agitation, excitement, or atypical features accompany the youth's depression. Therefore, when evaluating a depressed youth, it is imperative to screen for any past or current symptoms of mania/hypomania: for example, periods of abnormally elevated or irritable mood, grandiosity, decreased need for sleep, or episodic impulsivity that is uncharacteristic of their baseline. Involving parents in this history is crucial, as youths may not recognize or report hypomanic symptoms. If any such symptoms are present, or if there is a strong family history of bipolar disorder, the clinician should be cautious in diagnosing pure unipolar depression. A comprehensive psychiatric history that includes past mood episodes, even subtle ones, is needed for an accurate diagnosis. In summary, diagnosing depression in children and adolescents requires a broad differential and a longitudinal perspective to ensure the depressive episode is not part of another condition (like bipolar disorder or disruptive mood dysregulation disorder [DMDD], discussed below).

5.6 Course and Prognosis

The course of major depression in youth is often characterized by recovery within a year or two, but with a significant risk of recurrence and continuation into adulthood. Many depressed children will experience symptom remission within 1–2 years of the index depressive episode, especially with treatment. However, compared to adult-onset depression, early-onset depression has a higher likelihood of relapse and of eventually evolving into bipolar disorder (i.e., some children initially diagnosed with unipolar depression later manifest manic episodes) [36, 37]. Depressed children also tend to have longer episode durations than adults—pediatric depressive episodes frequently last 6 months or more, and in clinically referred samples, an episode often persists 5–8 months on average, versus 3–6 months in community samples. A sizeable subset of youth experience chronic depression: about 20% of depressed adolescents have episodes lasting 2 years or longer, meeting criteria for persistent depressive disorder or chronic MDD [38].

Childhood-onset MDD appears to carry at least as much risk of recurrence as adolescent- or adult-onset MDD. In one longitudinal study of depressed youth 8–13 years old, the probability of recurrence was approximately 40% within 2 years and 72% within 5 years of the initial episode [39]. Adolescent-onset major depression was found to have an intermediate outcome between childhood-onset and adult-onset in terms of chronicity. Recovery rates after a single depressive episode are relatively high in youth—roughly 80–90% of depressed children/adolescents will recover (no longer meet full criteria) within 1–2 years [38], and acute treatment (even placebo in trials) has a strong effect, with response or remission in about 85% by 1–2 years [40]. However, the relapse rates are also high, indicating that many youths who recover from one episode experience new episodes later. In follow-up studies, the majority of depressed adolescents go on to have at least one more depressive episode in adulthood [19]. Females tend to have a greater number of lifetime episodes and a longer duration of depressive illness than males, mirroring the adult pattern of depression being more recurrent in women.

Several features portend a worse prognosis or more chronic course: early age of onset, presence of comorbid psychiatric disorders (especially anxiety or disruptive behavior disorders), a history of severe psychosocial stress (like abuse), and depressive episodes with psychotic features or severe impairment. Notably, childhood-onset depression often delays access to treatment, as younger children are less likely to be brought to psychiatric care and early-onset disorders are often initially unrecognized or misattributed to developmental issues. This treatment delay can allow the illness to become more entrenched, contributing to a more chronic course. Indeed, depression beginning in childhood is more likely to persist as a chronic illness into adulthood, rather than being a transient developmental phase. This underscores the importance of early identification and continuous management.

On a positive note, aggressive maintenance treatment (continuing therapy and/or medication after remission) can significantly reduce relapse rates in youth depression. One controlled study showed that adolescents who continued on antidepressant medication after recovery had a substantially lower probability of relapse compared to those on placebo [41]. Thus, sustained treatment during the vulnerable period after remission can favorably alter the long-term trajectory of depression. Overall, while pediatric depression tends to remit, it should be viewed as a potentially chronic condition where ongoing monitoring and maintenance interventions are needed to prevent recurrence and to mitigate the impact on the child's development and functioning.

5.7 Treatment

Effective management of depression in children and adolescents requires a multimodal approach that takes into account the severity of depression, comorbid conditions, and the degree of psychosocial impairment. Before initiating a specific treatment, the clinician should assess these factors to guide the treatment plan. In young people, placebo response rates can be pretty high (up to ~60% in some studies). Therefore, for mild, brief depression—particularly if there are no active suicidal thoughts, no psychotic symptoms, and only mild functional impairment—it is reasonable to begin with conservative interventions such as supportive therapy, psychoeducation, and addressing problems in the family or school environment, while monitoring symptoms over about 4–6 weeks [28]. Supportive measures include ensuring the child has a stable daily routine, regular exercise and sleep, and that family members and teachers are aware of the situation and can provide appropriate support. Parental guidance and possibly family therapy can help address any familial conflicts or stressors contributing to the depression.

For mild to moderate episodes of depression, psychotherapy is typically considered first-line treatment [42]. Meta-analyses of controlled trials have demonstrated that psychosocial interventions can be effective for pediatric depression, particularly cognitive-behavioral therapy (CBT) and interpersonal psychotherapy (IPT) [43]. If a mild or moderate depressive episode does not respond adequately to psychotherapy alone, or if the depression is moderately severe to severe from the outset (e.g., marked by suicidal ideation, profound anhedonia, significant agitation or psychosis, or severe impairment in functioning), pharmacotherapy is usually indicated, often in combination with ongoing psychotherapy. In youth with chronic or recurrent depression, and certainly in those with severe episodes (e.g., nearly total social withdrawal, inability to attend school, or psychotic features), the evidence supports starting an antidepressant medication to achieve remission of symptoms.

Psychotherapy

A variety of psychotherapy modalities have been applied to depressed youth, but the ones with the strongest evidence base are cognitive-behavioral therapy (CBT) and interpersonal psychotherapy (IPT). Individual supportive or insight-oriented therapy can also be beneficial by providing the adolescent with a trusting relationship to explore issues of low self-esteem, guilt, hopelessness, and identity, as well as to address developmental or familial conflicts underlying the depression. Such therapy is often flexible in addressing a broad range of problems (family relationships, school stress, internal conflicts) and can be tailored to the youth's needs.

Cognitive-behavioral therapy (CBT) focuses on identifying and modifying negative thought patterns and behaviors that maintain depression. In CBT for adolescents, the therapist works with the youth to challenge distorted negative cognitions (e.g., "I am worthless" or catastrophic thinking about failures) and to engage in pleasant or rewarding activities to improve mood. Behavioral techniques (like activity scheduling or problem-solving training) are used alongside cognitive restructuring, aiming to break the self-perpetuating cycle of negative thoughts, low mood, and reduced activity. CBT is typically a time-limited, structured therapy (often ~12 to 16 sessions) and has been shown in numerous trials to reduce depressive symptoms in both children and adolescents, especially in mild–moderate cases.

Interpersonal psychotherapy for adolescents (IPT-A) is an adaptation of interpersonal psychotherapy (initially developed for adult depression) to the developmental needs of adolescents [44]. IPT conceptualizes depression as occurring in an interpersonal context, where depressive episodes are often triggered or sustained by problems in relationships or life role changes. IPT-A specifically targets interpersonal stressors that are common in adolescence. These may include conflicts with peers or family, grief over the loss of a loved one, difficulties due to role transitions (such as starting a new school or parental divorce), or social skills deficits leading to isolation. The therapy seeks to help the adolescent improve communication, build problem-solving skills for interpersonal issues, and form more supportive and conflict-free relationships. Research shows that IPT-A is an efficacious treatment: a landmark trial by Mufson et al. demonstrated that depressed adolescents receiving IPT had significantly higher recovery rates than those in control conditions [44].

Clinical guidelines often recommend IPT or CBT as first-line therapies for adolescent depression, and a recent network meta-analysis concluded that CBT and IPT are among the most efficacious and acceptable psychotherapies for youth depression [45].

Other therapeutic approaches, like family therapy or behavioral activation, can be helpful as adjuncts or alternatives in some instances (e.g., family therapy if familial conflict or parental depression is a contributing factor). For adolescents with depression and comorbid family issues, engaging the family in treatment can improve communication and support. Group therapy can also be considered, particularly CBT groups, which have the added benefit of peer support and reduced isolation.

It is important to note that in cases of mild depression, a period of supportive interventions and watchful waiting may result in improvement due to the high placebo effect. However, if a reasonable trial of psychotherapy (e.g., 6–8 weeks) yields insufficient improvement, or if the depression is moderate to severe, adding medication should be considered.

Pharmacotherapy

The use of antidepressant medications in children and adolescents should be carefully considered, weighing potential benefits against risks (such as side effects and the black-box warning about suicidal ideation). Selective serotonin reuptake inhibitors (SSRIs) are the first-line pharmacological treatment for pediatric depression due to their better tolerability and safety profile compared to older antidepressants. SSRIs in youth typically show response rates on the order of 40–60%, which is modestly higher than placebo in clinical trials [46]. According to current evidence and regulatory approvals, the two SSRIs officially approved by the U.S. Food and Drug Administration (FDA) for youth depression are fluoxetine and escitalopram. Fluoxetine is approved for children ≥8 years old, and escitalopram for adolescents ≥12 years old. Fluoxetine has the most robust evidence base, with multiple positive trials in both children and adolescents, and it is often considered the antidepressant of choice in this population. Sertraline has also shown efficacy over placebo in at least one trial, although the difference was small, and thus sertraline did not gain FDA approval for pediatric depression [47]. Paroxetine failed to demonstrate efficacy in adolescent trials and raised concerns about side effects, so it is not recommended for use in minors.

In practice, if an antidepressant is indicated, fluoxetine is commonly the first SSRI tried (starting at low doses, e.g., 10 mg daily, and titrating up as needed and tolerated). Escitalopram is another option, especially for older adolescents. If there is no response to one SSRI, switching to another SSRI or a different class (like an SNRI [serotonin-norepinephrine reuptake inhibitor] such as venlafaxine) can be considered. The Treatment for Adolescents with Depression Study (TADS) provided evidence supporting medication, especially fluoxetine: in TADS, adolescents treated with fluoxetine (10–40 mg/day) had higher response rates than those treated with CBT alone, and the combination of fluoxetine + CBT was more effective than either modality by itself [48]. Another pivotal trial showed that escitalopram (10–20 mg/day) was superior to placebo in 12–17-year-olds with MDD, confirming its efficacy in adolescents [49].

For adolescents who do not improve after an adequate SSRI trial, the Treatment of SSRI-Resistant Depression in Adolescents (TORDIA) study offers guidance [50]. TORDIA investigated switching medication (either to another SSRI or to venlafaxine) *with or without* CBT in teens who had not responded to an initial SSRI. The findings were that combining a switch in medication with CBT therapy yielded the highest response rates (~55% responded), significantly better than a medication switch alone (~41% responded). Notably, in TORDIA, there was no significant difference in response between switching to a second SSRI and switching to venlafaxine—both had roughly similar outcomes (~35% to 45% response range when given without CBT). However, venlafaxine was associated with more side effects (particularly elevated blood pressure) and, as later analyses suggested, possibly a higher risk of self-harm events. These results support the strategy of trying a different SSRI and adding psychotherapy when a first SSRI trial fails, rather than immediately moving to second-line antidepressants.

A major concern with antidepressant use in youth is the risk of suicidal ideation or behavior. In 2004, the FDA issued a black-box warning for all antidepressants in young people up to age 24, after meta-analyses of clinical trials found a slight increase (roughly 2–4 vs. 1–2% on placebo) in reports of suicidal thoughts/behaviors in those on antidepressants. Following the black-box warning and subsequent intense media coverage, there was a decline in antidepressant prescribing to youth, which corresponded with an uptick in youth suicide rates in the mid-2000s [51]. This temporal association raised concerns that under-treatment of depression might have contributed to the increased suicidality at the population level. A comprehensive meta-analysis of pediatric antidepressant trials (including both published and unpublished data) found that antidepressants *do* have a statistically significant beneficial effect in treating youth depression, and that while there is a slight increase in suicidal ideation, no increase in suicide deaths occurred in trials, and the overall benefits outweigh the risks for most patients. One meta-analysis reported that antidepressants as a class were efficacious in children and adolescents, and did not significantly increase the risk of suicide attempts or ideation when carefully monitored [46]. It is nonetheless imperative that clinicians monitor patients closely for suicidal thoughts, especially in the early phases of treatment or during dose changes, and to educate families about warning signs. Regular follow-up (weekly or biweekly in the first month) is recommended.

Recent large-scale analyses have refined our understanding of antidepressant efficacy in youth. The most comprehensive network meta-analysis to date (34 trials, over 5000 patients) comparing 14 antidepressants concluded that only fluoxetine (either alone or combined with

CBT) was more effective than placebo in alleviating depressive symptoms in children and teens [52]. Other antidepressants did not separate from placebo to a statistically significant degree, and some (like venlafaxine) were associated with more adverse effects, including higher rates of suicidal ideation. These findings reinforce fluoxetine's position as the antidepressant with the strongest evidence base in youth depression. They also highlight the need for caution and the importance of psychotherapy: many treatment guidelines recommend that psychotherapy should be the first-line treatment for mild–moderate depression, and even when medication is used, psychotherapy should be offered concurrently.

If an antidepressant is effective, it should be continued for a sufficient period. Typically, acute treatment lasts about 8–12 weeks to achieve remission. Once remission is achieved, a continuation phase of 6–12 months of the medication is recommended to consolidate gains and prevent relapse. Evidence supports that continued antidepressant treatment significantly reduces the risk of relapse compared to switching to a placebo. For those with recurrent or chronic depression, maintenance treatment beyond a year may be necessary, potentially lasting several years or through the high-risk period of later adolescence, in order to prevent recurrence.

In particularly severe cases, or if depression is accompanied by psychotic features, a combination of an antidepressant and an atypical antipsychotic may be required. Guidelines and algorithm-based treatments, including a Korean expert consensus algorithm, have suggested that for severe depression (even without psychotic features) in youth, an antidepressant plus an atypical antipsychotic can be considered to maximize response. This is partly extrapolated from adult practice and from evidence that atypical antipsychotics (like aripiprazole, quetiapine, or risperidone) can help with severe agitation or augment antidepressant effects. In psychotic depression, the combination is standard (typically an SSRI plus a second-generation antipsychotic such as aripiprazole). Clinicians must weigh the metabolic and extrapyramidal side effects of atypical antipsychotics against potential benefits.

Other pharmacological treatments occasionally used in youth depression include SNRIs (like venlafaxine or duloxetine) if multiple SSRIs fail—though as noted, venlafaxine carries a higher side effect burden and, in one study, a higher risk of suicidality. Bupropion or mirtazapine are sometimes tried off-label in adolescents, especially if there are comorbid conditions (e.g., ADHD in the case of bupropion, or severe insomnia/weight loss in the case of mirtazapine). These have less robust pediatric data. Tricyclic antidepressants (TCAs) are generally *not* used in children due to poor efficacy in trials (TCAs did not outperform placebo in prepubertal depression) and higher toxicity (e.g., cardiotoxicity risk in overdose). One exception might be imipramine for comorbid enuresis or specific pain syndromes, but otherwise TCAs are avoided for pediatric depression. Electroconvulsive therapy (ECT) is rarely used in adolescents, reserved only for life-threatening depression (e.g., depression with malignant catatonia or severe psychosis unresponsive to other treatments) in older adolescents, and requires significant safeguards.

In all cases, involvement of the family in treatment is important. Family psychoeducation about depression can improve compliance and support. If family conflict or parental depression is present, treating those concurrently (for example, family therapy or referring to a depressed parent for treatment) can improve the child's outcome. School involvement is also often necessary: schools can provide accommodation for a student struggling with concentration or attendance due to depression, such as flexible deadlines, reduced course load, or counseling services on site.

Finally, close monitoring for clinical changes—especially emergent suicidal ideation or manic symptoms—is needed throughout treatment. Antidepressant-treated youths should typically be seen within 1–2 weeks of starting medication, and frequently thereafter, to assess for side effects and mood changes. Psychotherapy provides a regular check-in as well, and therapists should communicate any safety concerns to the prescribing physician. With vigilant monitoring and a combination of therapeutic modalities, the prognosis for acute recovery in youth depression is good, though maintaining wellness remains a challenge requiring longer-term follow-up.

5.8 Disruptive Mood Dysregulation Disorder (DMDD)

Chronic, severe irritability in children—manifested by frequent temper outbursts and persistently irritable mood—has been recognized as a problematic clinical phenomenon that does not fit neatly into classic mood disorder categories. In DSM-5 (2013), the diagnosis of disruptive mood dysregulation disorder (DMDD) was introduced to capture this presentation, and it has been retained in DSM-5-TR. The DMDD category was created in part to address concerns about overdiagnosis of pediatric bipolar disorder in chronically irritable children. Prior to DSM-5, many of these children were mislabeled as "bipolar" due to their severe mood dysregulation, leading to inappropriate treatment (e.g., excessive use of antipsychotics or mood stabilizers). Research showed that children with chronic non-episodic irritability rarely progress to true bipolar disorder; instead, they are more likely to develop unipolar depression or anxiety disorders over time [53]. Thus, DMDD was placed in the depressive disorders section of DSM-5, reflecting that it is often a precursor to depression rather than mania. Despite its hallmark features of temper outbursts and anger, DMDD is not simply a behavioral issue—it is conceptualized as an affective disorder of youth.

Clinical features of DMDD include *recurrent temper tantrums* (verbal rages and/or physical aggression) that are grossly out of proportion to the situation and inconsistent with the child's developmental level. These outbursts can be triggered by frustration or stress and typically occur frequently (DSM-5 requires an average of ≥3 outbursts per week). In between the explosive episodes, the child's mood is persistently irritable or angry nearly every day, for most of the day, and this mood disturbance is observable by others (parents, teachers, peers). Importantly, the irritability in DMDD is chronic and non-episodic—it is not confined to discrete mood episodes (as irritability might be in bipolar mania). By definition, DMDD symptoms must be present for 12 or more months (with no symptom-free interval longer than 3 months) and must be evident in at least two settings (e.g., home and school). The onset of symptoms must be before age 10, and the diagnosis should not be made for the first time in children younger than 6 or older than 18. These age limits ensure DMDD is used in school-age children and early/mid-adolescents, as temper outbursts are developmentally normative in toddlers and irritability in late teens could indicate other disorders.

Taken together, DMDD is best understood as a chronic, cross-setting pattern of severe irritability rather than an episodic mood disorder. In clinical practice, the diagnosis rests on recurrent, developmentally inappropriate outbursts that are grossly disproportionate to the provoking situation, together with a persistently irritable or angry mood between episodes, and on evidence that this pattern is persistent, present across settings, and functionally impairing.

The diagnosis is further bounded by exclusion rules. DMDD should not be diagnosed when the presentation is better explained by another mental disorder, occurs exclusively during major depressive episodes, follows a distinct manic or hypomanic episode, or is attributable to a substance or another medical or neurological condition. It also cannot be assigned concurrently with oppositional defiant disorder, intermittent explosive disorder (IED), or bipolar disorder, although it may coexist with major depressive disorder, ADHD, conduct disorder, and substance use disorders.

Children and adolescents with DMDD typically have significant impairment in multiple domains. Due to their severe irritability and low frustration tolerance, they often experience frequent conflict in peer relationships and within the family. At school, these youth may exhibit poor behavioral control, leading to academic underachievement and disciplinary issues. They may be removed from classrooms or face suspensions due to aggressive outbursts. It is also important to monitor for risk-taking or self-harm behaviors in DMDD: studies indicate these youths can exhibit dangerous behavior, and rates of suicidal ideation and suicide attempts are not negligible, often related to the chronic distress and interpersonal difficulties they face.

The differential diagnosis of DMDD includes primarily ODD, intermittent explosive disorder (IED), and bipolar disorder. By definition, DMDD cannot be diagnosed alongside ODD or IED in the same individual; if criteria for DMDD are met, it subsumes ODD (which also involves irritability and temper outbursts). The difference is one of severity, chronicity, and mood pervasiveness: ODD has oppositional behavior and anger, but does not require the persistent angry mood between outbursts that DMDD does. If a child meets criteria for both, DMDD should be diagnosed, and ODD should not be given as a separate label. Likewise, if a child meets criteria for intermittent explosive disorder (which involves outbursts but not persistent mood disturbance) and DMDD, only DMDD is diagnosed. DMDD is also mutually exclusive with pediatric bipolar disorder: as per Criterion H and J, if a manic or hypomanic episode occurs, the diagnosis should be bipolar disorder, not DMDD. The intent is that DMDD captures non-episodic irritability, whereas bipolar disorder is episodic and includes classic manic symptoms.

It is critical to distinguish DMDD from bipolar disorder, as the treatments differ markedly. DMDD was explicitly added to provide an appropriate diagnosis (and thus more appropriate treatment) for a chronically irritable child who does not have episodic mania. Research has shown that children fitting DMDD criteria generally do not develop adult bipolar disorder; instead, in adolescence or adulthood, they are prone to unipolar depression or anxiety disorders. Thus, DMDD is conceptualized as a mood disorder closer to depression than to bipolar, albeit with prominent behavioral dyscontrol. Nevertheless, differentiating bipolar from DMDD can be challenging in some cases, and it relies on careful evaluation of longitudinal course: bipolar disorder requires distinct mood episodes with clear onset and offset (and the presence of manic symptoms like grandiosity, elated mood, decreased need for sleep, etc.), none of which occur in pure DMDD.

DMDD frequently has comorbidities. The most commonly co-occurring disorders include major depressive disorder, anxiety disorders (such as generalized anxiety or separation anxiety), ADHD, and autism spectrum disorder. Comorbidity is so common that one study found youth with DMDD had, on average, more comorbid diagnoses than youth with MDD or dysthymia. This underscores that DMDD often exists as part of a complex clinical picture [54]. Notably, if a child meets criteria for MDD or an anxiety disorder *and* has chronic irritability, both diagnoses can be given (unlike ODD/bipolar). However, if the severe irritability can be entirely explained by another diagnosis—for example, occurs only during major depressive episodes, or in an autistic child, only in reaction to routine disruption—then DMDD should not be diagnosed. This caveat is to avoid overlabeling transient or context-limited irritability as DMDD.

There has been some controversy and debate around the DMDD diagnosis. Critics point out the potential for DMDD to medicalize temper tantrums or to be inconsistently applied. Reflecting ongoing debate, the *International Classification of Diseases* (ICD)-11 (the World Health Organization's classification system) has chosen a different approach: instead of including DMDD as a mood disorder, ICD-11 places chronic irritability with frequent outbursts under the category of disruptive behavior disorders. Specifically, ICD-11 classifies it as a subtype of oppositional defiant disorder characterized by chronic irritability and anger (essentially merging DMDD features into ODD). This underscores that the conceptualization of chronic irritability is still evolving internationally.

Treatment of DMDD is challenging, as research is still limited and there are no treatments with strong evidence specifically for this disorder. Given the high rates of psychosocial stressors in these youths, a comprehensive psychosocial assessment is the first step—examining family dynamics (including parenting consistency and any abuse or maltreatment), academic setting (learning disabilities or peer problems), and other environmental stressors. Interventions are then tailored to findings: for instance, parent management training or family therapy can be helpful if there is parent–child conflict or inconsistent discipline. Behavioral therapy focusing on anger management and frustration tolerance can be beneficial for the child. Techniques might include cognitive-behavioral strategies to recognize when frustration is mounting, and skills to calm down (such as deep breathing, problem-solving alternatives, or removing oneself from triggering situations).

Medications are often considered in moderate to severe DMDD, but must be used cautiously (often off-label) and always in conjunction with psychosocial interventions. The choice of medication can target predominant symptom domains: for severe aggression and outbursts, atypical antipsychotics (like risperidone or aripiprazole) may reduce aggression and irritability in the short term—indeed, these are sometimes used in severe ODD or autism-related irritability, which overlaps with DMDD features. For persistent depressive or anxious mood that underlies the irritability, antidepressants (SSRIs) can be tried, with some reports of improvement in mood stability (e.g., an SSRI might reduce baseline anger and improve frustration tolerance). However, SSRIs and stimulants (for coexistent ADHD) must be used with care in DMDD because of the theoretical risk of inducing manic-like reactions, mainly if the child is later found to have bipolar diathesis. Clinicians often proceed by first treating any comorbid disorders: for example, if a child with DMDD has ADHD, a stimulant or atomoxetine might be prescribed; if there is an anxiety disorder, an SSRI might be used. Treating comorbidities can sometimes indirectly improve irritability.

There is a lack of robust trials to guide a "standard" pharmacotherapy for DMDD. Mood stabilizers (like divalproex or lithium) are used by some clinicians by extrapolation from treatment of bipolar irritability or aggression, but evidence in non-episodic irritability is sparse. Atypical antipsychotics have the strongest short-term evidence for reducing aggression in youth (e.g., risperidone is approved for irritability in autism). However, their side effects (weight gain, metabolic syndrome, extrapyramidal symptoms) make long-term use concerning, especially in children. Given these concerns, experts often recommend aiming for monotherapy when possible and using the lowest effective doses to minimize medication burden on the developing child. Polypharmacy may sometimes be necessary (for example, an SSRI for mood + a stimulant for ADHD), but one should add medications only when indicated.

The 2018–2021 Korean Medication Algorithm for Depressive Disorder included a section on DMDD, reflecting clinician experience due to the lack of solid evidence [55]. In that consensus, no medication strategy could be designated as first-line given the paucity of data. Instead, several strategies were listed as secondary options, including: SSRIs alone, atypical antipsychotics alone, or an SSRI + atypical antipsychotic combination. Notably, the algorithm identified escitalopram or fluoxetine as the preferred antidepressants, and aripiprazole or risperidone as the preferred antipsychotics for DMDD management. Clinicians might start with one of these (e.g., an SSRI) and gauge the effect on irritability over a couple of months; if inadequate, an antipsychotic could be added or substituted.

Current practice emphasizes addressing environmental factors and comorbidities, using psychosocial treatments as the foundation, and adding medications tailored to the individual's symptom profile and comorbid conditions. Any pharmacotherapy should be accompanied by close monitoring for side effects and any emergence of manic symptoms, since some DMDD kids might later be reclassified if bipolar symptoms appear.

5.9 Conclusion

Depression in children and adolescents is a prevalent, serious mental health condition that can substantially derail normal development and functioning—once thought to be rare or transient "moodiness," early-onset depression is now recognized as often having a more chronic and severe course than depression arising de novo in adulthood. Childhood-onset depressive episodes tend to be longer in duration, with higher rates of suicidal symptoms and psychiatric hospitalizations, compared to those with later onset. Moreover, depression that begins in youth frequently persists or recurs into adulthood, sometimes evolving into a lifelong affective illness. The cumulative burden—in terms of lost educational and social opportunities, impaired emotional development, and the risk of self-harm or substance abuse—can be devastating if the disorder is not adequately addressed early on.

Fortunately, growing knowledge of risk factors (such as genetic vulnerability, childhood adversities, and parental mental health) allows us to identify at-risk youths for preventive interventions. For instance, children with chronic medical illnesses or those who experience significant stress and trauma, as well as those whose mothers have severe depression, are known to be at higher risk of developing depression. Recognizing these risks provides an opportunity to implement preventive strategies, like resilience-building programs or early counseling, which have shown promise in delaying or reducing the onset of depression in high-risk youth. Indeed, childhood and early adolescence are increasingly seen as optimal periods for preventive intervention, before maladaptive patterns solidify.

For those youths who do develop depression, early detection and prompt treatment are paramount. Timely diagnosis (distinguishing depression from other look-alike conditions) and aggressive treatment that continues until full remission is achieved can alter the trajectory of the illness. The goal should extend beyond mere symptom reduction to achieving a full recovery (remission) and restoring normal functioning. Adequate treatment duration is essential—continuing therapy and/or medication for long enough to consolidate remission helps prevent a swift relapse. It can reduce the likelihood of the depression becoming chronic. As evidence-based guidelines suggest, a combination of psychotherapy and pharmacotherapy is often the most effective approach, especially in moderate to severe cases. Psychosocial treatments (CBT, IPT, family therapy) address developmental and interpersonal issues, while antidepressants (when indicated) tackle the neurochemical aspects of depression. Each has a role, and their integration is a cornerstone of practice.

In treating youth depression, clinicians must also focus on functional recovery—helping the young person re-engage with age-appropriate activities, resume academic progress, and rebuild social connections. This often means working closely with families and schools to create a supportive environment for the child's recovery. It is also crucial to address any comorbid disorders (anxiety, ADHD, etc.) simultaneously, as these can hinder recovery if left untreated.

Looking ahead, ongoing research continues to refine our understanding of pediatric depression. Advances in neurobiology might yield biomarkers to identify which children are most at risk or which treatments they are most likely to respond to. Psychosocial research is developing prevention programs to instill coping skills in at-risk youth, and new modalities (like computer-based CBT, or novel neuromodulatory techniques) are being explored for treatment-resistant cases. Long-term prospective studies are examining how early-onset depression unfolds over decades, which will inform strategies to prevent adolescent depression from becoming adult chronic depression.

In conclusion, childhood and adolescent depression is a treatable condition, but one that demands vigilant and comprehensive management. By combining early identification, evidence-based therapeutic interventions, and long-term follow-up, clinicians can substantially improve outcomes for depressed youth—reducing immediate suffering and helping to prevent a trajectory of recurrent depression into adult life. With continued research and improved implementation of known interventions, the field is moving toward more personalized and effective care, offering hope that more young people will recover and thrive despite an early encounter with depression.

Declarations

Competing Interests The author(s) has no competing interests to declare that are relevant to the content of this manuscript.

Ethics Approval The authors declare that this manuscript does not include primary research with human participants.

The authors also declare that this manuscript does not include primary studies involving animals.

References

1. Wesselhoeft RT. Childhood depressive disorders. Dan Med J. 2016;63(10)
2. Pataki C, Carlson GA. Major depressive disorder among children and adolescents. Focus (Am Psychiatr Publ). 2016;14(1):10–4.
3. Lewinsohn PM, Rohde P, Seeley JR, Klein DN, Gotlib IH. Natural course of adolescent major depressive disorder in a community sample: predictors of recurrence in young adults. Am J Psychiatry. 2000;157(10):1584–91.
4. Bujoreanu S, Benhayon D, Szigethy E. Treatment of depression in children and adolescents. Pediatr Ann. 2011;40(11):548–55.
5. Merry SN, Hetrick SE, Cox GR, Brudevold-Iversen T, Bir JJ, McDowell H. Psychological and educational interventions for preventing depression in children and adolescents. Cochrane Database Syst Rev 2011(12):CD003380.
6. Jane Costello E, Erkanli A, Angold A. Is there an epidemic of child or adolescent depression? J Child Psychol Psychiatry. 2006;47(12):1263–71.
7. Kim GE, Jo MW, Shin YW. Increased prevalence of depression in South Korea from 2002 to 2013. Sci Rep. 2020;10(1):16979.
8. Avenevoli S, Swendsen J, He JP, Burstein M, Merikangas KR. Major depression in the national comorbidity survey-adolescent supplement: prevalence, correlates, and treatment. J Am Acad Child Adolesc Psychiatry. 2015;54(1):37–44 e2.
9. Hutchison SM, Masse LC, Pawluski JL, Oberlander TF. Perinatal selective serotonin reuptake inhibitor (SSRI) and other antidepressant exposure effects on anxiety and depressive behaviors in offspring: a review of findings in humans and rodent models. Reprod Toxicol. 2021;99:80–95.
10. Green JG, McLaughlin KA, Berglund PA, Gruber MJ, Sampson NA, Zaslavsky AM, et al. Childhood adversities and adult psychiatric disorders in the national comorbidity survey replication I: associations with first onset of DSM-IV disorders. Arch Gen Psychiatry. 2010;67(2):113–23.
11. Nanni V, Uher R, Danese A. Childhood maltreatment predicts unfavorable course of illness and treatment outcome in depression: a meta-analysis. Am J Psychiatry. 2012;169(2):141–51.
12. Widom CS, DuMont K, Czaja SJ. A prospective investigation of major depressive disorder and comorbidity in abused and neglected children grown up. Arch Gen Psychiatry. 2007;64(1):49–56.
13. Vythilingam M, Heim C, Newport J, Miller AH, Anderson E, Bronen R, et al. Childhood trauma associated with smaller hippocampal volume in women with major depression. Am J Psychiatry. 2002;159(12):2072–80.
14. Tracy M, Zimmerman FJ, Galea S, McCauley E, Stoep AV. What explains the relation between family poverty and childhood depressive symptoms? J Psychiatr Res. 2008;42(14):1163–75.
15. Amato PR. The consequences of divorce for adults and children. J Marriage Fam. 2000;62(4):1269–87.
16. Kerestes R, Davey CG, Stephanou K, Whittle S, Harrison BJ. Functional brain imaging studies of youth depression: a systematic review. Neuroimage Clin. 2014;4:209–31.
17. Hulvershorn LA, Cullen K, Anand A. Toward dysfunctional connectivity: a review of neuroimaging findings in pediatric major depressive disorder. Brain Imaging Behav. 2011;5(4):307–28.
18. Redlich R, Opel N, Burger C, Dohm K, Grotegerd D, Forster K, et al. The limbic system in youth depression: brain structural and functional alterations in adolescent in-patients with severe depression. Neuropsychopharmacology. 2018;43(3):546–54.
19. Kim JH, Suh SI, Lee HJ, Lee JH, Lee MS. Cortical and subcortical gray matter alterations in first-episode drug-naive adolescents with major depressive disorder. Neuroreport. 2019;30(17):1172–8.
20. Augustinavicius JL, Zanjani A, Zakzanis KK, Shapiro CM. Polysomnographic features of early-onset depression: a meta-analysis. J Affect Disord. 2014;158:11–8.
21. Hammen C, Brennan PA. Severity, chronicity, and timing of maternal depression and risk for adolescent offspring diagnoses in a community sample. Arch Gen Psychiatry. 2003;60(3):253–8.
22. Gotlib IH, Joormann J, Foland-Ross LC. Understanding familial risk for depression: a 25-year perspective. Perspect Psychol Sci. 2014;9(1):94–108.
23. Mandelli L, Serretti A. Gene environment interaction studies in depression and suicidal behavior: an update. Neurosci Biobehav Rev. 2013;37(10 Pt 1):2375–97.
24. Dunn EC, Brown RC, Dai Y, Rosand J, Nugent NR, Amstadter AB, et al. Genetic determinants of depression: recent findings and future directions. Harv Rev Psychiatry. 2015;23(1):1–18.
25. Kaufman J, Yang BZ, Douglas-Palumberi H, Houshyar S, Lipschitz D, Krystal JH, et al. Social supports and serotonin transporter gene moderate depression in maltreated children. Proc Natl Acad Sci USA. 2004;101(49):17316–21.

26. Kaufman J, Yang BZ, Douglas-Palumberi H, Grasso D, Lipschitz D, Houshyar S, et al. Brain-derived neurotrophic factor-5-HTTLPR gene interactions and environmental modifiers of depression in children. Biol Psychiatry. 2006;59(8):673–80.
27. Stringaris A, Maughan B, Copeland WS, Costello EJ, Angold A. Irritable mood as a symptom of depression in youth: prevalence, developmental, and clinical correlates in the Great Smoky Mountains study. J Am Acad Child Adolesc Psychiatry. 2013;52(8):831–40.
28. Birmaher B, Brent D, Issues AWGoQ, Bernet W, Bukstein O, Walter H, et al. Practice parameter for the assessment and treatment of children and adolescents with depressive disorders. J Am Acad Child Adolesc Psychiatry. 2007;46(11):1503–26.
29. Weersing VR, Brent DA. Cognitive behavioral therapy for depression in youth. Child Adolesc Psychiatr Clin N Am. 2006;15(4):939–57. ix
30. Kovacs M, Rottenberg J, George C. Maladaptive mood repair responses distinguish young adults with early-onset depressive disorders and predict future depression outcomes. Psychol Med. 2009;39(11):1841–54.
31. Kaufman J, Birmaher B, Brent D, Rao U, Flynn C, Moreci P, et al. Schedule for affective disorders and schizophrenia for school-age children-present and lifetime version (K-SADS-PL): initial reliability and validity data. J Am Acad Child Adolesc Psychiatry. 1997;36(7):980–8.
32. Isa A, Bernstein I, Trivedi M, Mayes T, Kennard B, Emslie G. Childhood depression subscales using repeated sessions on children's depression rating scale – revised (CDRS-R) scores. J Child Adolesc Psychopharmacol. 2014;24(6):318–24.
33. Bang YR, Park JH, Kim SH. Cut-off scores of the children's depression inventory for screening and rating severity in Korean adolescents. Psychiatry Investig. 2015;12(1):23–8.
34. Ford T, Goodman R, Meltzer H. The British child and adolescent mental health survey 1999: the prevalence of DSM-IV disorders. J Am Acad Child Adolesc Psychiatry. 2003;42(10):1203–11.
35. Hettema JM. What is the genetic relationship between anxiety and depression? Am J Med Genet C Semin Med Genet. 2008;148C(2):140–6.
36. Geller B, Zimerman B, Williams M, Bolhofner K, Craney JL, Delbello MP, et al. Diagnostic characteristics of 93 cases of a prepubertal and early adolescent bipolar disorder phenotype by gender, puberty and comorbid attention deficit hyperactivity disorder. J Child Adolesc Psychopharmacol. 2000;10(3):157–64.
37. Kovacs M, Feinberg TL, Crouse-Novak MA, Paulauskas SL, Finkelstein R. Depressive disorders in childhood. I. A longitudinal prospective study of characteristics and recovery. Arch Gen Psychiatry. 1984;41(3):229–37.
38. Birmaher B, Arbelaez C, Brent D. Course and outcome of child and adolescent major depressive disorder. Child Adolesc Psychiatr Clin N Am. 2002;11(3):619–37. x
39. Kovacs M, Feinberg TL, Crouse-Novak M, Paulauskas SL, Pollock M, Finkelstein R. Depressive disorders in childhood. II. A longitudinal study of the risk for a subsequent major depression. Arch Gen Psychiatry. 1984;41(7):643–9.
40. Goodyer IM, Herbert J, Secher SM, Pearson J. Short-term outcome of major depression: I. Comorbidity and severity at presentation as predictors of persistent disorder. J Am Acad Child Adolesc Psychiatry. 1997;36(2):179–87.
41. Emslie GJ, Heiligenstein JH, Hoog SL, Wagner KD, Findling RL, McCracken JT, et al. Fluoxetine treatment for prevention of relapse of depression in children and adolescents: a double-blind, placebo-controlled study. J Am Acad Child Adolesc Psychiatry. 2004;43(11):1397–405.
42. David-Ferdon C, Kaslow NJ. Evidence-based psychosocial treatments for child and adolescent depression. J Clin Child Adolesc Psychol. 2008;37(1):62–104.
43. Weisz JR, McCarty CA, Valeri SM. Effects of psychotherapy for depression in children and adolescents: a meta-analysis. Psychol Bull. 2006;132(1):132–49.
44. Mufson L, Weissman MM, Moreau D, Garfinkel R. Efficacy of interpersonal psychotherapy for depressed adolescents. Arch Gen Psychiatry. 1999;56(6):573–9.
45. Zhou X, Hetrick SE, Cuijpers P, Qin B, Barth J, Whittington CJ, et al. Comparative efficacy and acceptability of psychotherapies for depression in children and adolescents: a systematic review and network meta-analysis. World Psychiatry. 2015;14(2):207–22.
46. Bridge JA, Iyengar S, Salary CB, Barbe RP, Birmaher B, Pincus HA, et al. Clinical response and risk for reported suicidal ideation and suicide attempts in pediatric antidepressant treatment: a meta-analysis of randomized controlled trials. JAMA. 2007;297(15):1683–96.
47. Wagner KD, Ambrosini P, Rynn M, Wohlberg C, Yang R, Greenbaum MS, et al. Efficacy of sertraline in the treatment of children and adolescents with major depressive disorder: two randomized controlled trials. JAMA. 2003;290(8):1033–41.
48. March J, Silva S, Petrycki S, Curry J, Wells K, Fairbank J, et al. Fluoxetine, cognitive-behavioral therapy, and their combination for adolescents with depression - treatment for adolescents with depression study (TADS) randomized controlled trial. JAMA. 2004;292(7):807–20.
49. Wagner KD, Jonas J, Findling RL, Ventura D, Saikali K. A double-blind, randomized, placebo-controlled trial of escitalopram in the treatment of pediatric depression. J Am Acad Child Adolesc Psychiatry. 2006;45(3):280–8.
50. Brent D, Emslie G, Clarke G, Wagner KD, Asarnow JR, Keller M, et al. Switching to another SSRI or to venlafaxine with or without cognitive behavioral therapy for adolescents with SSRI-resistant depression – the TORDIA randomized controlled trial. JAMA. 2008;299(8):901–13.

51. Gibbons RD, Brown CH, Hur K, Marcus SM, Bhaumik DK, Erkens JA, et al. Early evidence on the effects of regulators' suicidality warnings on SSRI prescriptions and suicide in children and adolescents. Am J Psychiatry. 2007;164(9):1356–63.
52. Cipriani A, Zhou X, Del Giovane C, Hetrick SE, Qin B, Whittington C, et al. Comparative efficacy and tolerability of antidepressants for major depressive disorder in children and adolescents: a network meta-analysis. Lancet. 2016;388(10047):881–90.
53. Stringaris A, Cohen P, Pine DS, Leibenluft E. Adult outcomes of youth irritability: a 20-year prospective community-based study. Am J Psychiatry. 2009;166(9):1048–54.
54. Benarous X, Renaud J, Breton JJ, Cohen D, Labelle R, Guile JM. Are youths with disruptive mood dysregulation disorder different from youths with major depressive disorder or persistent depressive disorder? J Affect Disord. 2020;265:207–15.
55. Seo JS, Bahk WM, Woo YS, Park YM, Kim W, Jeong JH, et al. Korean medication algorithm for depressive disorder 2021, fourth revision: an executive summary. Clin Psychopharmacol Neurosci. 2021;19(4):751–72.

Aging, Cognitive Decline, and Depression

6

IL Han Choo and Bo-Hyun Yoon

6.1 Aging

Up until the seventeenth century, the population aged 65 and older accounted for only about 1% of the total. However, by the nineteenth century, this proportion increased up to 4% [1]. In South Korea, the percentage of people aged 65 and older was 12.7% in 2014, 15.7% in 2020, 20% in 2024, and is expected to reach 24.3% by 2030. The suicide rate among elderly people, which is closely associated with depression, is at a very serious level. Old age is often divided into "young elderly" and "old elderly." Although the cutoff varies among researchers, the young elderly people are generally considered those between 60 and 75 years old, and the old elderly people are generally considered those aged 75 and older.

6.2 Definition of Aging

Aging refers to the mental and physical changes that occur from the completion of development until death. Aging occurs due to changes in cellular structure and function. One mechanism involves telomeres—the end parts of chromosomes—that shorten with each cell division, contributing to cellular aging. External factors such as lifestyle and environmental pollutants are believed to induce oxidative stress, which causes changes in cells. Aging differs depending on genetic factors, living environment, social life, health habits, and disease history. Thus, while chronological age generally correlates with aging, biological, functional, psychological, and socioeconomic characteristics cause significant individual variation.

I. H. Choo (✉)
Department of Neuropsychiatry, College of Medicine, Chosun University, Gwangju, Republic of Korea

Department of Psychiatry, Chosun University Hospital, Gwangju, Republic of Korea
e-mail: ilhan.choo@chosun.ac.kr

B.-H. Yoon
Department of Psychiatry, Naju National Hospital, Naju, Republic of Korea

6.3 Concepts of Normal, Successful, and Pathological Aging

The definition of normal aging is diverse and varies depending on how functional levels are determined. For example, it can be defined as the absence of disease, or having physical and mental functions within 1.5 standard deviations of the mean or below. However, applying a uniform definition is difficult due to differences in diseases and sociocultural backgrounds.

Successful aging refers to older individuals who are subjectively or objectively evaluated as leading happy lives in later years, considering their physical and mental function, social engagement, family, and financial status. Again, due to

W.-M. Bahk et al. (eds.), *Depressive Disorder*, https://doi.org/10.1007/978-981-92-1331-3_6

personal and societal differences, it is difficult to define uniformly.

Pathological aging may be defined as the presence of one or more illnesses in old age. However, since most older adults experience hypertension or diabetes—and many manage these well through treatment—there is debate over whether they should be included in pathological aging.

Prevalence of Depression in the Elderly

It is known that one in five people aged 65 and over experiences symptoms of depression. The most commonly used tool in epidemiological studies to assess depressive symptoms is the Center for Epidemiologic Studies Depression Scale (CES-D), a 20-item self-report scale [2]. Currently, the revised version (CESD-R) is mainly used [3]. According to the 2021 National Mental Health Survey, the lifetime prevalence of major depressive disorder across all ages was 7.7% (5.7% in men, 9.8% in women). The one-year prevalence was 1.7% (1.1% in men, 2.4% in women). For those aged 60–69, it was 1.7% (1.9% in men, 1.6% in women), and for those aged 70–79, it was 3.1% (0.3% in men, 5.4% in women), which is about 1.8 times higher than the overall average. In about half of all cases, depressive symptoms first appear before age 40, but in later life, depression is often related to recurrence or to physical and environmental changes.

6.4 Assessment of Depression in the Elderly

Psychiatric History Taking

In elderly individuals, depressive presentations frequently manifest as somatic complaints rather than overt sadness. It is critical to discern whether depressive symptoms are secondary to physical conditions or if physical illnesses are a consequence of depression. Clinicians should specifically inquire about disturbances in sleep, appetite, and a general loss of interest, as these are commonly observed in this population. A comprehensive history encompassing previous psychiatric and medical conditions is essential.

The patient's personal and psychosocial background should be thoroughly explored, including age, educational level, prior occupation, circumstances and timing of retirement or occupational change, marital status, and current living arrangements. It is important to determine whether the patient resides with a spouse.

Family history should address the stability of housing, household composition, frequency of family contact, institutionalization status, and the availability of caregiver support.

Given the prevalence of polypharmacy among elderly patients—often involving antihypertensives, antidiabetic agents, or hypnotics—a meticulous medication review is imperative. Potential drug interactions with newly prescribed medications must be carefully evaluated.

Mental Status Examination

General Appearance: Note the use of glasses, hearing aids, wheelchairs, or canes.

Attitude: Assess whether the patient is cooperative, guarded, defensive, angry, or tired during the interview.

Behavior: Observe for unusual movements, whether the patient needs help sitting, or if there are abnormal hand or foot movements while seated.

Mood and Affect: Evaluate if the patient can express emotions and shows interest in their surroundings.

Thought Content and Process: Assess comprehension, thought slowness, delusions, or paranoid thinking.

Perception: Identify any hallucinations related to self-harm or suicide.

Cognition: Start with a brief screening and follow with comprehensive neuropsychological testing.

Judgment and Insight: Determine the patient's understanding of their difficulties.

Neurocognitive Testing

Mini-Mental State Examination (MMSE) [4]: Various Korean versions exist (K-MMSE, MMSE-K, MMSE-KC, MMSE-DS). The test includes orientation, immediate and delayed recall, attention, naming, pentagon copying, repetition, and reading/writing comprehension, scored out of 30.

Clinical Dementia Rating (CDR) [5]: Evaluates six domains—memory, orientation, judgment/problem-solving, social activities, home/hobbies, and personal care—on a scale of 0–3. The global CDR score reflects dementia severity.

Global Deterioration Scale (GDS) [6]: Developed by Reisberg et al. in 1982, this tool assesses dementia severity on a 7-point scale ranging from no cognitive decline [1] to very severe decline [7].

Neuropsychiatric Inventory (NPI) [7]: Developed by Cummings et al. in 1994 to evaluate neuropsychiatric symptoms in patients with brain disorders. It includes 12 domains: delusions, hallucinations, agitation, depression, anxiety, euphoria, apathy, disinhibition, irritability, aberrant motor behavior, nighttime disturbances, and changes in appetite/eating. Scores are derived from frequency [1–4], severity [1–3], and caregiver distress (0–5), with total scores calculated as frequency × severity.

Comprehensive Cognitive Function Tests

Korean version of CERAD Neuropsychological Assessment Battery [8]: Assesses memory, orientation, language, visuospatial skills, and executive function over 30–40 min. Normative data are available for individuals aged 60–90.

Seoul Neuropsychological Screening Battery (SNSB) [9]: Measures attention, language, visuospatial function, and executive function in a two-hour test. Norms are available for ages 45–90.

Alzheimer's Disease Assessment Scale—Cognitive Subscale (ADAS-Cog) [10]: Includes word recall, following commands, constructional praxis, delayed recall, naming objects and fingers, ideational praxis, and orientation. Mainly used in clinical trials.

Neuroimaging

Neuroimaging is divided into structural imaging, functional imaging, and molecular imaging. Structural imaging includes computed tomography (CT) and magnetic resonance imaging (MRI) (T1/T2/fluid-attenuated inversion recovery [FLAIR] sequences). Functional imaging includes single-photon emission computed tomography [SPECT], fludeoxyglucose-18-positron emission tomography [FDG-PET], and functional magnetic resonance imaging (fMRI). Molecular imaging includes amyloid PET (florbetaben, florbetapir, flutemetamol PET) and tau PET (flortaucipir, [18F]-MK-6240 PET). In late-life depression, structural imaging, especially FLAIR MRI, is most commonly used to detect white matter hyperintensities (WMHs), which are strongly associated with depression in the elderly. Other imaging modalities are used for further evaluation or differential diagnosis.

Laboratory Tests

Tests may include a complete blood count with differential, erythrocyte sedimentation rate, serum chemistry, glucose, liver function tests, kidney function tests, electrolyte levels (calcium and magnesium), thyroid function tests, serum vitamin B_{12} and folate levels, syphilis screening, HIV testing, and urinalysis. The selection of tests should be based on the patient's history and physical examination.

Medication Review

In elderly patients, a medication review is essential due to the likelihood of multiple medications such as antihypertensives, antidiabetics, and hypnotics. Potential interactions between new and existing medications must be carefully considered.

Alcohol Use Assessment

The pattern of alcohol use—frequency, amount, duration, and cravings—should be evaluated. Tools such as the Cut down Annoyed Guilty Eyeopener (CAGE) questionnaire and the Alcohol Use Disorders Identification Test (AUDIT) can be used.

Evaluation of Daily Functioning

Assessment of Activities of Daily Living (ADL) [11] is important in evaluating depression in the elderly. This includes mobility, eating, dressing, personal hygiene, and toileting. Instrumental ADL assessment covers tasks such as transportation, shopping, financial management, meal preparation, housekeeping, communication, and medication management.

Geriatric Depression Scales

Hamilton Rating Scale for Depression (HRSD) [12]: Developed by Hamilton in 1967, this tool is widely used to assess depression and treatment response. The commonly used version includes 17 items scored from 0 to 52, with higher scores indicating greater severity.

Montgomery-Asberg Depression Rating Scale (MADRS) [13]: Developed in 1979, this 10-item scale assesses sadness, inner tension, reduced sleep and appetite, concentration, lassitude, inability to feel, pessimism, and suicidal thoughts. Items are scored from 0 to 6 with anchor points at even numbers.

Geriatric Depression Scale (GDS) [14]: Created by Yesavage in 1982, this 30-item self-report scale is useful for screening depression in the elderly. A 15-item short version (SGDS) [15] was later developed and standardized in Korean for primary screening use.

Beck Depression Inventory (BDI) [16]: Developed in 1961 by Beck et al., this self-report scale consists of 21 items, each scored from 0 to 3. Total scores range from 0 to 63, with higher scores indicating more severe depression.

Patient Health Questionnaire-9 (PHQ-9) [17]: Developed in 1999, the PHQ-9 consists of 9 items based on Diagnostic and Statistical Manual of Mental Disorders, Fourth edition (DSM-IV) criteria for major depressive episodes. Each item is scored from 0 to 3, with a total score above 10 indicating probable depression.

Clinical Assessment of Depression in Dementia (CADD) [18]: Developed by Zubenko in 2003 to assess depression in dementia patients. It uses the 17-item HRSD with evaluations based on self-report, observed behavior, and informant reports. Delusions and hallucinations from the NPI are also included.

6.5 Causes of Late-Life Depression

Biological factors include abnormalities in serotonin receptor genes, neurotransmitter imbalances (e.g., serotonin, dopamine, norepinephrine), increased cortisol levels, and comorbid psychiatric conditions like anxiety or substance abuse. Structural brain changes such as hippocampal atrophy are also involved.

Depression is more prevalent in elderly patients with hypertension, diabetes, coronary artery disease, and vascular dementia [19–22]. Studies show vascular disease is significantly more common in those with depression [23]. Patients with vascular dementia often exhibit more severe depression and anxiety symptoms than those with Alzheimer's disease [22]. Moreover, depression may increase the risk of cerebrovascular disease [24].

Depressed individuals have higher rates of hypertension and type 2 diabetes [25, 26]. Among hypertensive patients, those with depression have a 2.3–2.7 times higher risk of stroke [27]. Depression can reduce adherence to treatments like diet, medication, and exercise, further increasing vascular risk [28]. Autonomic nervous system changes and side effects of antidepressants (e.g., hypotension, metabolic effects, platelet aggregation) may also elevate stroke risk [29].

Stroke and Depression

About 20–60% of stroke patients develop depression [30, 31]. Depression after stroke is associated with poorer rehabilitation outcomes [32, 33] and higher long-term mortality [34, 35].

There is ongoing debate on whether post-stroke depression results from biological damage or psychological stress [36]. Left hemisphere lesions [37, 38], particularly in the frontal lobe or basal ganglia, are more associated with early-onset post-stroke depression [39–43]. Post-stroke depression occurring 6 months after a stroke is closely associated with functional, physical, cognitive impairments, and social functioning. In contrast, early-onset post-stroke depression, which develops within the first month after stroke, is reported to be strongly associated with left anterior brain lesions [31, 44]. However, some systematic reviews found no clear link between lesion location and depression [45, 46]. Variations in study design, patient population, diagnostic criteria, and follow-up duration may explain these inconsistencies [47].

In addition to the location of lesions, psychosocial factors such as physical disability, loss of independence, diminished quality of life, and heightened stress levels also play contributory roles in the development of depression [36]. MRI studies show a strong association between white matter hyperintensities (WMHs)—especially periventricular and deep white matter lesions—and late-life depression [48–50]. WMHs are more frequently seen in depressed elders than in controls [51–54]. WMH volumes are also related to depression [55]. WMHs influence the worsening of depressive symptoms. WMHs not only show a significant association with the severity of depressive symptoms at a specific point in time [56, 57], but also predict an increased risk of developing depression in the future as their severity increases [58, 59]. The directionality of this relationship indicates that WMHs predict the subsequent severity of depressive symptoms, whereas the reverse direction does not hold [60]. WMHs are also significantly associated with cognitive decline. Higher WMH severity is linked to more pronounced cognitive impairment [61], and a faster subsequent decline in cognitive function [62, 63]. The impact of WMH differs depending on their location: cognitive function is more strongly associated with periventricular WMH (Fig. 6.1) than with deep white matter WMH, whereas depressive symptoms show the opposite pattern [64]. In summary, WMHs are likely to have a causal relationship with both cognitive decline and the worsening of depressive symptoms [60, 65]. Furthermore, WMHs may have a direct effect on cognitive decline, and also exert an indirect effect through depressive symptoms. This relationship is illustrated in Fig. 6.2. Meanwhile, patients with depression accompanied by WMHs tend to have a poor response to pharmacological treatment and a higher incidence of side effects [43].

Clinical Significance of White Matter Hyperintensities (WMHs)

White matter hyperintensities (WMHs) observed in periventricular and deep white matter areas on FLAIR or T2-weighted MRI are highly associated with late-life depression. WMHs are more frequently found in elderly patients with depression compared to healthy controls. WMH volume is significantly associated with depression onset and severity. WMHs also impact cognitive function: greater WMH burden is linked to more severe cognitive decline and faster deterioration over time. The location of WMHs matters—those near the ventricles are more strongly related to cognitive impairment, while deep WMHs are more associated with depressive symptoms. WMHs may directly affect cognition but also exert indirect effects via depressive symptoms. Additionally, depression with WMHs is more resistant to medication and has a higher rate of adverse effects (Table 6.1).

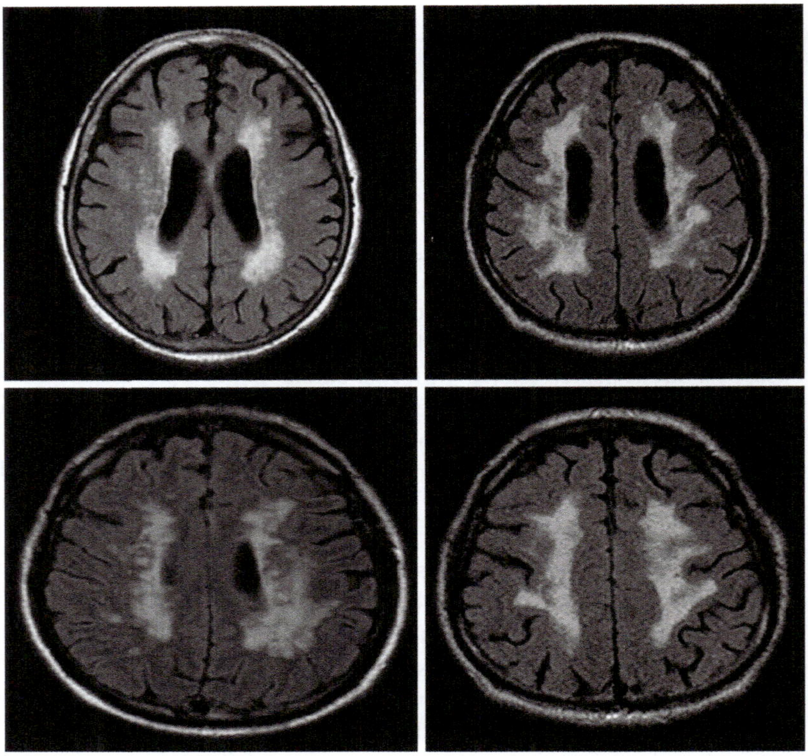

Fig. 6.1 Various forms of white matter hyperintensities observed in periventricular regions

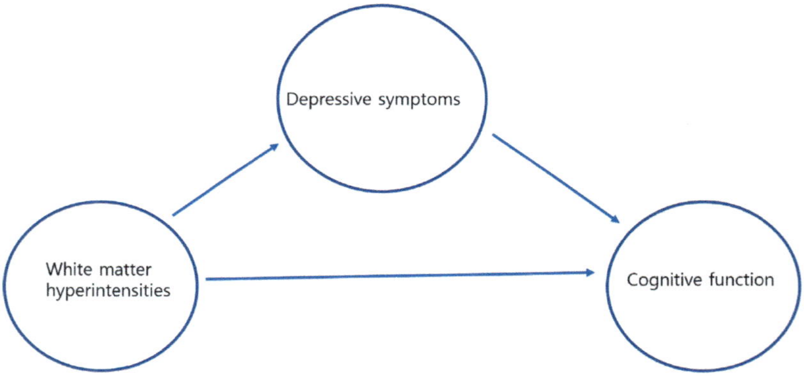

Fig. 6.2 The relationship among white matter lesions, depressive symptoms, and cognition

Psychosocial Risk Factors

Significant life events, including bereavement, interpersonal conflicts with close relations, retirement, physical decline associated with aging or illness, financial setbacks, and institutionalization, are all recognized contributors to depression in the elderly population. Bereavement is considered the most impactful life event, whereas having a spouse serves as a major protective factor against depression among older adults. Notably, more than half of caregivers for individuals with Alzheimer's disease meet the criteria for depression.

Table 6.1 Clinical implications of white matter hyperintensities

Factors related to subcortical white matter hyperintensities	
	Normal aging
	More severe late-life depressive symptoms compared to adult-onset depression or non-depressed older adults
	Loss of interest or apathy
	Psychomotor retardation
	The presence of systemic atherosclerosis and vascular risk factors (hypertension, diabetes, and coronary artery disease)
	Reduced cognitive processing speed on neuropsychological testing
	Reduced treatment response to antidepressants
Factors related to basal ganglia white matter hyperintensities	
	More severe late-life depressive symptoms compared to adult-onset depression or non-depressed older adults
	Increased incidence of delirium with antidepressant or electroconvulsive therapy

6.6 Clinical Features and Differential Diagnosis

Depressed elderly individuals often present with somatic complaints, changes in sleep and appetite, or general loss of interest, rather than overt sadness [66]. The severity and persistence of depressive symptoms are linked to hippocampal atrophy [67]. Compared to early-onset major depression, late-onset depression is less likely to have a family history of mood disorders [68] and shows more frequent WMHs on MRI [51, 54]. Salloway et al. (1996) measured WMH in 15 individuals with late-onset major depressive disorder (MDD) over the age of 60 and 15 individuals with early-onset MDD under the age of 60, and reported that the late-onset group had twice as many subcortical hyperintensities (SCH) compared to the early-onset group [69].

Suicide risk increases with age, and while older adults attempt suicide less often, their attempts are more likely to be fatal. Up to 80% of suicide victims aged 74 and older had depression [70].

6.7 Cognitive Decline and Depression

Pseudodementia describes cognitive impairment resembling dementia caused by depression [71]. It is characterized by: (1) cognitive decline occurring with psychiatric illness; (2) resemblance to neurodegenerative patterns; (3) improvement with psychiatric treatment; and (4) absence of evidence for primary neurological disease [72].

Depression in Alzheimer's Disease

The prevalence of major depression in Alzheimer's disease patients ranges widely (2–85%) [73], but many studies report rates of 30–50% [74]. The prevalence of dysthymia in Alzheimer's disease has been reported to be between 25% and 50% [73, 75]. Factors such as diagnostic criteria, selection methods, and follow-up duration contribute to variability. Depression is the most common psychiatric comorbidity in Alzheimer's disease [76–78]. Some studies suggest that individuals with depression may have an increased risk of developing Alzheimer's disease, especially when depression occurs prior to the onset of cognitive decline [79, 80].

Hippocampal atrophy has been found in patients with untreated depression [81]. Elevated long-term cortisol levels due to chronic stress negatively affect hippocampal structure and function, impairing memory and cognition [82]. Meta-analyses suggest depression doubles the risk of developing Alzheimer's disease [83]. Depression is associated with cognitive decline [84, 85] and may further accelerate cognitive deterioration in patients with dementia [86]. In a 10-year longitudinal study of 3325 individuals aged 78 and older, Mirza et al. (2016) found that the risk of developing dementia increased as depressive symptoms worsened over time [87]. A study that observed changes in depressive symptoms over a 28-year period also reported that late-life depressive symptoms increase the risk of dementia [88]. Korean national dementia surveys conducted every four years since 2008 show that people with a score ≥8 on the GDS have a 2.67–4.6 times higher risk of dementia compared to those without depressive symptoms.

Depression in Alzheimer's disease is often characterized by less overt mood symptoms but includes social withdrawal, irritability, reduced interest, and anhedonia [74]. Rapp et al. (2006) reported that patients with Alzheimer's disease dementia who had a history of depression showed significantly more neuritic plaques and neurofibrillary tangles in the hippocampus compared to those without a history of depression [89]. Butters et al. (2008) reported that half of older adults treated for major depression with escitalopram had brain amyloid deposits [90]. One study reported that, in patients with depression, the plasma Aβ40/Aβ42 ratio was associated with memory, visuospatial working performance, and executive function [91]. Longitudinal studies have also shown that elevated plasma Aβ42 levels in older adults increase the likelihood of developing future depression, and that the Aβ42/Aβ40 ratio is associated with a higher risk of depression onset [92].

A biomarker study published in 2017 by the Washington University Alzheimer's Disease Research Center found a significant association between mood changes and brain amyloid deposition in 118 cognitively normal older adults [93]. Similarly, the Mayo Clinic in the U.S. reported that individuals who frequently experienced depressive and anxious symptoms showed higher levels of brain amyloid deposition in a study of 1038 cognitively normal elderly individuals [94]. A 2016 study from Harvard University also found that among 79 cognitively normal older adults, those who experienced greater feelings of loneliness had higher levels of cerebral amyloid deposition [95]. This was further supported by a 2018 study involving 270 cognitively normal older adults, which reported a significant association between anxiety-depression symptoms and cerebral amyloid deposition [96]. However, in a study of 301 cognitively normal older adults with a mean age of 70 years, tau, but not amyloid, was associated with a depression diagnosis [97]. A recent biomarker study found that, in a baseline cohort previously diagnosed with major depressive disorder, elevated levels of GFAP (glial fibrillary acidic protein), NFL (neurofilament light chain), and PSG1 (pregnancy-specific beta-1-glycoprotein 1) were associated with an increased risk of Alzheimer's disease-related disorders over a mean follow-up period of 13.3 years [98].

Medication and Depression

Older adults with depression tend to take more medications compared to younger adults with depression, increasing the risk of drug-induced depression. Therefore, evaluating concomitant medications is crucial. The following are examples of drugs known to induce depression [99].

> Steroids, Methyldopa, Benzodiazepines, Propranolol, Reserpine, Stimulants, anti-Parkinsonian drugs, calcium channel blockers, beta-blockers, Cimetidine Clonidine, Disulfiram, Hydralazine, Estrogens, Progesterone, Tamoxifen, Vinblastine, Vincristine, Dextropropoxyphene.

6.8 Treatment of Elderly Depression

Treatment of late-life depression includes pharmacotherapy, psychotherapy, electroconvulsive therapy (ECT), and transcranial magnetic stimulation (TMS). In pharmacological treatment for older adults, it is important to consider age-related changes in pharmacokinetics and pharmacodynamics, comorbid medical conditions, potential drug-drug interactions due to polypharmacy, and medication adherence. The same dosage of antidepressants used during the acute treatment phase should be maintained for at least 6 months. ECT is known to be an effective treatment in cases where there is no response to medication, when severe side effects occur, or when there are recurrent suicidal thoughts or attempts.

6.9 Prognosis of Elderly Depression

It has been reported that among older adults with depression, one-third recover or maintain recovery within a year, one-third experience a relapse, and the remaining one-third do not recover [100]. Several studies have shown that executive dysfunction in late-life depression is associated with a poor response to antidepressant treatment [101–106]. Executive dysfunction is also linked to higher relapse rates [107]. Approximately 50% of late-life depression cases are first-onset; however, when individuals who experienced their first depressive episode in early or middle adulthood relapse in later life, they tend to respond poorly to treatment and are more likely to develop chronic depression. Risk factors for recurrence include a history of frequent depressive episodes, late-onset depression, chronic medical conditions, disability, stroke, neurodegenerative diseases, and chronic insomnia.

Declarations

Competing Interests The author(s) has no competing interests to declare that are relevant to the content of this manuscript.

Ethics Approval The author(s) declares that this manuscript does not include primary research with human participants.

The author(s) declares that this manuscript does not include primary studies involving animals.

References

1. Cowgil D. The demography of aging. Hoffman AM, editor. Springfield: Thomas, C. C.; 1970.
2. Radloff LS. The CES-D scale a self-report depression scale for research in the general population. Appl Psychol Meas. 1977;1(3):385–401.
3. Van Dam NT, Earleywine M. Validation of the Center for Epidemiologic Studies Depression Scale–Revised (CESD-R): pragmatic depression assessment in the general population. Psychiatry Res. 2011;186(1):128–32.
4. Folstein MF, Folstein SE, McHugh PR. "Mini-mental state". A practical method for grading the cognitive state of patients for the clinician. J Psychiatr Res. 1975;12(3):189–98.
5. Hughes CP, Berg L, Danziger WL, Coben LA, Martin RL. A new clinical scale for the staging of dementia. Br J Psychiatry. 1982;140:566–72.
6. Reisberg B, Ferris SH, de Leon MJ, Crook T. The global deterioration scale for assessment of primary degenerative dementia. Am J Psychiatry. 1982;139(9):1136–9.
7. Cummings JL, Mega M, Gray K, Rosenberg-Thompson S, Carusi DA, Gornbein J. The neuropsychiatric inventory: comprehensive assessment of psychopathology in dementia. Neurology. 1994;44(12):2308–14.
8. Lee DY, Lee KU, Lee JH, Kim KW, Jhoo JH, Kim SY, et al. A normative study of the CERAD neuropsychological assessment battery in the Korean elderly. J Int Neuropsychol Soc. 2004;10(1):72–81.
9. Kang Y, Na D, Hahn S. Seoul neuropsychological screening battery. Incheon: Human Brain Research & Consulting Co.; 2003.
10. Graham DP, Cully JA, Snow AL, Massman P, Doody R. The Alzheimer's disease assessment scale-cognitive subscale: normative data for older adult controls. Alzheimer Dis Assoc Disord. 2004;18(4):236–40.
11. Katz S. Assessing self-maintenance: activities of daily living, mobility, and instrumental activities of daily living. J Am Geriatr Soc. 1983;31(12):721–7.
12. Hamilton M. Development of a rating scale for primary depressive illness. Br J Soc Clin Psychol. 1967;6(4):278–96.
13. Montgomery SA, Asberg M. A new depression scale designed to be sensitive to change. Br J Psychiatry. 1979;134:382–9.
14. Yesavage JA, Brink TL, Rose TL, Lum O, Huang V, Adey M, et al. Development and validation of a geriatric depression screening scale: a preliminary report. J Psychiatr Res. 1982;17(1):37–49.
15. Sheikh JI, Yesavage JA. Geriatric depression scale (GDS): recent evidence and development of a shorter version. Clin Gerontol. 1986;5:165–73.
16. Beck AT, Ward CH, Mendelson M, Mock J, Erbaugh J. An inventory for measuring depression. Arch Gen Psychiatry. 1961;4:561–71.
17. Spitzer RL, Kroenke K, Williams JB. Validation and utility of a self-report version of PRIME-MD: the PHQ primary care study. Primary care evaluation of mental disorders. Patient health questionnaire. JAMA. 1999;282(18):1737–44.
18. Zubenko GS, Zubenko WN, McPherson S, Spoor E, Marin DB, Farlow MR, et al. A collaborative study of the emergence and clinical features of the major depressive syndrome of Alzheimer's disease. Am J Psychiatry. 2003;160(5):857–66.

19. Rabkin JG, Charles E, Kass F. Hypertension and DSM-III depression in psychiatric outpatients. Am J Psychiatry. 1983;140(8):1072–4.
20. Carney RM, Rich MW, Tevelde A, Saini J, Clark K, Jaffe AS. Major depressive disorder in coronary artery disease. Am J Cardiol. 1987;60(16):1273–5.
21. Gavard JA, Lustman PJ, Clouse RE. Prevalence of depression in adults with diabetes. An epidemiological evaluation. Diabetes Care. 1993;16(8):1167–78.
22. Sultzer DL, Levin HS, Mahler ME, High WM, Cummings JL. A comparison of psychiatric symptoms in vascular dementia and Alzheimer's disease. Am J Psychiatry. 1993;150(12):1806–12.
23. Alexopoulos GS, Meyers BS, Young RC, Campbell S, Silbersweig D, Charlson M. 'Vascular depression' hypothesis. Arch Gen Psychiatry. 1997;54(10):915–22.
24. Ramasubbu R. Relationship between depression and cerebrovascular disease: conceptual issues. J Affect Disord. 2000;57(1–3):1–11.
25. Eaton WW, Armenian H, Gallo J, Pratt L, Ford DE. Depression and risk for onset of type II diabetes. A prospective population-based study. Diabetes Care. 1996;19(10):1097–102.
26. Jonas BS, Franks P, Ingram DD. Are symptoms of anxiety and depression risk factors for hypertension? Longitudinal evidence from the National Health and nutrition examination survey I epidemiologic follow-up study. Arch Fam Med. 1997;6(1):43–9.
27. Simonsick EM, Wallace RB, Blazer DG, Berkman LF. Depressive symptomatology and hypertension-associated morbidity and mortality in older adults. Psychosom Med. 1995;57(5):427–35.
28. Van den Berg MD, Oldehinkel AJ, Bouhuys AL, Brilman EI, Beekman AT, Ormel J. Depression in later life: three etiologically different subgroups. J Affect Disord. 2001;65(1):19–26.
29. Sackeim HA, Prohovnik I, Moeller JR, Brown RP, Apter S, Prudic J, et al. Regional cerebral blood flow in mood disorders. I. Comparison of major depressives and normal controls at rest. Arch Gen Psychiatry. 1990;47(1):60–70.
30. Wade DT, Legh-Smith J, Hewer RA. Depressed mood after stroke. A community study of its frequency. Br J Psychiatry. 1987;151:200–5.
31. Astrom M, Adolfsson R, Asplund K. Major depression in stroke patients. A 3-year longitudinal study. Stroke. 1993;24(7):976–82.
32. Agrell B, Dehlin O. Comparison of six depression rating scales in geriatric stroke patients. Stroke. 1989;20(9):1190–4.
33. Starkstein SE, Robinson RG. Affective disorders and cerebral vascular disease. Br J Psychiatry. 1989;154:170–82.
34. Morris PL, Robinson RG, Andrzejewski P, Samuels J, Price TR. Association of depression with 10-year poststroke mortality. Am J Psychiatry. 1993;150(1):124–9.
35. Morris PL, Robinson RG, Samuels J. Depression, introversion and mortality following stroke. Aust N Z J Psychiatry. 1993;27(3):443–9.
36. Aben I, Verhey F, Honig A, Lodder J, Lousberg R, Maes M. Research into the specificity of depression after stroke: a review on an unresolved issue. Prog Neuro-Psychopharmacol Biol Psychiatry. 2001;25(4):671–89.
37. Robinson RG, Price TR. Post-stroke depressive disorders: a follow-up study of 103 patients. Stroke. 1982;13(5):635–41.
38. Robinson RG, Kubos KL, Starr LB, Rao K, Price TR. Mood changes in stroke patients: relationship to lesion location. Compr Psychiatry. 1983;24(6):555–66.
39. Lipsey JR, Robinson RG, Pearlson GD, Rao K, Price TR. Mood change following bilateral hemisphere brain injury. Br J Psychiatry. 1983;143:266–73.
40. Robinson RG, Kubos KL, Starr LB, Rao K, Price TR. Mood disorders in stroke patients. Importance of location of lesion. Brain. 1984;107(Pt 1):81–93.
41. Robinson RG, Starkstein SE, Price TR. Post-stroke depression and lesion location. Stroke. 1988;19(1):125–6.
42. Greenwald BS, Kramer-Ginsberg E, Krishnan KR, Ashtari M, Auerbach C, Patel M. Neuroanatomic localization of magnetic resonance imaging signal hyperintensities in geriatric depression. Stroke. 1998;29(3):613–7.
43. Steffens DC, Krishnan KR. Structural neuroimaging and mood disorders: recent findings, implications for classification, and future directions. Biol Psychiatry. 1998;43(10):705–12.
44. Robinson RG, Starr LB, Lipsey JR, Rao K, Price TR. A two-year longitudinal study of post-stroke mood disorders: dynamic changes in associated variables over the first six months of follow-up. Stroke. 1984;15(3):510–7.
45. Singh A, Herrmann N, Black SE. The importance of lesion location in poststroke depression: a critical review. Can J Psychiatr. 1998;43(9):921–7.
46. Carson AJ, MacHale S, Allen K, Lawrie SM, Dennis M, House A, et al. Depression after stroke and lesion location: a systematic review. Lancet. 2000;356(9224):122–6.
47. Soares JC, Mann JJ. The anatomy of mood disorders–review of structural neuroimaging studies. Biol Psychiatry. 1997;41(1):86–106.
48. Coffey CE, Figiel GS, Djang WT, Weiner RD. Subcortical hyperintensity on magnetic resonance imaging: a comparison of normal and depressed elderly subjects. Am J Psychiatry. 1990;147(2):187–9.
49. Brown FW, Lewine RJ, Hudgins PA, Risch SC. White matter hyperintensity signals in psychiatric and nonpsychiatric subjects. Am J Psychiatry. 1992;149(5):620–5.
50. Krishnan KR, Hays JC, Blazer DG. MRI-defined vascular depression. Am J Psychiatry. 1997;154(4):497–501.

51. Taylor WD, MacFall JR, Payne ME, McQuoid DR, Steffens DC, Provenzale JM, et al. Greater MRI lesion volumes in elderly depressed subjects than in control subjects. Psychiatry Res. 2005;139(1):1–7.
52. Shimony JS, Sheline YI, D'Angelo G, Epstein AA, Benzinger TL, Mintun MA, et al. Diffuse microstructural abnormalities of normal-appearing white matter in late life depression: a diffusion tensor imaging study. Biol Psychiatry. 2009;66(3):245–52.
53. Colloby SJ, Firbank MJ, Thomas AJ, Vasudev A, Parry SW, O'Brien JT. White matter changes in late-life depression: a diffusion tensor imaging study. J Affect Disord. 2011;135(1–3):216–20.
54. Wang L, Leonards CO, Sterzer P, Ebinger M. White matter lesions and depression: a systematic review and meta-analysis. J Psychiatr Res. 2014;56:56–64.
55. Godin O, Dufouil C, Maillard P, Delcroix N, Mazoyer B, Crivello F, et al. White matter lesions as a predictor of depression in the elderly: the 3C-Dijon study. Biol Psychiatry. 2008;63(7):663–9.
56. Son SJ, Lee KS, Na DL, Seo SW, Kim CH, Kim JH, et al. Anemia associated with depressive symptoms in mild cognitive impairment with severe white matter hyperintensities. J Geriatr Psychiatry Neurol. 2011;24(3):161–7.
57. Cole J, Chaddock CA, Farmer AE, Aitchison KJ, Simmons A, McGuffin P, et al. White matter abnormalities and illness severity in major depressive disorder. Br J Psychiatry. 2012;201(1):33–9.
58. Teodorczuk A, Firbank MJ, Pantoni L, Poggesi A, Erkinjuntti T, Wallin A, et al. Relationship between baseline white-matter changes and development of late-life depressive symptoms: 3-year results from the LADIS study. Psychol Med. 2010;40(4):603–10.
59. Park JH, Lee SB, Lee JJ, Yoon JC, Han JW, Kim TH, et al. Epidemiology of MRI-defined vascular depression: a longitudinal, community-based study in Korean elders. J Affect Disord. 2015;180:200–6.
60. Firbank MJ, Teodorczuk A, van der Flier WM, Gouw AA, Wallin A, Erkinjuntti T, et al. Relationship between progression of brain white matter changes and late-life depression: 3-year results from the LADIS study. Br J Psychiatry. 2012;201(1):40–5.
61. Mungas D, Jagust WJ, Reed BR, Kramer JH, Weiner MW, Schuff N, et al. MRI predictors of cognition in subcortical ischemic vascular disease and Alzheimer's disease. Neurology. 2001;57(12):2229–35.
62. Brickman AM, Honig LS, Scarmeas N, Tatarina O, Sanders L, Albert MS, et al. Measuring cerebral atrophy and white matter hyperintensity burden to predict the rate of cognitive decline in Alzheimer disease. Arch Neurol. 2008;65(9):1202–8.
63. Carmichael O, Schwarz C, Drucker D, Fletcher E, Harvey D, Beckett L, et al. Longitudinal changes in white matter disease and cognition in the first year of the Alzheimer disease neuroimaging initiative. Arch Neurol. 2010;67(11):1370–8.
64. Kim KW, MacFall JR, Payne ME. Classification of white matter lesions on magnetic resonance imaging in elderly persons. Biol Psychiatry. 2008;64(4):273–80.
65. Prins ND, Scheltens P. White matter hyperintensities, cognitive impairment and dementia: an update. Nat Rev Neurol. 2015;11(3):157–65.
66. Gallo JJ, Anthony JC, Muthen BO. Age differences in the symptoms of depression: a latent trait analysis. J Gerontol. 1994;49(6):P251–64.
67. Taylor WD, McQuoid DR, Payne ME, Zannas AS, MacFall JR, Steffens DC. Hippocampus atrophy and the longitudinal course of late-life depression. Am J Geriatr Psychiatry. 2014;22(12):1504–12.
68. Devanand DP, Adorno E, Cheng J, Burt T, Pelton GH, Roose SP, et al. Late onset dysthymic disorder and major depression differ from early onset dysthymic disorder and major depression in elderly outpatients. J Affect Disord. 2004;78(3):259–67.
69. Salloway S, Malloy P, Kohn R, Gillard E, Duffy J, Rogg J, et al. MRI and neuropsychological differences in early- and late-life-onset geriatric depression. Neurology. 1996;46(6):1567–74.
70. Conwell Y, Duberstein PR, Cox C, Herrmann JH, Forbes NT, Caine ED. Relationships of age and axis I diagnoses in victims of completed suicide: a psychological autopsy study. Am J Psychiatry. 1996;153(8):1001–8.
71. Kiloh LG. Pseudo-dementia. Acta Psychiatr Scand. 1961;37(4):336–51.
72. Caine ED. Pseudodementia. Current concepts and future directions. Arch Gen Psychiatry. 1981;38(12):1359–64.
73. Cummings JL. Cognitive and behavioral heterogeneity in Alzheimer's disease: seeking the neurobiological basis. Neurobiol Aging. 2000;21(6):845–61.
74. Olin JT, Katz IR, Meyers BS, Schneider LS, Lebowitz BD. Provisional diagnostic criteria for depression of Alzheimer disease: rationale and background. Am J Geriatr Psychiatry. 2002;10(2):129–41.
75. Lyketsos CG, Steele C, Baker L, Galik E, Kopunek S, Steinberg M, et al. Major and minor depression in Alzheimer's disease: prevalence and impact. J Neuropsychiatry Clin Neurosci. 1997;9(4):556–61.
76. Steffens DC, Potter GG. Geriatric depression and cognitive impairment. Psychol Med. 2008;38(2):163–75.
77. Diniz BS, Butters MA, Albert SM, Dew MA, Reynolds CF 3rd. Late-life depression and risk of vascular dementia and Alzheimer's disease: systematic review and meta-analysis of community-based cohort studies. Br J Psychiatry. 2013;202(5):329–35.
78. Thielscher C, Thielscher S, Kostev K. The risk of developing depression when suffering from neurological diseases. Ger Med Sci. 2013;11:Doc02.
79. Saiz-Vazquez O, Gracia-Garcia P, Ubillos-Landa S, Puente-Martinez A, Casado-Yusta S, Olaya B, et al. Depression as a risk factor for Alzheimer's disease: a systematic review of longitudinal meta-analyses. J Clin Med. 2021;10(9)
80. Modrego PJ, de Cerio LD, Lobo A. The Interface between depression and Alzheimer's disease. A

comprehensive approach. Ann Indian Acad Neurol. 2023;26(4):315–25.
81. Sheline YI, Gado MH, Kraemer HC. Untreated depression and hippocampal volume loss. Am J Psychiatry. 2003;160(8):1516–8.
82. Joels M. Corticosteroid actions in the hippocampus. J Neuroendocrinol. 2001;13(8):657–69.
83. Ownby RL, Crocco E, Acevedo A, John V, Loewenstein D. Depression and risk for Alzheimer disease: systematic review, meta-analysis, and metaregression analysis. Arch Gen Psychiatry. 2006;63(5):530–8.
84. Wilson RS, Barnes LL, Mendes de Leon CF, Aggarwal NT, Schneider JS, Bach J, et al. Depressive symptoms, cognitive decline, and risk of AD in older persons. Neurology. 2002;59(3):364–70.
85. Kohler S, Thomas AJ, Barnett NA, O'Brien JT. The pattern and course of cognitive impairment in late-life depression. Psychol Med. 2010;40(4):591–602.
86. Wilson RS, Capuano AW, Boyle PA, Hoganson GM, Hizel LP, Shah RC, et al. Clinical-pathologic study of depressive symptoms and cognitive decline in old age. Neurology. 2014;83(8):702–9.
87. Mirza SS, Wolters FJ, Swanson SA, Koudstaal PJ, Hofman A, Tiemeier H, et al. 10-year trajectories of depressive symptoms and risk of dementia: a population-based study. Lancet Psychiatry. 2016;3(7):628–35.
88. Singh-Manoux A, Dugravot A, Fournier A, Abell J, Ebmeier K, Kivimaki M, et al. Trajectories of depressive symptoms before diagnosis of dementia: a 28-year follow-up study. JAMA Psychiatry. 2017;74(7):712–8.
89. Rapp MA, Schnaider-Beeri M, Grossman HT, Sano M, Perl DP, Purohit DP, et al. Increased hippocampal plaques and tangles in patients with Alzheimer disease with a lifetime history of major depression. Arch Gen Psychiatry. 2006;63(2):161–7.
90. Butters MA, Klunk WE, Mathis CA, Price JC, Ziolko SK, Hoge JA, et al. Imaging Alzheimer pathology in late-life depression with PET and Pittsburgh compound-B. Alzheimer Dis Assoc Disord. 2008;22(3):261–8.
91. Sun X, Steffens DC, Au R, Folstein M, Summergrad P, Yee J, et al. Amyloid-associated depression: a prodromal depression of Alzheimer disease? Arch Gen Psychiatry. 2008;65(5):542–50.
92. Metti AL, Cauley JA, Newman AB, Ayonayon HN, Barry LC, Kuller LM, et al. Plasma beta amyloid level and depression in older adults. J Gerontol A Biol Sci Med Sci. 2013;68(1):74–9.
93. Babulal GM, Ghoshal N, Head D, Vernon EK, Holtzman DM, Benzinger TLS, et al. Mood changes in cognitively normal older adults are linked to Alzheimer disease biomarker levels. Am J Geriatr Psychiatry. 2016;24(11):1095–104.
94. Krell-Roesch J, Lowe VJ, Neureiter J, Pink A, Roberts RO, Mielke MM, et al. Depressive and anxiety symptoms and cortical amyloid deposition among cognitively normal elderly persons: the Mayo Clinic study of aging. Int Psychogeriatr. 2018;30(2):245–51.
95. Donovan NJ, Okereke OI, Vannini P, Amariglio RE, Rentz DM, Marshall GA, et al. Association of Higher Cortical Amyloid burden with loneliness in cognitively normal older adults. JAMA Psychiatry. 2016;73(12):1230–7.
96. Donovan NJ, Locascio JJ, Marshall GA, Gatchel J, Hanseeuw BJ, Rentz DM, et al. Longitudinal association of amyloid beta and anxious-depressive symptoms in cognitively normal older adults. Am J Psychiatry. 2018;175(6):530–7.
97. Babulal GM, Roe CM, Stout SH, Rajasekar G, Wisch JK, Benzinger TLS, et al. Depression is associated with Tau and not amyloid positron emission tomography in cognitively normal adults. J Alzheimer's Dis. 2020;74(4):1045–55.
98. Diniz BS, Chen Z, Steffens DC, Pilling L, Fortinsky RH, Kuchel GA, et al. Proteogenomic signature of risk of Alzheimer's disease and related dementia risk in individuals with a history of major depression disorder. medRxiv. 2024;
99. Patten SB, Barbui C. Drug-induced depression: a systematic review to inform clinical practice. Psychother Psychosom. 2004;73(4):207–15.
100. Alexopoulos GS, Meyers BS, Young RC, Kakuma T, Feder M, Einhorn A, et al. Recovery in geriatric depression. Arch Gen Psychiatry. 1996;53(4):305–12.
101. Kalayam B, Alexopoulos GS. Prefrontal dysfunction and treatment response in geriatric depression. Arch Gen Psychiatry. 1999;56(8):713–8.
102. Alexopoulos GS, Kiosses DN, Murphy C, Heo M. Executive dysfunction, heart disease burden, and remission of geriatric depression. Neuropsychopharmacology. 2004;29(12):2278–84.
103. Baldwin R, Jeffries S, Jackson A, Sutcliffe C, Thacker N, Scott M, et al. Treatment response in late-onset depression: relationship to neuropsychological, neuroradiological and vascular risk factors. Psychol Med. 2004;34(1):125–36.
104. Alexopoulos GS, Kiosses DN, Heo M, Murphy CF, Shanmugham B, Gunning-Dixon F. Executive dysfunction and the course of geriatric depression. Biol Psychiatry. 2005;58(3):204–10.
105. Sneed JR, Roose SP, Keilp JG, Krishnan KR, Alexopoulos GS, Sackeim HA. Response inhibition predicts poor antidepressant treatment response in very old depressed patients. Am J Geriatr Psychiatry. 2007;15(7):553–63.
106. Bella R, Pennisi G, Cantone M, Palermo F, Pennisi M, Lanza G, et al. Clinical presentation and outcome of geriatric depression in subcortical ischemic vascular disease. Gerontology. 2010;56(3):298–302.
107. Alexopoulos GS, Meyers BS, Young RC, Kalayam B, Kakuma T, Gabrielle M, et al. Executive dysfunction and long-term outcomes of geriatric depression. Arch Gen Psychiatry. 2000;57(3):285–90.

Physical Illnesses and Depression

7

Seung-Ho Jang and Saeheon Jang

7.1 Depression in Various Physical Illnesses

A study conducted in South Korea found that 34% of individuals diagnosed with depression have at least one comorbid physical illness. The most frequently observed comorbidities include hypertension (16%), diabetes (7%), peptic ulcers (4%), coronary artery disease (3%), and thyroid disorders (3%) [1]. Treatment outcomes tend to be poorer when depression co-occurs with a physical illness compared to when it occurs alone. Functional recovery is often delayed, and the associated socioeconomic burden is substantially increased [2]. Because depression and chronic physical illnesses have a bidirectional relationship, appropriate management of coexisting physical conditions can improve the effectiveness of depression treatment (Fig. 7.1) [3].

Neurological Disorders

Parkinson's Disease

Parkinson's disease (PD) is a neurodegenerative disorder of the central nervous system characterized by the progressive degeneration of dopaminergic neurons in the substantia nigra of the midbrain. This degeneration, influenced by both genetic and environmental factors, leads to impaired dopamine production [4]. Depression is a frequently observed non-motor symptom of PD, affecting approximately 30% of patients and substantially impairing daily functioning. It tends to occur more frequently during the early and late stages of the disease [5]. Non-motor symptoms such as apathy, reduced concentration, and memory impairment—often linked to Parkinson's dementia—can complicate the differential diagnosis of depression, necessitating comprehensive clinical evaluation [6]. Due to conspicuous motor manifestations such as tremors and rigidity, patients with PD often experience significant stigma, which may result in profound social isolation.

Stroke

Post-stroke depression (PSD) is a frequent neuropsychiatric complication that substantially impairs daily functioning, cognitive performance, and overall clinical prognosis. Despite its clinical significance, PSD is often difficult to recognize and diagnose due to overlapping physical symptoms, cognitive and language impairments, anosognosia, and difficulties in emotional expression. Somatic or cognitive symptoms of stroke may mimic depressive features, leading to misdiagnosis, while true depressive symptoms may be

S.-H. Jang
Jeil Psychiatry Clinic, Gimje, Republic of Korea

S. Jang (✉)
Department of Psychiatry, Bong Seng Memorial Hospital, Busan, Republic of Korea
e-mail: powernp@nate.com

W.-M. Bahk et al. (eds.), *Depressive Disorder*, https://doi.org/10.1007/978-981-92-1331-3_7

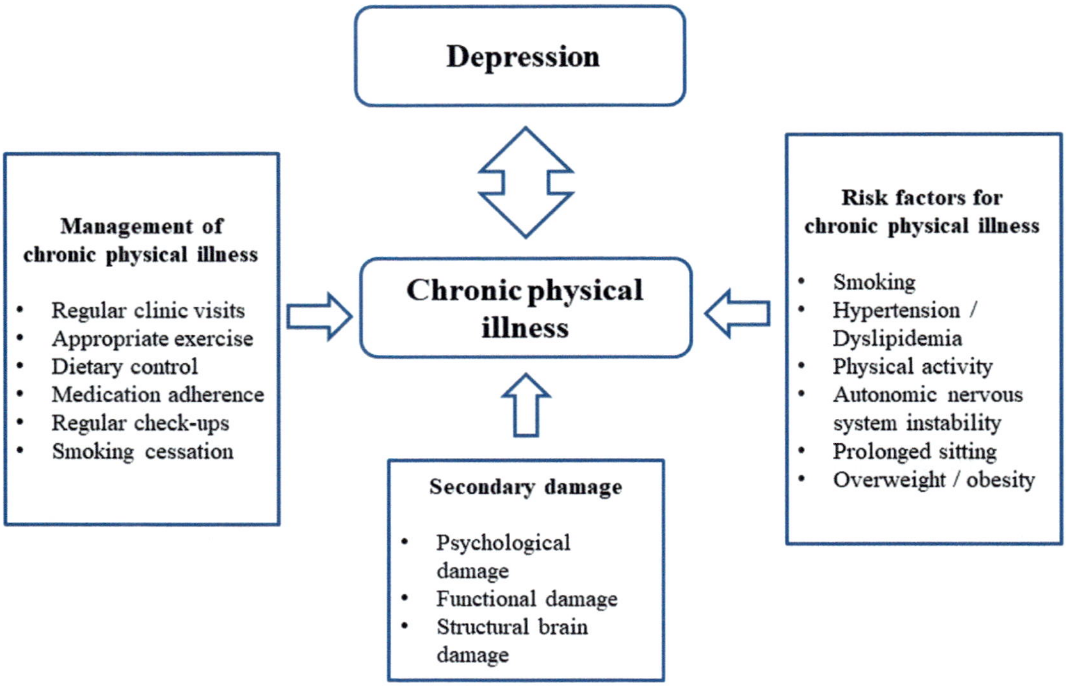

Fig. 7.1 Bidirectional interaction between depression and chronic physical illness

overlooked. PSD is reported to occur in 5.6–55% of stroke survivors, depending on the population studied and diagnostic criteria used, as shown in systematic reviews. Early-onset PSD typically shows a more favorable prognosis and may be resolved within 1 year, whereas late-onset PSD tends to be more chronic. Therefore, timely identification and early intervention are critical for improving long-term outcomes [7].

Epilepsy

Patients with epilepsy, characterized by recurrent seizures due to neuronal hyperexcitability, often experience considerable physical and psychological distress beyond the seizures themselves [8]. Among this population, depression is one of the most prevalent psychiatric comorbidities, affecting approximately 24% [9]. The relationship between epilepsy and depression is bidirectional: individuals with depression are at increased risk of developing epilepsy, and vice versa [10]. Depression in epilepsy increases the risk of suicide and contributes to stigmatization. It also exacerbates medication-related side effects, reduces responsiveness to treatment, and significantly impairs quality of life (QOL) [11]. Moreover, depression is associated with increased healthcare costs in patients with epilepsy, regardless of seizure type or duration. This underscores the importance of systematic screening and timely intervention [12]. Therefore, clinicians should routinely assess depressive symptoms and integrate psychiatric care into the comprehensive treatment of epilepsy.

Cardiovascular Diseases

Depression is a significant risk factor for the development of coronary artery disease (CAD) and other cardiovascular diseases (CVDs), as well as for increased cardiovascular mortality [13]. It is also strongly linked to hypertension, both as a comorbidity and a contributing risk factor [14]. A study of office workers found that individuals with depression had a 1.41 times higher likelihood of developing hypertension compared to those without depression [15]. The 2018 European Society of Cardiology guidelines recognize depression in patients with CAD as an independent risk factor for both mortality and recurrence [16]. Depression compromises both prognosis and quality of life (QOL) in cardiovascular patients by contributing to unhealthy behaviors (e.g., smoking, physical inactivity) and delaying treatment-seeking. Additionally, shared biological mechanisms between depression and ischemic heart disease contribute to increased recurrence and mortality in affected patients [17]. Jee et al. reported that individuals with depression had nearly twice the risk of developing ischemic heart disease and, among those already diagnosed, a 1.5 to 1.8-fold higher risk of mortality compared to non-depressed counterparts [18].

Gastrointestinal Diseases and Functional Gastrointestinal Disorders

Functional Gastrointestinal Disorders

Functional gastrointestinal disorders (FGIDs) are defined by chronic symptoms that impair eating and bowel habits—such as abdominal pain, nausea, dyspepsia, diarrhea, and constipation—yet occur in the absence of identifiable structural or biochemical abnormalities [19]. This diagnostic ambiguity poses significant challenges for both clinical evaluation and treatment. Emerging evidence highlights the critical role of psychosocial factors in the pathophysiology and clinical expression of FGIDs. One study found that 25% of outpatients with dysthymia and 39% of inpatients with affective disorders met diagnostic criteria for irritable bowel syndrome (IBS) [20]. Depression frequently precedes the onset of gastrointestinal symptoms or exacerbates their severity. Similarly, anxiety has a well-documented impact on gastrointestinal function. Specifically, anxiety is closely associated with the severity of dyspeptic symptoms and may disrupt adaptive stress-coping mechanisms, thereby contributing to increased healthcare utilization [21, 22].

Inflammatory Bowel Disease

Ulcerative colitis is a chronic inflammatory condition that extends proximally in a continuous manner from the rectum to the colon. It involves only the mucosal and submucosal layers and can be definitively treated with total colectomy. In contrast, Crohn's disease is characterized by transmural inflammation that affects all layers of the intestinal wall and may result in fistula formation involving adjacent organs. Common clinical manifestations include diarrhea, abdominal pain, anorexia, and low-grade fever. Extraintestinal manifestations are not uncommon and may affect the musculoskeletal, dermatologic, ocular, hepatobiliary, and renal systems [23]. Their type and severity vary significantly across individuals. The prevalence of depression in patients with Crohn's disease is estimated to be 24–28% [24]. This is comparable to rates observed in patients with rheumatic diseases and notably higher than in those with ulcerative colitis or the general population. Various factors are associated with depression in Crohn's disease, including sex, age, educational attainment, disease duration, extraintestinal symptoms, corticosteroid or immunosuppressant use, disease activity, prior intestinal surgeries, and the location of inflammation. When depression coexists with inflammatory bowel disease, physical symptoms such as pain and fatigue tend to worsen [25]. Negative emotional states, including anxiety and suicidal ideation, may also intensify, significantly impairing daily functioning. These outcomes underscore the need for timely psychiatric evaluation and integrated care approaches.

7.2 Endocrine Diseases

Diabetes Mellitus

Patients with diabetes mellitus have a twofold increased risk of developing depression relative to the general population. A meta-analysis reported that the prevalence of depression in patients with either type 1 or type 2 diabetes was 29.5%, indicating that nearly one-third of individuals with diabetes experience depressive symptoms [26]. Prevalence rates are especially high among older adults, reaching up to 58%, likely due to more pronounced cognitive decline, including impairments in memory, information processing, and concentration [27]. Depression in individuals with diabetes is associated with reduced quality of life (QOL) and impaired daily functioning, both of which can worsen glycemic control and exacerbate diabetes-related symptoms. In addition, depression decreases treatment adherence and is linked to higher rates of complications and mortality. Therefore, early detection and management of depression in patients with diabetes mellitus are essential to improve both psychological and metabolic outcomes [28]. The mechanisms linking diabetes and depression are generally classified into proximal and distal factors. Proximal factors include alterations in hypothalamic–pituitary–adrenal (HPA) axis activity, neurotransmitter imbalances (e.g., norepinephrine and serotonin), and organic brain changes secondary to diabetic complications such as cerebrovascular disease [29]. Distal factors involve the long-term burden of chronic illness, which can erode social support systems and lead to a loss of self-esteem (Fig. 7.2) [30].

Thyroid Diseases

The relationship between thyroid dysfunction and depression remains inconclusive. Notably, elevated thyroid-stimulating hormone (TSH) levels were reported in 54.5% of patients with severe depression. In older adults, an observed association between elevated TSH levels and depressive symptoms suggests that thyroid dysfunction may contribute to the development of depression [31]. One study found that individuals with subclinical hypothyroidism had a 2.33-fold increased incidence of depression compared to healthy controls [32]. By contrast, several studies found no significant association between subclinical hypothyroidism and depression, highlighting the need for further large-scale, longitudinal research [33].

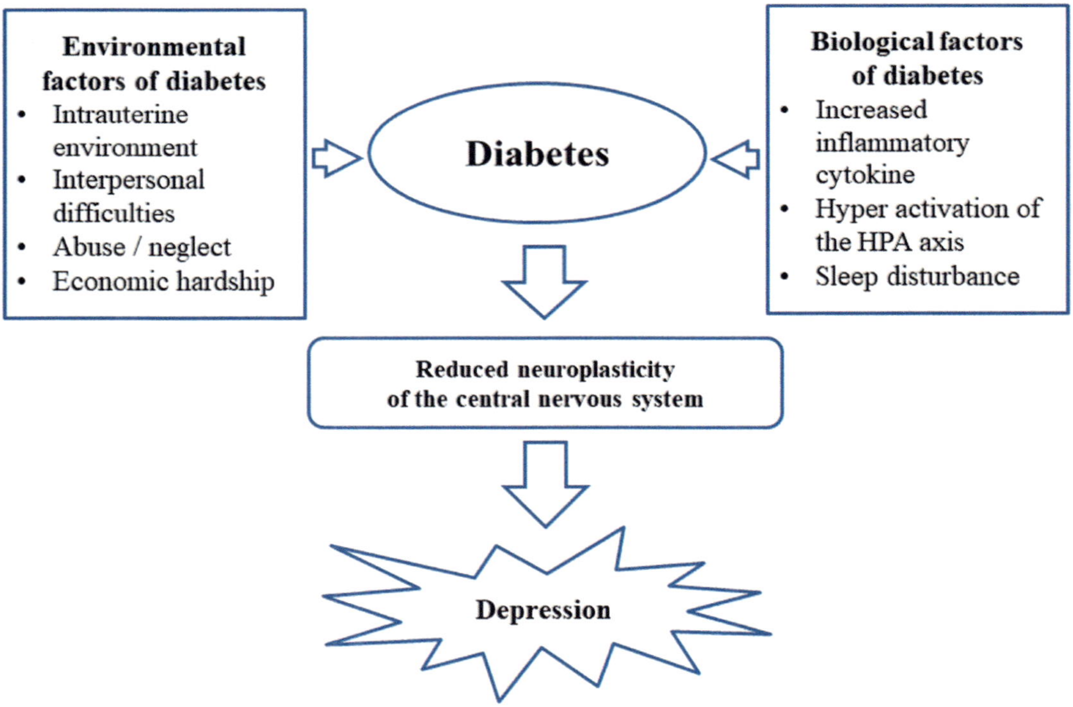

Fig. 7.2 Biological commonalities between depression and diabetes

7.3 Respiratory Diseases

Asthma

Patients with asthma have an increased prevalence of psychiatric comorbidities, particularly depression, anxiety, and panic disorders, compared to the general population. Additionally, asthma has been linked to attention-deficit/hyperactivity disorder (ADHD), especially in children and adolescents. The relationship between asthma and psychiatric disorders is bidirectional: anxiety and depression increase the risk of developing asthma, while asthma, in turn, elevates the risk for these psychiatric conditions. Specifically, panic disorder is associated with a 6.3-fold increased risk of asthma onset, whereas asthma raises the risk of panic disorder by a factor of 4.5 [34]. Symptom severity in asthma increases by a factor of 3.7 in the presence of anxiety and 2.4 with depression [35]. These psychiatric comorbidities are also associated with significantly higher healthcare utilization. Depression further impairs asthma management, particularly among older adults. Proposed mechanisms by which depression contributes to the onset or exacerbation of asthma include:

1. Impaired recognition and self-monitoring of asthma control [36].
2. Reduced adherence to medication regimens in patients with comorbid psychiatric conditions [37].
3. Increased secretion of inflammatory cytokines due to psychological stress, exacerbating airway inflammation [38].
4. Enhanced corticosteroid resistance, resulting in poorer treatment response [39].

Chronic Obstructive Pulmonary Disease

Chronic obstructive pulmonary disease (COPD) is characterized by irreversible airflow limitation resulting from chronic inflammation and structural damage to the airways and lung parenchyma. Depression is a frequent psychiatric comorbidity in patients with COPD, occurring at substantially higher rates than in the general population [40]. Reported prevalence rates of depression in COPD patients range from 10% to 57%, depending on assessment methods and study populations [41]. Depression impairs treatment adherence and adversely affects the clinical course of COPD. It also contributes to increased morbidity and mortality and substantially impairs quality of life (QOL).

7.4 Musculoskeletal Diseases

Osteoarthritis

Numerous studies across different countries have consistently reported a higher prevalence of depression among patients with osteoarthritis compared to the general population [42]. Although prevalence estimates vary depending on population characteristics and assessment tools, data from the U.S. National Health and Nutrition Examination Survey indicated that 13.9% of patients with osteoarthritis had depression—approximately 1.6 times higher than the general population [43]. Furthermore, depression prevalence was positively correlated with the severity of arthritic symptoms. Similarly, Korean studies have shown that adults over 45 years of age with osteoarthritis experience a 1.5-fold higher prevalence of depression compared to the general population. The prevalence of depression in patients with osteoarthritis has been reported as 11.2%, which is comparable to that in patients with cancer (11.1%) and higher than in those with diabetes (8.7%) or hypertension (8.3%) [44]. Pain and joint deformities in osteoarthritis contribute to functional impairment and reduced physical activity. These mobility limitations may, in turn, exacerbate feelings of loneliness and social isolation, increasing the risk of depression.

Rheumatoid Arthritis (RA)

Rheumatoid arthritis (RA) is a chronic progressive autoimmune disease that requires lifelong treatment. It is characterized by joint pain, swelling, morning stiffness, and progressive functional decline, often resulting in substantial limitations in daily life and socioeconomic participation [45]. These physical burdens are frequently accompanied by mental health challenges, including anxiety, depression, and psychological distress [46]. Comorbid anxiety and depression are particularly prevalent in individuals with RA [47]. The fluctuating course of the disease, along with chronic pain and mobility restrictions, can significantly exacerbate emotional instability. Such experiences elevate the risk of depression and may contribute to suicidal ideation, underscoring the need for timely psychological interventions and integrated care. Persistent pain perception in RA can lead to fatigue, feelings of helplessness, and sleep disturbances, all of which contribute to depressive symptomatology. Epidemiological studies estimate that 13–47% of RA patients experience anxiety and/or depression [48]. Due to the chronic and unpredictable nature of RA, quality of life deteriorates across physical, psychological, and social domains. Anxiety and depression are associated with reduced treatment adherence and poorer clinical outcomes in RA, highlighting the importance of ongoing mental health monitoring and support.

7.5 Other Physical Diseases

Atopic Dermatitis

Atopic dermatitis is a chronic, relapsing inflammatory skin disorder characterized by intense pruritus and eczematous lesions. It typically begins in infancy and often persists into or progresses during adulthood [49]. Adults with atopic dermatitis frequently report chronic anxiety and difficulties with anger management [50]. Visible lesions in exposed areas of the body can lead to negative body image, diminished self-esteem, and interpersonal difficulties [51]. These psychosocial burdens contribute to increased risks of depression, anxiety, and suicidal ideation. Among adolescents with atopic dermatitis, the risk of suicidal ideation is 1.14-fold higher than in peers without the condition [52], with approximately 14.8% reporting such thoughts [53].

Pain

Pain and depression often coexist in a bidirectional, mutually reinforcing relationship. They share common neurobiological pathways and neurotransmitters, further supporting their clinical and mechanistic association [54]. The lifetime prevalence of depression among individuals with chronic pain ranges from 32.4% to 56.8% [55]. Conversely, 15–100% of individuals with depression report pain symptoms, with an average prevalence of approximately 65%, highlighting the high comorbidity of pain in this population. Individuals experiencing multiple types of pain have a three- to fivefold increased risk of developing depression compared to those without pain. Similarly, patients with depression report pain at approximately twice the rate of those without depression [56].

7.6 Diagnosis of Depression in Patients with Physical Illness

Diagnosing depression in patients with comorbid physical illnesses presents several challenges:

1. Many symptoms of physical illnesses—such as fatigue, appetite or weight loss, psychomotor slowing, and reduced concentration—overlap with those of depression, making differential diagnosis difficult. For example, post-stroke symptoms like pathological crying, emotional lability, apathy, and fatigue may be misinterpreted as depressive features [57].
2. Thoughts or wishes related to death may occur in patients with advanced physical illnesses, even in the absence of depressed

mood. For instance, subtle suicidal ideation—such as a desire to hasten death—has been reported in 4% of hospitalized cancer patients and 17% of patients with only a few weeks to live. While such thoughts are associated with depression, despair, and uncontrolled pain, they may also occur independently of clinical depression. Therefore, a diminished will to live alone may not be a reliable indicator of depression in patients with severe medical conditions [58].

3. Even without clinical depression, physical illness and pain can reduce the capacity to experience pleasure in daily activities. While anhedonia is a hallmark symptom of depression, severe physical symptoms may independently diminish enjoyment and motivation. Without adequate control of pain and physical discomfort, patients may remain disengaged from meaningful activities. Consequently, a disproportionately reduced level of social or physical activity—relative to mood or physical impairment—may suggest comorbid depression.
4. In clinical populations, depression may present atypically or covertly—through excessive somatic complaints, irritability, or nonadherence to medical treatment. Physical illness may, therefore, contribute to both underdiagnosis and overdiagnosis of depression, depending on the clinical context.

Given these diagnostic challenges, several screening instruments have been validated for detecting depression in medically ill populations and may help improve diagnostic accuracy in complex cases.

- The Center for Epidemiologic Studies Depression Scale (CES-D) is a 20-item self-report questionnaire that includes only four somatic items, making it suitable for medically ill populations. It takes approximately 5 min to complete and shows high sensitivity and specificity, with a commonly used cut-off score between 16 and 17 [59].
- The Hospital Anxiety and Depression Scale (HADS) is a 14-item self-report instrument developed specifically to assess anxiety and depression in patients with physical illnesses. It avoids somatic symptom overlaps and takes less than 5 min to administer. Its psychometric properties are comparable to those of the CES-D [60].
- The Patient Health Questionnaire-9 (PHQ-9) comprises nine items and was initially developed to screen for depression, anxiety, and eating disorders in primary care. It is widely used due to its brevity, ease of scoring, and strong psychometric performance, including high sensitivity, specificity, and positive predictive value—even in physically ill populations [61].
- The Beck Depression Inventory (BDI) is one of the most widely used tools for depression screening. However, it requires more time to complete (10–15 min) and includes a greater number of somatic items. This limits its utility in patients with comorbid physical conditions, where distinguishing depressive symptoms from physical illness-related symptoms is critical [62].

7.7 Treatment of Depression Accompanied by Physical Illness

General Principles of Treatment

Effective treatment of depression comorbid with physical illness requires close collaboration with the medical team overseeing the underlying condition. Priority should be given to comprehensive evaluation and management of medical illnesses, including a thorough review of current and past treatments for efficacy and adverse effects. Ineffective interventions should be discontinued, as they may contribute to additional functional impairments such as impaired concentration and disrupted sleep. In addition, medications used for treating physical illnesses should be evaluated for their potential to induce or exacerbate depressive symptoms. Notably, corticosteroids, interferon-alpha, interleukin-2, gonadotropin-releasing hormone (GnRH) agonists, β-blockers, and certain anticonvulsants such as topiramate have been associated with depression [63]. Given the frequent occurrence of sleep disturbances in this population, patient education on basic sleep hygiene practices is often beneficial. Prolonged periods of inactivity or enforced rest due to physical illness may also contribute to rapid emotional decline, including loss of motivation and feelings of helplessness. Accordingly, implementing a structured physical activity program adapted to the individual's functional abilities can help enhance both physical and emotional well-being [64].

Specialized Principles of Treatment

Although standard treatment modalities for depression are applicable in patients with comorbid physical illness, they should be carefully tailored to the stage of illness, symptom profile, treatment side-effect risks, and the patient's overall medical condition. Both psychotherapeutic and pharmacological approaches may be employed with appropriate adjustments.

Psychotherapy

Psychotherapeutic interventions for patients with depression and coexisting physical illness should be tailored to the severity of depressive symptoms, the nature of the medical condition, and the patient's capacity for engagement in treatment. For patients with severe cognitive impairment, communication difficulties, or limited mobility, intensive psychotherapy may not be feasible. In such cases, lower-intensity interventions—such as group-based physical activity or supportive programs—may serve as preferable alternatives. For patients with mild-to-moderate depression, a variety of psychotherapeutic approaches have demonstrated clinical effectiveness. In particular, numerous studies on cancer patients have shown that cognitive behavioral therapy (CBT), delivered either individually or in group settings, yields favorable outcomes [65].

Pharmacological Treatment

When prescribing antidepressants to patients with depression comorbid with physical illness, clinicians must carefully consider drug–drug interactions and pharmacokinetic alterations caused by the underlying medical condition. In patients with hepatic impairment, the initial antidepressant dose should be reduced by at least 50%, and adverse effects should be closely monitored, especially during dose titration. Cardiovascular safety is a major concern in patients with arrhythmia or cardiovascular diseases (CVDs). Among antidepressants, sertraline has been shown to be both effective and well-tolerated in this population. Depression negatively affects the prognosis of coronary artery disease (CAD) and heart failure, and some antidepressants may exacerbate cardiovascular symptoms [66]. Tricyclic antidepressants (TCAs) are known to prolong the QT interval and increase the risk of arrhythmias. In contrast, serotonin-norepinephrine reuptake inhibitors (SNRIs) have minimal cardiovascular effects, and selective serotonin reuptake inhibitors (SSRIs) are generally considered safer [67]. However, caution is warranted with escitalopram and citalopram, which have been associated with QT prolongation, particularly in women and older adults [68]. In patients with comorbid chronic pain, SNRIs are preferred. Duloxetine is indicated for major depressive disorder and is also effective for fibromyalgia, diabetic peripheral neuropathy, and osteoarthritis unresponsive to nonsteroidal anti-inflammatory drugs (NSAIDs). A systematic review found that 12 weeks of duloxetine (60 mg/day) resulted in ≥50% pain reduction in 1.73 times more patients with diabetic neuropathy than placebo, and in 1.57 times more patients with fibromyalgia. These effects were sustained beyond 28 weeks of treatment [69]. In the context of asthma, early studies (since 1965) suggested bronchodilatory effects of doxepin, a TCA. Subsequent research has shown that antidepressants may benefit inflammatory conditions by inhibiting proinflammatory cytokines, modulating immune responses, and suppressing HPA axis hyperactivity. These mechanisms support the therapeutic potential of TCAs and SSRIs in inflammatory diseases such as rheumatoid arthritis and atopic dermatitis [70]. Given the widespread distribution of serotonin receptors in the gastrointestinal tract, serotonergic antidepressants may also help manage irritable bowel syndrome (IBS). Although evidence is limited, paroxetine has shown some benefit [71]. Among TCAs, amitriptyline (10–25 mg) and desipramine (50 mg) have demonstrated efficacy in IBS treatment [72]. In stress urinary incontinence, duloxetine has been shown to improve bladder control by enhancing the activity of the external urethral sphincter and is approved for therapeutic use [73]. In cases of overactive bladder, agents such as imipramine or SSRIs may reduce bladder contractility and improve symptoms [74].

7.8 Summary

In patients with physical illnesses, diagnosing depression requires concurrent assessment of both medical and psychiatric conditions, ideally through a multidimensional approach. In certain cases, psychological assessment tools can provide valuable diagnostic support.

The treatment of depression in this population should follow several key principles:

1. Identify and manage underlying organic causes as a primary step.
2. Reduce resistance to psychiatric treatment by addressing common emotional responses to physical illness, such as fear and helplessness.
3. Select appropriate pharmacological treatment based on individual needs.

When prescribing antidepressants for patients with comorbid medical conditions, clinicians should consider the severity of depressive symptoms, the pharmacokinetics and pharmacodynamics of the chosen medication, and the risk of adverse effects. Special caution is necessary to monitor for drug–disease and drug–drug interactions.

Among available options, selective serotonin reuptake inhibitors (SSRIs) and serotonin-norepinephrine reuptake inhibitors (SNRIs) are generally preferred. In patients with prominent pain symptoms, tricyclic antidepressants (TCAs) may also be considered.

Declarations

Competing Interests The author(s) has no competing interests to declare that are relevant to the content of this manuscript.

Ethics Approval The author(s) declares that this manuscript does not include primary research with human participants.

The author(s) declares that this manuscript does not include primary studies involving animals.

References

1. Kim JM, Stewart R, Bae KY, Yang SJ, Yoon JS, Jung SW, et al. Physical comorbidities and 12-week treatment outcomes in Korean patients with depressive disorders: the CRESCENT study. J Psychosom Res. 2011;71:311–8.
2. Stommel M, Given CW. Depression and functional status as predictors of death in patients with cancer. Cancer. 2002;94:2719–27.
3. Thase ME. Managing medical comorbidities in patients with depression to improve prognosis. J Clin Psychiatry. 2016;77(Suppl 1):22–7.
4. Pandya MI, Kubu CS, Giroux ML. Parkinson's disease: not just a movement disorder. Cleve Clin J Med. 2008;75(12):856–64.
5. McDonald WM, Righard IH, DeLong MR. Prevalence, etiology, and treatment of depression in Parkinson's disease. Biol Psychiatry. 2003;54(3):363–75.
6. Starkstein S, Dragovic M, Jorge R, Brockman S, Merello M, Robinson RG, et al. Diagnostic criteria for depression in Parkinson's disease: a study of symptom patterns using latent class analysis. Mov Disord. 2011;26:2239–45.
7. Robinson RG, Starr LB, Lipsey JR, Rao K, Price TR. A two-year longitudinal study of post-stroke mood disorders: dynamic changes in associated variables over the first six months of follow-up. Stroke. 1984;15(3):510–7.
8. Gaitatzis A, Carroll K, Majeed A, Wsander J. Epidemiology of epilepsy comorbidities in the general population. Epilepsia. 2004;45:1613–22.
9. Fiest KM, Dykeman J, et al. Depression in patients with epilepsy: a systematic review and meta-analysis. Neurology. 2013;80:590–9.

10. Hesdorffer DC, Ishihara L, Mynepalli L, Webb DJ, Weil J, Hauser WA. Epilepsy, suicidality, and psychiatric disorders: a bidirectional association. Ann Neurol. 2012;72:184–91.
11. Kwon OY, Park SP. Depression and anxiety in people with epilepsy. J Clin Neurol. 2014;10:175–88.
12. Cramer JA, Blum D, Fanning K, et al.; Epilepsy impact project group. Impact of comorbid depression on health resource utilization in a community sample of patients with epilepsy. Epilepsy Behav. 2004;5:337–42.
13. Carney RM, Freedland KE. Depression and coronary heart disease. Nat Rev Cardiol. 2017;14(9):493–505.
14. Meng L, Chen D, Yang Y, Zheng Y, Hui R. Depression increases the risk of hypertension incidence: a meta-analysis of prospective cohort studies. J Hypertens. 2012;30(5):842–51.
15. Choi JW, Cho JJ, Chang HM, Kim CW, Paek YJ, et al. Association between depression and cardiovascular risk factors in workers undergoing comprehensive medical examinations at a university-based hospital. J Korean Acad Fam Med. 2008;29(9):645–50.
16. Vaccarino V, Badimon L, Bremner JD, Cenko E, Cubedo J, Dorobantu M, et al. Depression and coronary heart disease: a 2018 position paper of the ESC Working Group on Coronary Pathophysiology and Microcirculation. Eur Heart J. 2020;41(17):1687–96.
17. Lichtman JH, Froelicher ES, Blumenthal JA, Carney RM, Doering LV, et al. Depression as a risk factor for poor prognosis among patients with acute coronary syndrome: a systematic review and recommendation: a scientific statement from the American Heart Association. Circulation. 2014;129(12):1350–69.
18. Jee YH, Chang H, Jung KJ, et al. A cohort study on the effects of depression on atherosclerotic cardiovascular disease risk in Korea. BMJ Open. 2019;9(3):e026913.
19. Drossman DA. Functional gastrointestinal disorders and Rome III process. Gastroenterology. 2006;130:1377–90.
20. Gomborone JE, Gorard DA, Dewsnap PA, Libby GW, et al. Prevalence of IBS symptoms in acute psychiatric inpatients with an affective diagnosis. Psychosomatics. 1996;37:385–9.
21. Jones MP. Evaluation and treatment of dyspepsia. Postgrad Med J. 2003;79:25–9.
22. Kroenke K, Jackson JL, Chamberlin J. Depressive and anxiety disorders in patients presenting with physical complaints: clinical predictors and outcome. Am J Med. 1997;107:1040–9.
23. Scheper HJ, Brand HS. Oral aspects of Crohn's disease. Int Dent J. 2002;52:163–72.
24. Graff LA, Walker JR, Bernstein CN, et al. Depression and anxiety in inflammatory bowel disease: a review of comorbidities and management. Inflamm Bowel Dis. 2009;15:1105–18.
25. Ephgrave K. Extraintestinal manifestations of Crohn's. Surg Clin North Am. 2007;87:673–80.
26. Anderson RJ, RE FKEC, Lustman PJ. Prevalence of comorbid depression in adults with diabetes: a meta-analysis. Diabetes Care. 2001;24:1069–78.
27. Trief PM, Teresi JA, Izquierdo R, Morin PC, Goland R, Field L, et al. Psychosocial outcomes of telemedicine case management for elderly patients with diabetes: a randomized IDEATel trial. Diabetes Care. 2007;30:1266–8.
28. Lustman PJ, Clouse RE. Depression in patients with diabetes: the relationship between mood and glycemic control. J Diabetes Complicat. 2005;19:113–22.
29. Alexopoulos GS, Meyers BS, Young RG, et al. Vascular depression hypothesis. Arch Gen Psychiatry. 1997;54:915–22.
30. Jacobson AM, Hauser ST, Willett JB, Wolfsdorf JI, Dvorak R, Herman L, de Groot M. Psychological adjustment to IDDM: 10-year follow-up of an onset cohort of child and adolescent patients. Diabetes Care. 1997;20:811–34.
31. Chueire VB, Romaldini JH, et al. Subclinical hypothyroidism increases the risk of depression in the elderly. Arch Gerontol Geriatr. 2007;44(1):21–8.
32. Almeida C, Brasil MA, Costa AJ, Reis FA, Reuters V, Teixeira P, et al. Subclinical hypothyroidism: psychiatric disorders and symptoms. Rev Bras Psiquiatr. 2007;29(2):157–9.
33. Fjaellegaard K, Kvetny J, Allerup PN, Bech P, Ellervik C. Well-being and depression in individuals with subclinical hypothyroidism and thyroid autoimmunity—a general population study. Nord J Psychiatry. 2015;69(1):73–8.
34. Hasler G, Gergen PJ, Kleinbaum DG, Ajdacic V, Gamma A, et al. Asthma and panic in young adults: a 20-year prospective community study. Am J Respir Crit Care Med. 2005;171:1224–30.
35. Di Marco F, Verga M, Santus P, Giovannelli F, et al. Close correlations among anxiety, depression, and asthma control. Respir Med. 2010;104:22–8.
36. Kuehn BM. Asthma linked to psychiatric disorders. JAMA. 2008;299:158–60.
37. Krauskopf KA, Sofianou A, Goel MS, Wolf MS, Wilson EA, et al. Depressive symptoms, low adherence, and poor asthma outcomes in the elderly population. J Asthma. 2013;50:260–6.
38. Wright RJ, Finn P, Contreras JP, Cohen S, Wright RO, Staudenmayer J, et al. Chronic caregiver stress, IgE expression, allergen-induced proliferation, and cytokine profiles in a birth cohort predisposed to atopy. J Allergy Clin Immunol. 2004;113:1051–7.
39. Haczku A, Panettieri RA Jr. Social stress and asthma: role of corticosteroid insensitivity. J Allergy Clin Immunol. 2010;125:550–8.
40. Hynninen KM, Breitve MH, Wiborg AG, Pallesen S, Nordhus IH. Psychological characteristics of patients with chronic obstructive pulmonary disease: a review. J Psychosom Res. 2005;59:429–43.
41. Atlantis E, Fahey P, Cochrane B, Smith S. Bidirectional associations between clinically relevant depression or anxiety and COPD: a systematic review and meta-analysis. Chest. 2013;144:766–77.

42. Han SB, Lee SH, Ha IH, Kim EJ. Association between the severity of depressive symptoms and chronic knee pain in Korean adults aged > 50 years: a cross-sectional study using nationally representative data. BMJ Open. 2019;9(12):e032451.
43. Brooks JM, Petersen C, Kelly SM, Reid MC. Likelihood of depressive symptoms in US older adults by prescribed opioid potency: National Health and Nutrition Examination Survey 2005–2013. Int J Geriatr Psychiatry. 2019;34(10):1481–9.
44. Kim YH, Kwon M. Factors affecting depression in female patients with osteoarthritis. J Korean Acad Fundam Nurs. 2017;24(2):138–45.
45. Ko HJ, Kim HY. Recent advances in rheumatoid treatment. Korean J Intern Med. 2009;52(7):657–64.
46. Haroon N, Aggarwal A, Lawrence A, et al. Impact of rheumatoid arthritis on quality of life. Mod Rheumatol. 2007;17(4):290–5.
47. Sheegy C, Murphy E, Barry M. Depression in rheumatoid arthritis: underscoring the problem. Rheumatology. 2006;45(11):1325–7.
48. Dickens C, Creed F. The burden of depression in patients with rheumatoid arthritis. Rheumatology. 2001;40(12):1327–30.
49. Lee YM, Hwang SW. Prevalence and risk factors of atopic dermatitis in preschool and school-aged children. J Korean Acad Nurs. 2008;14(3):285–94.
50. Ginsburg IH, Prystowsky JH, Kornfeld DS, et al. Role of emotional factors in adults with atopic dermatitis. Int J Dermatol. 1993;32(9):656–60.
51. Piardi A, Lega I, Tarolla E. Suicide risk in skin disorders. Clin Dermatol. 2013;31(1):47–56.
52. Seo JY, Lee DY, Lee CS, Park CS, Kim BJ, Cha BS, et al. Depressive symptoms and suicidal ideation in adolescents with allergic diseases. J Korean Soc Biol Ther Psychiatry. 2015;21(3):167–73.
53. Lee HJ. Factors influencing allergic diseases in Korean adolescents. Seoul: Chung-Ang University; 2016. p. 113.
54. Blier P, Abbott FV. Putative mechanisms of action of antidepressant drugs in affective and anxiety disorders and pain. J Psychiatry Neurosci. 2001;26:37–43.
55. Katon W, Egan K, Miller D. Chronic pain: lifetime psychiatric diagnoses and family history. Am J Psychiatry. 1985;142:1156–60.
56. Wessely S, Powell R. Fatigue syndrome: a comparison of chronic "postviral" fatigue with neuromuscular and affective disorders. J Neurol Neurosurg Psychiatry. 1989;52:940–8.
57. Bogousslavsky J. William Feinberg lecture 2002. Emotions, mood and behavior after stroke. Stroke. 2003;34:1046–50.
58. Breitbart W, Rosenfeld B, Pessin H, Kaim M, Funesti-Esch J, Galietta M, et al. Depression, hopelessness and desire for hastened death in terminally ill patients with cancer. JAMA. 2000;284:2907–11.
59. Radloff LS. The CES-D scale: a self-report depression scale for research in the general population. Appl Psychol Meas. 1977;1:385–401.
60. Zigmond AS, Snaith RP. The hospital anxiety and depression scale. Acta Psychiatr Scand. 1983;67:361–70.
61. Kroenke K, Spitzer R, Williams J. The PHQ-9: validity of a brief depression severity measure. J Gen Intern Med. 2001;16:606–13.
62. Schwab J, Bialow M, Clemmons R, Martic P, Holzer C. The Beck depression inventory with medical inpatients. Acta Psychiatr Scand. 1967;43:255–66.
63. Patten SB, Barbui C. Drug-induced depression: a systematic review to inform clinical practice. Psychother Psychosom. 2004;73:207–15.
64. Herring MP, Puetz TW, Dishman RK. Effect of exercise training on depressive symptoms among patients with a chronic illness: a systematic review and meta-analysis of randomized controlled trials. Arch Intern Med. 2012;172:101–11.
65. Beltman MW, Voshaar RCO, Speckens AE. Cognitive-behavioral therapy for depression in people with a somatic disease: meta-analysis of randomized controlled trials. Br J Psychiatry. 2010;197:11–9.
66. Nezafati MH, Vojdanparast M, Nezafati P. Antidepressants and cardiovascular adverse events: a narrative review. ARYA Atheroscler. 2015;11:295–304.
67. Pather P, Ungvari Z, Nanasi PP, Furst S, Kecskemeti V. Speculations on difference between tricyclic and selective serotonin reuptake inhibitor antidepressants on their cardiac effects. Is there any? Curr Med Chem. 1999;6:469–80.
68. Ojero-Senard A, Benevent J, Bondon-Guitton E, Durrieu G, Chebane L, Araujo M, et al. A comparative study of QT prolongation with serotonin reuptake inhibitors. Psychopharmacology. 2017;234:3075–81.
69. Lunn MP, Hughes RA, Wiffen PJ. Duloxetine for treating painful neuropathy, chronic pain or fibromyalgia. Cochrane Database Syst Rev. 2014;1:CD007115.
70. Krommydas G, Gourgoulianis KI, Karamitsos K, Krapis K, Kotrotsiou E, Molyvdas PA. Therapeutic value of antidepressants in asthma. Med Hypotheses. 2005;64:938–40.
71. Tabas G, Beaves M, Wang J, Friday P, Mardini H, Arnold G. Paroxetine to treat irritable bowel syndrome not responding to high-fiber diet: a double-blind, placebo-controlled trial. Am J Gastroenterol. 2004;99:914–20.
72. Hislop IG. Psychological significance of the irritable colon syndrome. Gut. 1971;12:452–7.
73. Yang SK. Psycho-urology: possible links between stress, anxiety, depression and bladder function. J Korean Continence Soc. 2006;10:1–8.
74. Gstleden CM, George GF, Renwick AG, Asher MJ. Imipramine possible alternative to current therapy for urinary incontinence in the elderly. J Urol. 1981;125:318–20.

8 Depression in Cancer Patients

In Hee Shim and Kwanghun Lee

8.1 Introduction: Distress and Depression in Cancer Patients

Cancer can affect various organs and often metastasizes to others. In psycho-oncology, the field addressing the mental health of cancer patients, it is often metaphorically stated that the one organ consistently affected across all types of cancer is the mind [1]. This reflects the high prevalence of both physical and psychological symptoms experienced by cancer patients. The psychological suffering associated with cancer is commonly referred to as distress [2].

Distress may emerge at any stage of the disease trajectory—including at the time of diagnosis, during initiation or completion of treatment, upon recurrence, or throughout palliative care. The National Comprehensive Cancer Network (NCCN) in the United States defines distress as an unpleasant experience of a mental, physical, social, or spiritual nature that encompasses common feelings like sadness, worry, and anger but is much broader [2].

I. H. Shim (✉)
Department of Psychiatry, Dongnam Institute of Radiological & Medical Sciences, Busan, Republic of Korea
e-mail: ihshim1224@gmail.com

K. Lee
Lee KwangHun Mental Health Clinic, Gyeongju, Republic of Korea

For instance, upon receiving a cancer diagnosis, individuals may experience a shift in self-identity, adopting the role of a "cancer patient." Depending on the cancer type and stage, they may be confronted with the prospect of death. Cancer can alter one's familial or occupational roles, and changes in appearance due to surgery or chemotherapy may result in diminished self-confidence. Physical symptoms—such as pain, nausea, and fatigue—may contribute to the onset of depressive symptoms. Additionally, frequent medical visits and concerns about recurrence or metastasis often lead to chronic anxiety. Cancer patients often face issues such as uncertainty, a lack of control, and increased dependency at any point in their illness. As their condition progresses, many cancer patients experience a fear of future suffering, including the loss of relationships and roles, as well as the painful prospect of death.

While most patients feel emotions such as sadness, grief, and anxiety, these feelings are often resolved naturally when the physician clearly outlines a treatment plan that provides hope and alleviates suffering, and when supported by family and friends. Therefore, the depression and anxiety felt by cancer patients can be considered normal reactions to some extent. However, excessive or prolonged distress can impact daily functioning and necessitates evaluation and intervention. Developing major depressive disorder (MDD) is not a typical course of

W.-M. Bahk et al. (eds.), *Depressive Disorder*, https://doi.org/10.1007/978-981-92-1331-3_8

cancer, but rather a psychiatric condition that requires individualized assessment and treatment in order to improve quality of life, enhance treatment adherence, and prevent suicide. This is an important complication that must be addressed.

8.2 Prevalence of Depression in Cancer Patients

It is reported that approximately 7.9–32.4% of all cancer patients are diagnosed with depression [3]. Specifically, the prevalence of MDD, as defined by the Diagnostic and Statistical Manual of Mental Disorders (DSM) or International Statistical Classification of Diseases and Related Health Problems (ICD), is around 16%, while the prevalence of subthreshold depression and dysthymia is 22% [4]. Depression is most common within the first year following a cancer diagnosis, with prevalence rates estimated to be three to four times higher than those observed in the general population.

The variation in reported prevalence across studies can be attributed to various factors, including differences in cancer type, stage, treatment methods, age and sex distribution, and sociocultural factors such as religious affiliation and educational level. Differences in healthcare systems and diagnostic approaches (such as the use of screening questionnaires or face-to-face versus virtual interviews) can also contribute to varying prevalence estimates.

8.3 Assessment of Depression

Screening

When selecting depression screening tools for cancer patients, several factors must be considered, including the format, length, administration time, and the effort required for scoring and interpretation. In oncology settings, where the primary focus is on cancer diagnosis and treatment, limited time and resources are available for mental health assessment. To address this, brief screening tools with only one or two items have been developed. Both the American Society of Clinical Oncology (ASCO) and the Pan Canadian guidelines recommend regular and periodic distress screening at key points in cancer care, including diagnosis, during and after treatment, and throughout survivorship. These guidelines prioritize the use of brief and repeatable measures such as the Edmonton Symptom Assessment System (ESAS) or the Distress Thermometer (DT). For example, a DT score of 4 or higher should prompt further evaluation.

These short tools are advantageous in busy clinical environments because they are quick to administer and sensitive for detecting distress, although they may have limited specificity and capture only a narrow spectrum of depressive symptoms. On the other hand, longer screening tools may be more time-consuming and incur additional costs, making them less practical in certain clinical settings.

As a result, the choice of screening tool may vary depending on the clinical setting; however, brief screening tools—such as the ESAS or a 1–2 item DT—are used first; patients who screen positive are then assessed with more comprehensive instruments like the Hospital Anxiety and Depression Scale (HADS), Patient Health Questionnaire-9 (PHQ-9), or Beck Depression Inventory (BDI), which is, generally recommended for cancer patients [5]. Table 8.1 pres-

Table 8.1 Commonly used screening tools for depression in cancer patients

Beck Depression Inventory (BDI)
Beck Depression Inventory—Short Form (BDI-SF)
Brief Symptom Inventory (BSI)
Brief Version, Zung Self-Rating Depression Scale (BZSDRS)
Center for Epidemiologic Studies Depression Scale (CES-D)
Distress Thermometer (DT)
Edmonton Symptom Assessment System (ESAS)
General Health Questionnaire (GHQ)
Hamilton Rating Scale for Depression (HAM-D)
Hospital Anxiety and Depression Scale (HADS)
Montgomery–Åsberg Depression Rating Scale (MADRS)
Patient Health Questionnaire-9 (PHQ-9)

ents commonly used screening tools for depression in cancer patients [6, 7].

HADS, while commonly used, has variable cut-off points across studies and may be less reliable in advanced cancer or palliative care. The BDI is generally applicable across different cancer types and stages, making it particularly useful for screening [8]. The CES-D is often preferred for assessing treatment response.

Thus, the selection of a depression screening tool must align with the clinical context and the intended purpose of assessment. Because screening tests alone can be insufficient for accurately diagnosing and managing depression, any positive result in cancer patients should be confirmed through a formal diagnostic interview to establish a depression diagnosis [9, 10].

Diagnosis

To diagnose depression in cancer patients, it is often necessary to differentiate between depressive disorders accompanied by mood changes, such as adjustment disorder with depressed mood, mood disorders due to cancer, and medication- or substance-induced mood disorders (see Table 8.2).

This process requires not only an understanding of the psychosocial aspects of cancer but also an evaluation of symptoms that may arise during the course of the illness. It is crucial to recognize the neuropsychiatric sequelae of cancer treatments or other biological cancer therapies [11].

A depressive episode is diagnosed when an individual experiences a persistent depressed mood or anhedonia nearly every day for a period of 2 weeks, along with at least four other symptoms, such as changes in appetite (either increase or decrease), insomnia or excessive sleep, psychomotor agitation or retardation, fatigue, feelings of guilt or worthlessness, difficulty concentrating, and thoughts of death or suicidal ideation.

The physical symptoms of depression, such as changes in sleep, appetite, energy levels, mental activity, and concentration, often overlap with symptoms of cancer itself or those induced by

Table 8.2 Differential diagnosis of depressive symptoms in cancer patients

Cancer-related depressive syndromes	Secondary depressive syndrome	Primary psychiatric disorders
Brain tumors, brain metastasis Paraneoplastic syndrome: Endocrine/cytokine/autoimmune factors Cancer-related physical symptoms: Pain/fatigue, etc. Substance-induced depression: Cancer treatments, etc. Hypoactive delirium Adjustment disorder with depressed mood Demoralization syndrome Maladaptive coping: Substance abuse, suicide attempts, etc. Major depressive disorder: First onset	Comorbid conditions unrelated to cancer	Major depressive disorder: History of depression or family history Bipolar disorder: Depressive episodes or with mixed features Other psychiatric disorders with depressive mood

cancer treatments. Therefore, caution is required to avoid misdiagnosing depression as a natural progression of cancer symptoms or the effects of treatment. Additionally, in the context of a life-threatening illness, depression may be underestimated and misinterpreted as an expected reaction, such as adjustment disorder.

The persistence, type, severity of symptoms, and the resulting functional impairment are crucial factors in distinguishing MDD from adjustment disorder. Although not included in the DSM diagnostic system, demoralization syndrome is described by existential despair, helplessness, and a loss of meaning and purpose in life, and differs from depression in that it does not include anhedonia [12].

It has been reported to occur in 13–18% of cancer patients, and there has been a call to classify it as a depressive spectrum syndrome [13]. Cancer patients with demoralization syndrome are found to have a stronger association with depression compared to those without the syndrome, and they also have a higher suicide rate, necessitating clinical attention [14].

Substance-induced depression can often occur during cancer treatment, especially when exogenous cytokines or corticosteroids are used (Table 8.3). Since it is not always feasible to reduce or discontinue the medication, adjunctive antidepressants may sometimes be prescribed.

Mood disorder due to cancer is diagnosed when a depressive episode is caused by the direct physiological effects of the illness itself, such as in cases involving primary or metastatic brain tumors. Additionally, inflammatory cytokines or autoimmune processes associated with cancer may contribute to the development of depressive episodes accompanied by prominent somatic symptoms. When depression arises during the acute course of cancer progression, this diagnostic category should be considered.

However, the relationship between depression and physical symptoms in cancer patients—particularly pain and fatigue—is complex. Patients experiencing acute pain may report feelings of sadness, hopelessness, or suicidal ideation, but these cannot be taken as definitive indicators of depression until the pain is adequately managed. Fatigue is a common side effect of both cancer and its treatment and may mimic depressive symptoms by affecting concentration, activity level, and sleep. Distinguishing between the two is essential for effective intervention. If somatic symptoms are clinically well-managed yet psychological distress persists and the patient exhibits symptoms consistent with a depressive episode, the diagnosis of depression due to cancer may be warranted.

Hypoactive delirium can present with symptoms that closely resemble depression, as patients may exhibit diminished interest and motivation toward previously enjoyed activities and may even report suicidal ideation. However, delirium is characterized by disturbances in attention, cognition, consciousness, and perception. Since the clinical management of delirium differs markedly from that of depression, it is crucial to distinguish delirium when evaluating depression in cancer patients. Although underlying depressive symptoms may coexist in patients with delirium, priority should be given to treating the delirium, followed by a reassessment of mood symptoms once the delirium resolves.

Lastly, clinicians should remain vigilant for the possibility of bipolar disorder. In patients with a personal or family history of mania or hypomania, it is essential to assess for manic or mixed features, as these would significantly alter both the diagnosis and the course of treatment.

8.4 Risk Factors for Depression in Cancer Patients

The most significant risk factors for the development of depression in cancer patients include a lack of social support, a personal history of depression, and pre-existing immature personality traits [15]. According to the biopsychosocial model, psychosocial factors tend to play a more substantial role than cancer-related physical or treatment factors in influencing depression risk.

While major depressive disorder is generally more prevalent among women in the general population, studies on gender differences in depression among cancer patients have yielded inconsistent results [16]. As noted previously in the discussion of differential diagnosis, cancer treatments such as corticosteroids, exogenous cytokines, hormone therapy, and chemotherapy can all contribute to the manifestation of depressive symptoms [6, 17–19].

Although certain cancer types—such as pancreatic or lung cancer—have been reported to be associated with a higher risk of depression, meta-analytic findings that aggregate high-quality

Table 8.3 Chemotherapy drugs associated with substance-induced depression

Corticosteroids	Interferon-alpha	Interleukin 2	Tamoxifen	Cyproterone
Leuprolide	Vincristine	Vinorelbine	Procarbazine	Asparaginase
Vinblastine	Paclitaxel	Docetaxel		

Table 8.4 Biopsychosocial risk factors for depression in cancer patients

Cancer-related factors
Diagnosis at a younger age
Advanced or progressive disease
Decline in physical functioning
Physical symptoms (e.g., pain, fatigue, nausea)
Certain cancer types: pancreatic, head and neck, lung
Psychological and personal history factors
Personal or family history of depression
Maladaptive coping strategies (e.g., hopelessness, substance abuse)
Recent experience of loss
Exposure to stressful life events
History of trauma or abuse
Low self-esteem
Anxious or avoidant attachment style
Less optimistic outlook
Ambivalence toward expressing negative emotions
Social factors
Lack of family or social support (e.g., divorced, separated, single)
Poor social functioning
Financial difficulties

studies have not consistently supported a significant correlation, warranting cautious interpretation of such associations [20]. Table 8.4 presents the biological, psychological, and social risk factors known to influence the development of depression in cancer patients.

8.5 Biological Mechanisms of Depression in Cancer Patients

Pathophysiological studies on depression in cancer patients have focused primarily on psychoneuroimmunological pathways. Reduced activity of natural killer (NK) cells has been associated with depressive symptoms. Moreover, common factors in cancer patients such as life stress, smoking, psychomotor retardation, insomnia, anxiety, and alcohol dependence—also frequently observed in depression—contribute to decreased NK cell activity [21]. One study reported that patients with biliary tract cancer who exhibited depressive symptoms had significantly lower NK cell counts compared to non-depressed cancer patients [22]. Antidepressant use and group therapy have been shown to enhance NK cell activity in individuals with depression. The activation of proinflammatory cytokines has also been implicated in the development of symptoms such as anhedonia, fatigue, anorexia, weight loss, insomnia, cognitive impairment, psychomotor retardation, and hyperalgesia, which overlap substantially with symptoms of MDD [23].

A recent meta-analysis in cancer patients found that elevated levels of proinflammatory markers—including interleukin-6 (IL-6), tumor necrosis factor-alpha (TNF-α), and C-reactive protein (CRP)—were significantly associated with depressive symptoms, and IL-6, in particular, emerged as a potential predictor of depression in specific cancer types [24]. These cytokines may induce depression by stimulating the hypothalamic-pituitary-adrenal (HPA) axis via activation of corticotropin-releasing factor (CRF) and by altering the metabolism of monoamines, tryptophan, and thyroid-stimulating hormone [25]. Furthermore, in response to stress, the release of catecholamines, glucocorticoids, and other stress hormones from the adrenal glands, brain, and sympathetic nerve terminals can modulate various components of the tumor microenvironment. This modulation can activate oncogenic viruses and alter immune functions such as antibody production, cytokine release, and cellular trafficking. As a result, increased cytokine production may promote tumor cell proliferation, migration, invasion, and angiogenesis.

Therefore, future therapeutic strategies should adopt an integrative approach by incorporating anti-inflammatory agents alongside stress-reduction interventions. A growing body of evidence highlights psychoneuroimmunological mechanisms as central to the comorbidity of cancer and depression. Consequently, clinical and preclinical research has started exploring cytokine antagonists—such as TNF-α inhibitors and IL-6 blockers—as potential dual-action treatments targeting both tumor biology and mood regulation [26].

8.6 Impact of Depression on Cancer Outcomes

Cancer patients with comorbid depression exhibit lower quality of life, reduced adherence to medical treatments, and prolonged hospital stays [27]. A meta-analysis examining the influence of depression on treatment adherence revealed that patients with depression are approximately three times less likely to adhere to medical treatment compared to those without depression [28].

Numerous studies have investigated whether depression and other psychological factors influence cancer incidence, progression, and prognosis. Earlier literature generally concluded that psychological factors, including depression, do not have a direct effect on cancer development or progression [29]. However, in terms of prognosis, multiple studies have demonstrated that cancer patients with depression have higher mortality rates than those without depression [30–32]. This finding has been consistently observed in studies evaluating both cancer-specific mortality and all-cause mortality [33–35].

These results may be explained by the pathophysiological mechanisms through which depression and stress stimulate tumor growth and metastasis—such as hypersecretion of cortisol and elevated levels of proinflammatory cytokines. Additionally, depression may impair patients' ability to comprehend and process prognostic information, resulting in poor treatment compliance and potentially suboptimal cancer care. Behavioral mechanisms associated with depression, including maladaptive coping strategies such as smoking, alcohol use, and suicidal behavior, may further negatively impact outcomes.

Although there is currently insufficient prospective evidence to confirm that treating depression directly improves survival in cancer patients, it is important to recognize that untreated depression may adversely affect prognosis. Treating depression may improve adherence to cancer treatment and offer an opportunity to enhance patients' quality of life. At the same time, recent randomized controlled trials have suggested that effective depression management can improve treatment adherence, which may indirectly contribute to better cancer outcomes and potentially prolong survival [36].

8.7 Suicide Risk and Prevention in Cancer Patients

Depression is the most common psychiatric disorder associated with suicide. In cancer patients, suicide is frequently linked to persistent depressive symptoms and pre-existing psychiatric conditions. Notably, depression has been reported as a significant risk factor in approximately 75% of suicide cases among cancer patients [37]. According to Asian studies, the suicide mortality rate among cancer patients is about 1.5 times higher than that of the general population [38]. Furthermore, among cancer patients with depression, up to one-third report symptoms consistent with the DSM-5 criterion of "thoughts of death or suicide" [39].

Suicide rates are particularly elevated among patients with cancers such as oral and head and neck cancer, pancreatic cancer, and lung cancer [38]. Other factors associated with heightened suicide risk include physical impairment or pain due to cancer, being within the first year of diagnosis, having advanced or terminal-stage cancer, perceived loss of dignity, and being a childhood or adolescent cancer survivor [40]. Conversely, protective factors against suicide in cancer patients include active treatment for psychiatric and medical conditions, supportive family and social environments, effective coping skills, and cultural or religious beliefs that discourage suicide [40].

It is essential to distinguish between suicidal ideation driven by depression and the desire to alleviate unmanageable physical pain, as this differentiation critically informs therapeutic interventions. Management of suicidal cancer patients requires careful assessment of the context surrounding the ideation, with a focus on identifying and alleviating both physical distress (e.g., pain, nausea, fatigue) and emotional suffering (e.g., depression, anxiety, sleep disturbances). Reassuring patients that there are still ways to improve their quality of life—even in the face of poor prognosis—can offer hope and comfort. Providing consistent, empathetic support and being present when patients and families need help can reduce anxiety related to abandonment and assist patients in enduring periods of heightened vulnerability.

When considering hospitalization for patients with suicidal ideation, it is important to evaluate the presence and lethality of any suicide plans and any history of suicide attempts. If no physiological condition is significantly contributing to the psychiatric symptoms, psychiatric admission should be considered. However, if the patient is in the terminal stage and is too medically compromised for psychiatric hospitalization, admission to an oncology ward, palliative care unit, or hospice facility where 24-h monitoring and therapeutic support are available may be more appropriate. As depression is a strong predictor of both suicide and the desire for hastened death (DHD), it remains a critical target for suicide prevention interventions at the time of hospitalization.

8.8 Treatment Approaches for Depression in Cancer Patients

As with the general population, the most effective approach to treating depression in cancer patients involves a combination of pharmacologic and non-pharmacologic interventions, including psychosocial support. This combined approach has been shown to yield the most significant improvement in depressive symptoms over a 12-month period [41]. Although short-term (12-week) treatment using either pharmacotherapy or psychosocial interventions alone may be effective, these monotherapies have not demonstrated sustained long-term benefits. This finding underscores the importance of understanding depression in cancer patients from a biopsychosocial perspective, as with non-cancer patients with depression. Optimal treatment can be achieved by assessing not only psychiatric symptoms but also coexisting physical symptoms. A careful exploration of the patient's understanding of their illness and prognosis, personal experiences since diagnosis, perceived losses, stressful life events, and level of social support can aid in developing an individualized psychosocial treatment plan.

However, well-designed intervention studies targeting this population remain limited [42, 43]. Both pharmacologic and non-pharmacologic studies often suffer from small sample sizes, high dropout rates, and issues such as selection bias and confounding variables. This highlights the need for a more integrated healthcare system that addresses both the physical and psychological symptoms of cancer patients, and for standardizing this approach within oncological care to strengthen mental health support for cancer patients.

Pharmacological Treatment

When selecting antidepressants for the treatment of depression, it is essential to consider the presence of comorbid medical conditions, potential drug–drug interactions, and the mode of administration—especially since many cancer patients may have difficulty taking oral medications. Additional considerations include the time required for the therapeutic effect to emerge in relation to the patient's prognosis, the nature of physical symptoms (e.g., pain, sleep disturbance, agitation, hot flashes), and the side effect profiles of the medications.

All antidepressants carry a risk of serious adverse effects. For instance, they may increase the risk of osteoporosis and fractures in older adults, as well as significantly elevate the likelihood of gastrointestinal bleeding and hyponatremia. Although rare, serotonin toxicity—commonly referred to as serotonin syndrome—can occur and is a potentially life-threatening complication. The risk increases when antidepressants are combined with certain medications such as analgesics (e.g., fentanyl, tramadol) and antiemetics (e.g., metoclopramide, ondansetron). Signs of serotonin toxicity include acute autonomic instability, confusion, and tremors.

SSRIs and SNRIs

Despite the high prevalence of depression among cancer patients, high-quality studies on pharmacologic treatments in this population remain limited. The choice of antidepressants is typically guided by patient-specific factors, safety profiles, and tolerability, as no conclusive evidence supports the superiority of one class over another [44]. As such, selective serotonin reuptake inhibitors (SSRIs) and serotonin-norepinephrine reuptake inhibitors (SNRIs) are commonly used as first-line treatments for depression. Both classes have demonstrated efficacy in alleviating depressive symptoms, with clinical improvement generally observed within 2–4 weeks of appropriate dosing. However, as with the general population, many cancer patients exhibit either no response or only partial response to these medications.

SSRIs and venlafaxine have been shown to not only alleviate depressive and anxiety symptoms in breast cancer patients but also reduce hot flashes by approximately 50% (range: 37–61%), depending on dosage [45]. However, caution is warranted when prescribing strong cytochrome P450 2D6 inhibitors such as fluoxetine and paroxetine to breast cancer patients taking tamoxifen. Tamoxifen is metabolized by CYP2D6 into its active metabolite, 4-hydroxy-N-desmethyl-tamoxifen (endoxifen), which exerts antiestrogenic effects. Concomitant use of CYP2D6-inhibiting antidepressants may interfere with this metabolic conversion, potentially increasing the risk of breast cancer recurrence [46, 47]. Therefore, antidepressants with minimal CYP2D6 inhibition—such as escitalopram, venlafaxine, and mirtazapine—are preferred for these patients [48].

SSRIs are associated with a number of similar adverse effects, including gastrointestinal disturbances, headache, fatigue, insomnia, and sexual dysfunction. They may also increase anxiety during the initial phase of treatment. Fluoxetine, with its long half-life, requires caution in patients anticipating changes in chemotherapy regimens, as interactions may arise due to shared metabolism via the CYP450 system. Other SSRIs generally have shorter half-lives (approximately 24 h), and abrupt discontinuation—for example, following surgery or in cases of acute bowel obstruction that prevent oral intake—may result in psychiatric, gastrointestinal, or neurological symptoms. Among SSRIs, sertraline and escitalopram are favored for their low interaction potential and good tolerability.

Hyponatremia associated with antidepressant use has been reported in case studies, retrospective chart reviews, case–control studies, and prospective observational studies [49]. All SSRIs, along with venlafaxine and mirtazapine, have been implicated in hyponatremia. Therefore, routine monitoring of serum electrolytes is recommended, particularly for cancer patients who may have additional risk factors.

Increased bleeding risk is another well-documented adverse effect of SSRIs, with gastrointestinal bleeding being the most common manifestation [50]. Uterine bleeding has also been reported, though less frequently. This is believed to result from SSRIs' effect on serotonin receptors, which leads to depletion of platelet serotonin and impaired hemostasis. Patients taking acetylsalicylic acid (ASA) or nonsteroidal anti-inflammatory drugs (NSAIDs) may be particularly vulnerable to this effect. While the extent to which this risk applies to patients undergoing chemotherapy or those with thrombocytopenia is unclear, heightened caution is warranted.

Venlafaxine may cause dose-dependent increases in blood pressure. Both duloxetine and venlafaxine have demonstrated efficacy in relieving neuropathic pain.

Other Antidepressants

Bupropion is a norepinephrine and dopamine reuptake inhibitor, known to improve sexual function and alleviate fatigue in cancer patients [51, 52]. Mirtazapine is an antidepressant that activates norepinephrine and serotonin, with a high affinity for histamine (H1) receptors, and acts as an antagonist at 5HT2 and 5HT3 receptors. It has effects in reducing depression and anxiety, inducing sedation, stimulating appetite, and providing antiemetic effects. These properties make mirtazapine particularly beneficial for treating both depression and associated weight loss and insomnia in cancer patients.

Trazodone, a weak but selective serotonin reuptake inhibitor and postsynaptic serotonin receptor antagonist, is used in the treatment of insomnia in cancer patients. It is typically prescribed in doses of 100 mg or less. Due to its alpha-receptor blockade effects, trazodone may cause orthostatic hypotension and dizziness, and caution is advised in elderly patients, as there is an increased risk of falls.

Tricyclic antidepressants (TCAs) are generally not considered as first-line treatments due to their side effect profiles. However, they are used in smaller doses for the management of neuropathic pain. In elderly patients, TCAs require careful monitoring due to their anticholinergic side effects, which may lead to constipation, urinary retention, and confusion. Additionally, the alpha-receptor blockade effect of TCAs can cause orthostatic hypotension, increasing the risk of falls. Due to their antimuscarinic effects, TCAs may also impact cardiac conduction, and caution is advised in patients with a history of arrhythmias.

Stimulants

Stimulants such as methylphenidate and dextroamphetamine are sometimes used to elevate the mood and energize depressed cancer patients due to their rapid onset of action. They are particularly used in patients with advanced or terminal cancer. However, there is only one randomized controlled trial providing evidence for their effect on reducing depression. Very rarely, high doses of these medications have been associated with the development of paranoid psychosis. Due to their cardiovascular stimulating effects, these drugs should not be used in patients with hypertension or arrhythmias.

Non-pharmacological Treatment

Psychosocial interventions, including non-pharmacological treatments for depression in cancer patients, do not improve the cancer's progression or survival rates. Moreover, systematic reviews have shown insufficient evidence that psychosocial interventions improve depression itself or depressive symptoms [53].

Interventions known to be effective for depression include counseling/psychotherapy (e.g., self-help groups, mindfulness cognitive therapy, telephone/web-based counseling, family-centered counseling), yoga and exercise therapy, healthcare provider-led interventions (e.g., psychosocial education, problem-solving, integrated care through consultation between oncology and psychiatry), and art therapy [54–64]. These interventions can reduce depression and anxiety symptoms, positively impact daily functioning such as eating, sleeping, and physical activity, and improve adherence to cancer treatment, which may indirectly contribute to better cancer progression and survival. However, when looking at the body of research, there is insufficient evidence to fully support the effectiveness of psychosocial interventions alone in treating depression in advanced cancer patients.

As mentioned earlier, psychosocial interventions may be delivered individually, in groups, or with families [65]. For pediatric cancer patients, family-based psychosocial interventions are particularly beneficial. Additionally, various models, including interpersonal and psychodynamic approaches, should be considered. For advanced or terminal cancer patients, existential and meaning-centered interventions have been found effective [66]. Supportive, non-judgmental environments that provide realistic reassurance and emphasize strengths and coping mechanisms are therapeutically beneficial. Thus, it is essential to develop intervention programs that focus on finding alleviating factors within sociodemographic, disease-related, and psycho-environmental factors for recovery in cancer patients [67]. For depressed cancer patients, maintaining a balance between hope and despair, managing uncertainty, and providing continuous messages to live in the face of these challenges is crucial. Supportive and behavioral interventions can be applied to achieve these goals.

8.9 Conclusion

Depression is one of the most common psychiatric disorders in cancer patients and negatively affects prognosis and suicide risk. Therefore, proper screening, differential diagnosis, and timely treatment of depression in cancer patients are crucial. Based on a comprehensive understanding of depression and recent research findings, a biopsychosocial approach is essential in managing depression in cancer patients. Combined use of pharmacological and non-pharmacological treatments is beneficial in providing effective care.

Declarations

Competing Interests The author(s) has no competing interests to declare that are relevant to the content of this manuscript.

Ethics Approval The author(s) declares that this manuscript does not include primary research with human participants.

The author(s) declares that this manuscript does not include primary studies involving animals.

References

1. Holland JC, Lewis S. The human side of cancer. New York: Harper Collins; 2001.
2. National Comprehensive Cancer Network. NCCN guidelines for patients: distress; 2024. Available from: https://www.nccn.org/patients/guidelines/content/PDF/distress-patient.pdf
3. Ostovar S, Modarresi Chahardehi A, Mohd Hashim IH, Othman A, Kruk J, Griffiths MD. Prevalence of psychological distress among cancer patients in Southeast Asian countries: a systematic review. Eur J Cancer Care (Engl). 2022;31:e13669. https://doi.org/10.1111/ecc.13669.
4. Mitchell AJ, Chan M, Bhatti H, Halton M, Grassi L, Johansen C, et al. Prevalence of depression, anxiety, and adjustment disorder in oncological, haematological, and palliative-care settings: a meta-analysis of 94 interview-based studies. Lancet Oncol. 2011;12:160–74. https://doi.org/10.1016/S1470-2045(10)70256-5.
5. Mitchell AJ, Vahabzadeh A, Magruder K. Screening for distress and depression in cancer settings: 10 lessons from 40 years of primary-care research. Psychooncology. 2011;20(6):572–84. https://doi.org/10.1002/pon.1984.
6. Holland JC, Breitbart WS, Jacobsen PB, Lederberg MS, Loscalzo MJ, McCorkle R. Psycho-oncology. 2nd ed. New York: Oxford University Press; 2010.
7. Whooley MA, Avins AL, Miranda J, Browner WS. Case-finding instruments for depression. Two questions are as good as many. J Gen Intern Med. 1997;12:439–45. https://doi.org/10.1046/j.1525-1497.1997.00076.x.
8. Wakefield CE, Butow PN, Aaronson NA, Hack TF, Hulbert-Williams NJ, Jacobsen PB. Patient-reported depression measures in cancer: a meta-review. Lancet Psychiatry. 2015;2:635–47. https://doi.org/10.1016/S2215-0366(15)00168-6.
9. Hoffman MA, Weiner JS. Is Mrs S depressed? Diagnosing depression in the cancer patient. J Clin Oncol. 2007;25:2853–6. https://doi.org/10.1200/JCO.2006.10.0821.
10. Gilbody S, Sheldon T, House A. Screening and case-finding instruments for depression: a meta-analysis. CMAJ. 2008;178:997–1003. https://doi.org/10.1503/cmaj.070281.
11. Irwin KE, Freudenreich O, Peppercorn J, Taghian AG, Freer PE, Gudewicz TM, Case Records of the Massachusetts General Hospital. Case 30-2016. A 63-year-old woman with bipolar disorder, cancer, and worsening depression. N Engl J Med. 2016;375:1270–81. https://doi.org/10.1056/NEJMcpc1601432.
12. Clarke DM, Kissane DW. Demoralization: its phenomenology and importance. Aust N Z J Psychiatry. 2002;36:733–42. https://doi.org/10.1046/j.1440-1614.2002.01086.x.
13. Robinson S, Kissane DW, Brooker J, Burney S. A systematic review of the demoralization syndrome in individuals with progressive disease and cancer: a decade of research. J Pain Symptom Manag. 2015;49:595–610. https://doi.org/10.1016/j.jpainsymman.2014.07.008.
14. Tang PL, Wang HH, Chou FH. A systematic review and meta-analysis of demoralization and depression in patients with cancer. Psychosomatics. 2015;56:634–43. https://doi.org/10.1016/j.psym.2015.06.003.
15. Riedl D, Schusler G. Factors associated with and risk factors for depression in cancer patients—a systematic literature review. Transl Oncol. 2022;16:101328. https://doi.org/10.1016/j.tranon.2021.101328.
16. Bailey RK, Geyen DJ, Scott-Gurnell K, Hipolito MM, Bailey TA, Beal JM. Understanding and treating depression among cancer patients. Int J Gynecol Cancer. 2005;15:203–8. https://doi.org/10.1111/j.1525-1438.2005.15204.x.
17. Ibrahim EY, Domenicano I, Nyhan K, Elfil M, Mougalian SS, Cartmel B, et al. Cognitive effects and depression associated with taxane-based chemotherapy in breast cancer survivors: a meta-analysis. Front Oncol. 2021;11:642382. https://doi.org/10.3389/fonc.2021.642382.
18. Carmassi C, Cordone A, Dell'Oste V, Pedrinelli V, Pardini F, Simoncini M, et al. Prescribing tamoxifen in patients with mood disorders: a systematic review of potential antimanic versus depressive effects. J Clin Psychopharmacol. 2021;41:450–60. https://doi.org/10.1097/JCP.0000000000001413.
19. Ismail MF, Lavelle C, Cassidy EM. Steroid-induced mental disorders in cancer patients: a systematic review. Future Oncol. 2017;13:2719–31. https://doi.org/10.2217/fon-2017-0343.
20. Ahn HK, Bae JH, Ahn HY, Hwang IC. Risk of cancer among patients with depressive disorder: a meta-analysis and implications. Psychooncology. 2016;25:1393–9. https://doi.org/10.1002/pon.4044.

21. Irwin MR, Miller AH. Depressive disorders and immunity: 20 years of progress and discovery. Brain Behav Immun. 2007;21:374–83. https://doi.org/10.1016/j.bbi.2007.01.010.
22. Steel JL, Geller DA, Gamblin TC, Olek MC, Carr BI. Depression, immunity, and survival in patients with hepatobiliary carcinoma. J Clin Oncol. 2007;25:2397–405. https://doi.org/10.1200/JCO.2006.08.7235.
23. Raison CL, Miller AH. Depression in cancer: new developments regarding diagnosis and treatment. Biol Psychiatry. 2003;54:283–94. https://doi.org/10.1016/S0006-3223(03)00413-X.
24. Manigault AW, Ganz PA, Irwin MR, et al. Moderators of inflammation-related depression: a prospective study of breast cancer survivors. Transl Psychiatry. 2021;11:615. https://doi.org/10.1038/s41398-021-01716-2.
25. Musselman DL, Lawson DH, Gumnick JF, Manatunga AK, Penna S, Goodkin RS, et al. Paroxetine for the prevention of depression induced by high-dose interferon alfa. N Engl J Med. 2001;344:961–6. https://doi.org/10.1056/NEJM200103293441303.
26. Kappelmann N, Lewis G, Dantzer R, Jones PB, Khandaker GM. Antidepressant activity of anti-cytokine treatment: a systematic review and meta-analysis of clinical trials of chronic inflammatory conditions. Mol Psychiatry. 2018;23:335–43. https://doi.org/10.1038/mp.2016.167.
27. Kissane DW. Unrecognised and untreated depression in cancer care. Lancet Psychiatry. 2014;1:320–1. https://doi.org/10.1016/S2215-0366(14)70379-8.
28. DiMatteo MR, Lepper HS, Croghan TW. Depression is a risk factor for noncompliance with medical treatment: meta-analysis of the effects of anxiety and depression on patient adherence. Arch Intern Med. 2000;160:2101–7. https://doi.org/10.1001/archinte.160.14.2101.
29. Garssen B. Psychological factors and cancer development: evidence after 30 years of research. Clin Psychol Rev. 2004;24:315–38. https://doi.org/10.1016/j.cpr.2004.01.002.
30. Walker J, Mulick A, Magill N, Symeonides S, Gourley C, Burke K, et al. Major depression and survival in people with cancer. Psychosom Med. 2021;83:410–6. https://doi.org/10.1097/PSY.0000000000000908.
31. Holland JC, Andersen B, Breitbart WS, Buchmann LO, Compas B, Deshields TL, et al. Distress management. J Natl Compr Cancer Netw. 2013;11:190–209. https://doi.org/10.6004/jnccn.2013.0027.
32. Pinquart M, Duberstein PR. Depression and cancer mortality: a meta-analysis. Psychol Med. 2010;40:1797–810. https://doi.org/10.1017/S0033291709992285.
33. Satin JR, Linden W, Phillips MJ. Depression as a predictor of disease progression and mortality in cancer patients: a meta-analysis. Cancer. 2009;115:5349–61. https://doi.org/10.1002/cncr.24561.
34. Mols F, Husson O, Roukema JA, van de Poll-Franse LV. Depressive symptoms are a risk factor for all-cause mortality: results from a prospective population-based study among 3,080 cancer survivors from the PROFILES registry. J Cancer Surviv. 2013;7:484–92. https://doi.org/10.1007/s11764-013-0286-0.
35. Vodermaier A, Linden W, Rnic K, Young SN, Ng A, Ditsch N, et al. Prospective associations of depression with survival: a population-based cohort study in patients with newly diagnosed breast cancer. Breast Cancer Res Treat. 2014;143:373–85. https://doi.org/10.1007/s10549-013-2800-8.
36. Bazrafshan S, et al. Effect of depression treatment on adherence and survival in cancer patients: a randomized controlled trial. J Clin Oncol. 2024;42(10):1234–45.
37. de la Grandmaison GL, Watier L, Cavard S, Charlier P. Are suicide rates higher in the cancer population? An investigation using forensic autopsy data. Med Hypotheses. 2014;82:16–9. https://doi.org/10.1016/j.mehy.2013.10.027.
38. Choi Y, Park EC. Suicide after cancer diagnosis in South Korea: a population-based cohort study. BMJ Open. 2021;11:e049358. https://doi.org/10.1136/bmjopen-2021-049358.
39. Walker J, Magill N, Rosenstein DL, Frost C, Sharpe M. Suicidal thoughts in patients with cancer and comorbid major depression: findings from a depression screening program. J Acad Consult Liaison Psychiatry. 2022;63:251–9. https://doi.org/10.1016/j.jaclp.2022.03.002.
40. McFarland DC, Walsh L, Napolitano S, Morita J, Jaiswal R. Suicide in patients with cancer: identifying the risk factors. Oncology (Williston Park). 2019;33:221–6.
41. Li M, Kennedy EB, Byrne N, Gerin-Lajoie C, Katz MR, Keshavarz H, et al. Systematic review and meta-analysis of collaborative care interventions for depression in patients with cancer. Psychooncology. 2017;26:573–87. https://doi.org/10.1002/pon.4443.
42. Turner J, Zapart S, Pedersen K, Rankin N, Luxford K, Fletcher J. Clinical practice guidelines for the psychosocial care of adults with cancer. Psychooncology. 2005;14:159–73. https://doi.org/10.1002/pon.889.
43. Rodin G, Katz M, Lloyd N, Green E, Mackay JA, Wong RK. Treatment of depression in cancer patients. Curr Oncol. 2007;14:180–8. https://doi.org/10.3747/co.v14i5.154.
44. Ostuzzi G, Matcham F, Dauchy S, Barbui C, Hotopf M. Antidepressants for the treatment of depression in people with cancer. Cochrane Database Syst Rev. 2018;4:Cd011006. https://doi.org/10.1002/14651858.CD011006.pub2.
45. Bordeleau L, Pritchard K, Goodwin P, Loprinzi C. Therapeutic options for the management of hot flashes in breast cancer survivors: an evidence-based review. Clin Ther. 2007;29:230–41. https://doi.org/10.1016/j.clinthera.2007.02.005.
46. Jin Y, Desta Z, Stearns V, Ward B, Ho H, Lee KH, et al. CYP2D6 genotype, antidepressant use, and tamoxifen metabolism during adjuvant breast can-

cer treatment. J Natl Cancer Inst. 2005;97:30–9. https://doi.org/10.1093/jnci/dji005.
47. Stearns V, Johnson MD, Rae JM, Morocho A, Novielli A, Bhargava P, et al. Active tamoxifen metabolite plasma concentrations after coadministration of tamoxifen and the selective serotonin reuptake inhibitor paroxetine. J Natl Cancer Inst. 2003;95:1758–64. https://doi.org/10.1093/jnci/djg107.
48. Kelly CM, Juurlink DN, Gomes T, Duong-Hua M, Pritchard KI, Austin PC, et al. Selective serotonin reuptake inhibitors and breast cancer mortality in women receiving tamoxifen: a population based cohort study. BMJ. 2010;340:c693. https://doi.org/10.1136/bmj.c693.
49. Jacob S, Spinler SA. Hyponatremia associated with selective serotonin-reuptake inhibitors in older adults. Ann Pharmacother. 2006;40:1618–22. https://doi.org/10.1345/aph.1G658.
50. Looper KJ. Potential medical and surgical complications of serotonergic antidepressant medications. Psychosomatics. 2007;48:1–9. https://doi.org/10.1176/appi.psy.48.1.1.
51. Mathias C, Cardeal Mendes CM, Ponde de Sena E, Dias de Moraes E, Bastos C, Braghiroli MI, et al. An open-label, fixed-dose study of bupropion effect on sexual function scores in women treated for breast cancer. Ann Oncol. 2006;17(12):1792–6.
52. Moss EL, Simpson JS, Pelletier G, Forsyth P. An open-label study of the effects of bupropion SR on fatigue, depression and quality of life of mixed-site cancer patients and their partners. Psychooncology. 2006;15:259–67. https://doi.org/10.1002/pon.945.
53. Zhu RY, Chen H, Gao YJ, Pan ZH, Wang JY. Effects of psychological nursing care on anxiety and depression in perioperative patients with lung cancer: a systematic review and meta-analysis. Medicine (Baltimore). 2022;101:e29914. https://doi.org/10.1097/MD.0000000000029914.
54. Coutino-Escamilla L, Pina-Pozas M, Tobias Garces A, Gamboa-Loira B, Lopez-Carrillo L. Non-pharmacological therapies for depressive symptoms in breast cancer patients: systematic review and meta-analysis of randomized clinical trials. Breast. 2019;44:135–43. https://doi.org/10.1016/j.breast.2019.01.002.
55. Xia JL, Zeng YW, Zhao XM, Hou LL. Psychological intervention for negative emotion and quality of life of patients with head and neck cancer (HNC): a meta-analysis. Shanghai Kou Qiang Yi Xue. 2022;31:330–6.
56. Wan SW, Chng YJD, Lim SH, Chong CS, Pikkarainen M, He HG. A systematic review and meta-analysis on the effectiveness of web-based psychosocial interventions among patients with colorectal cancer. J Adv Nurs. 2022;78:1883–96. https://doi.org/10.1111/jan.15164.
57. McCloy K, Hughes C, Dunwoody L, Marley J, Gracey J. Effects of mindfulness-based interventions on fatigue and psychological well-being in women with cancer: a systematic review and meta-analysis of randomised control trials. Psychooncology. 2022;31:1821–34. https://doi.org/10.1002/pon.5982.
58. Chayadi E, Baes N, Kiropoulos L. The effects of mindfulness-based interventions on symptoms of depression, anxiety, and cancer-related fatigue in oncology patients: a systematic review and meta-analysis. PLoS One. 2022;17:e0269519. https://doi.org/10.1371/journal.pone.0269519.
59. Zhang X, Zhang D, Yu P, Li X. Effects of continuous care combined with evidence-based nursing on mental status and quality of life and self-care ability in patients with liver from breast cancer: a single-center randomized controlled study. Comput Math Methods Med. 2022;2022:3637792. https://doi.org/10.1155/2022/3637792.
60. Xu S, Wang X, Wang R. The effects of integrated palliative care on quality of life and psychological distress in patients with advanced cancer: a systematic review and meta-analysis. Ann Palliat Med. 2022;11:2586–99. https://doi.org/10.21037/apm-21-3566.
61. Zhang K, Ma J, Chen J, Xu L, Gu C. Effects of drawing therapy on pediatric oncology patients: a systematic review. Cancer Nurs. 2022;45:E397–406. https://doi.org/10.1097/NCC.0000000000001090.
62. Vasilopoulou K, Skoutari A, Siomos K, Christodoulou N. The effects of family therapeutic interventions on mental health and quality of life of children with cancer: a systematic review. Clin Child Psychol Psychiatry. 2022;27:911–28. https://doi.org/10.1177/13591045211051681.
63. Park M, Choi EK, Lee HJ, Park HE, Chinbayar A. Resilience-promoting programs in families of children with cancer: a systematic review. J Pediatr Hematol Oncol Nurs. 2022;39:185–201. https://doi.org/10.1177/27527530221079863.
64. Yang W, Geng G, Hua J, Cui M, Geng Z. Informational support for depression and quality of life improvements in older patients with cancer: a systematic review and meta-analysis. Support Care Cancer. 2022;30:1065–77. https://doi.org/10.1007/s00520-021-06454-2.
65. Zhang S, Li J, Hu X. Peer support interventions on quality of life, depression, anxiety, and self-efficacy among patients with cancer: a systematic review and meta-analysis. Patient Educ Couns. 2022;105:3213–24. https://doi.org/10.1016/j.pec.2022.06.002.
66. Zhang Y, Li J, Hu X. The effectiveness of dignity therapy on hope, quality of life, anxiety, and depression in cancer patients: a meta-analysis of randomized controlled trials. Int J Nurs Stud. 2022;132:104273. https://doi.org/10.1016/j.ijnurstu.2022.104273.
67. Zhu P, Chen C, Liu X, Gu W, Shang X. Factors associated with benefit finding and mental health of patients with cancer: a systematic review. Support Care Cancer. 2022;30:6483–96. https://doi.org/10.1007/s00520-022-07139-8.

9 The Relationship Between Pain and Depression

Cheolmin Shin and Jong-Hyun Jeong

9.1 Introduction

Depression and pain frequently co-occur and have a simultaneous detrimental impact on an individual's health, functioning, and quality of life. One study reported that approximately 100 million people in the United States suffer from pain, resulting in 200 million days of work absenteeism and an estimated economic burden of $635 billion [1]. Depression is also one of the most common psychiatric disorders, with a 1-year prevalence of 6.6% and a lifetime prevalence of 16.2% globally. It is projected to become the leading cause of disease burden worldwide by 2030 [2]. Pain can be regarded as a syndrome, yet its symptomatology and pathophysiological mechanisms remain incompletely understood. However, recent studies suggest a strong association between depression and pain. According to the World Health Organization, one in five patients in primary care settings suffers from persistent, debilitating pain, and these patients are four to five times more likely to develop anxiety or depressive disorders than those without pain [3]. Patients with depression frequently report pain and functional impairments. In particular, the presence of multiple pain sites is associated with an increased risk of depression and a greater impact on quality of life [4, 5]. Serotonin (5-hydroxytryptamine, 5-HT) and norepinephrine, neurotransmitters located in key pain pathways, have been shown in both preclinical and clinical studies to play important roles in the occurrence and treatment of pain [6]. In fact, antidepressants such as selective serotonin reuptake inhibitors (SSRIs), noradrenergic and specific serotonergic antidepressants (NaSSAs), and serotonin-norepinephrine reuptake inhibitors (SNRIs), which influence the transmission of serotonin and norepinephrine, are widely used to treat pain regardless of psychiatric diagnoses [6]. This chapter explores the complex interplay between depression and pain, examining their shared pathophysiological mechanisms and approaches to treatment.

9.2 Clinical Association Between Pain and Depression

Pain and depression are both prevalent medical conditions. The prevalence of pain among patients with depression, and conversely the prevalence of depression among patients with pain, is significantly higher than the prevalence of either condition in the general population. A

C. Shin (✉)
Department of Psychiatry, Korea University Ansan Hospital, Korea University College of Medicine, Ansan, Republic of Korea
e-mail: shincm@korea.ac.kr

J.-H. Jeong
Department of Psychiatry, St. Vincent's Hospital, College of Medicine, The Catholic University of Korea, Suwon, Republic of Korea

W.-M. Bahk et al. (eds.), *Depressive Disorder*, https://doi.org/10.1007/978-981-92-1331-3_9

literature review that synthesized findings from multiple clinical studies reported that approximately 65% of patients with depression experience comorbid pain [7]. Depressive symptoms are particularly associated with a higher incidence of low back pain, neck-shoulder pain, and musculoskeletal complaints. A Korean study found that somatic symptom scales, including pain, effectively predicted remission status in patients with depression [8]. In the U.S. STAR*D (Sequenced Treatment Alternatives to Relieve Depression) study, 80% of patients with depression reported physical pain, and the presence of pain was associated with lower remission rates [9]. Additionally, patients with depression frequently report specific types of pain, such as headaches, abdominal pain, joint pain, chest pain, and back pain [10–12]. Similarly, individuals with chronic pain show a significantly higher likelihood of developing depressive symptoms. For instance, patients experiencing one or more types of pain (e.g., low back pain, headache, abdominal pain, chest pain, facial pain) have been reported to have a three- to fivefold increased risk of depression compared to those without such symptoms [13]. Moreover, patients with chronic pain are over three times more likely to meet diagnostic criteria for depression than those without pain [14]. The bidirectional relationship between depression and pain has been consistently observed across various pain conditions. A longitudinal 12-month study in primary care settings demonstrated that depression has been identified as a significant predictor of intense and persistent pain, and conversely, chronic pain is a significant predictor of severe depressive symptoms [15]. Clinically, patients with pain and those with depression exhibit overlapping symptoms, including depressed mood, alexithymia, irritability, decreased energy and fatigue, cognitive impairment, increased vulnerability to stress, altered heart rate variability, and abnormal sleep patterns (e.g., reduced rapid eye movement [REM] latency) [16]. The severity of pain is strongly correlated with depressive mood, fatigue, functional impairment, suicidal ideation, poor general health, and somatic symptoms [7]. Despite numerous studies supporting the bidirectionality of pain and depression, it remains unclear whether specific neurobiological changes cause pain or depression, or whether these are merely biological consequences of each condition. Interestingly, some clinicians interpret chronic pain as a psychological disorder or a nonverbal expression of depressive states, although evidence supporting this interpretation is limited.

Another important clinical point to consider is the relationship between pain and suicide. Suicide risk is elevated not only in patients with depression but also in those with chronic pain, suggesting that pain may serve as a shared risk factor or contributing factor for both depression and suicidal behavior. Several clinical reports have linked serious medical conditions such as cancer or cardiovascular disease, as well as chronic headaches, to increased suicide attempts. For example, patients with migraine have a 2.2–4.0 times higher likelihood of developing depression and a 1.68 times higher risk of death by suicide. When depression is comorbid, the risk of suicidal ideation or attempts increases substantially [17]. Therefore, clinicians should pay close attention to the interactions between pain and depression, especially in cases like migraine, given their significance in both the occurrence and prevention of suicide.

9.3 Shared Pathophysiological Mechanisms Between Pain and Depression

Although the exact etiological and pathological mechanisms underlying pain are not yet fully understood, several clinical and biological factors have been implicated in the development of pain. These include changes in neuromodulation [18], alterations in immune-genetic systems such as proinflammatory cytokine activity and gene expression [19–21], fluctuations in melatonin levels, abnormalities in platelet 3H-imipramine binding sites [22], oxidative stress responses [20], neurotransmitter system imbalances [23], increased sensitivity to stress [24], dysregulation of the hypothalamic–pituitary–adrenal (HPA) axis [25], and cognitive vulnerabilities [26]. In addition to these biological factors, psychosocial elements such as self-esteem, self-efficacy, anger, personality traits, history of sexual or childhood abuse have been reported to significantly impact the onset of pain [16]. Interestingly, many of these clinical and biological factors are also implicated in the pathogenesis of depression. However, it is important to distinguish between the associations of depression with acute versus chronic pain. The clinical features of these two pain types are quite distinct: acute pain typically arises from a specific disease or injury and is self-limiting, whereas chronic pain is considered a disease entity in itself, with a substantial contribution from psychological factors [27]. Chronic pain is thought to be associated with persistent signaling in the somatosensory pathway, due to biochemical changes in specific brain regions and functional reorganization driven by central nervous system plasticity [28]. Therefore, understanding the differences between acute and chronic pain in relation to depression is essential for accurate diagnosis and treatment.

9.4 Genetic Factors

A key question regarding genetics is whether there is an inherent vulnerability that predisposes individuals to both pain and depression. Genetic studies in this field are still in their early stages, and findings have often been inconsistent. However, recent evidence suggests that genes regulating the synthesis, degradation, or receptor binding of neurotransmitters and cytokines may contribute to the pathophysiology of both conditions. For example, individuals with chronic pain have a higher prevalence of depression in first-degree relatives compared to the general population, and even among families of chronic pain patients without a personal history of depression, rates of depression are elevated [3, 22]. Genes such as galanin-2 and the μ-opioid receptor have been reported to interact with pain-related genes and are hypothesized to mediate the impact of pain on mood [29]. A study found that polymorphisms in the promoter regions of the serotonin 1A and 2A receptor genes were associated with gender-dependent differences in depressive symptoms and physical functioning among chronic pain patients [30]. These findings support the hypothesis that depression and pain share a genetic basis, particularly involving genes that regulate pain sensitivity, stress reactivity, and mood regulation.

9.5 Biochemical Factors

Descending pathways in the central nervous system that inhibit nociception extend from the brainstem nuclei to the dorsal horn of the spinal cord via the dorsolateral funiculus (DLF). The DLF comprises serotonergic fibers from the raphe nuclei, dopaminergic fibers from the ventral tegmental area (VTA), and noradrenergic fibers from the locus coeruleus [16]. These descending fibers utilize endogenous opioids, serotonin, and norepinephrine as key inhibitory mediators that hyperpolarize afferent sensory neurons and suppress nociceptive transmission originating in spinal pain neurons [16]. Notably, the activation of nociceptors and pain pathways itself does not constitute the experience of pain. It is pain perception in the central nervous system that defines it. Although the pathophysiology of chronic pain remains unclear, neurotransmitters such as gamma-aminobutyric acid (GABA), glutamate, norepinephrine, serotonin, neurokinin-1, nitric oxide, substance P, glycine, and endogenous opioids are believed to be involved [31]. The biochemical mechanisms linking pain and depression primarily center on serotonin and norepinephrine. These neurotransmitter pathways originate in brainstem nuclei and project to the somatosensory cortex, intralaminar nuclei, and ventral posterior nuclei of the thalamus [32]. Descending serotonergic and noradrenergic projections terminate in the dorsal horn of the spinal cord, where various neurotransmitters modulate pain processing [32]. Preclinical and experimental studies suggest that dopamine may be involved in the modulation of depressive symptoms and pain. The VTA, known for its role in motor regulation, has also been implicated in pain processing. Rodent studies have shown that lesions in the VTA enhance self-injurious behavior, while electrical stimulation of the VTA after a nociceptive stimulus promotes analgesia [33]. These findings support the hypothesis that the VTA may contribute to pain processing and affective modulation and that dopamine homeostasis may influence both depression and pain perception (see Fig. 9.1).

In patients with chronic pain, both central and peripheral pain mechanisms undergo changes that amplify pain signaling [34]. Continuous stimulation of the pain pathway—particularly the C-fibers—leads to overactivation of N-methyl-D-aspartate (NMDA) receptors in the dorsal horn of the spinal cord [35, 36]. In studies involving patients with irritable bowel syndrome (IBS), repeated stimulation of the colon was used to sensitize the central nervous system, and subsequent administration of dextromethorphan, an NMDA receptor antagonist, was shown to prevent pain. These findings suggest that NMDA receptor mediated mechanisms may contribute to central sensitization and pain amplification [36]. Increased secretion of excitatory neuromodulators such as substance P, along with psychological factors, further exacerbates pain. As a result, patients with chronic pain often enter a state of central sensitization, experiencing severe pain in response to even non-noxious stimuli. In such individuals, cerebral blood flow is decreased in brain areas involved in central pain processing, such as the caudate nucleus and thalamus. Elevated cerebrospinal fluid levels of substance P and brain-derived neuro-

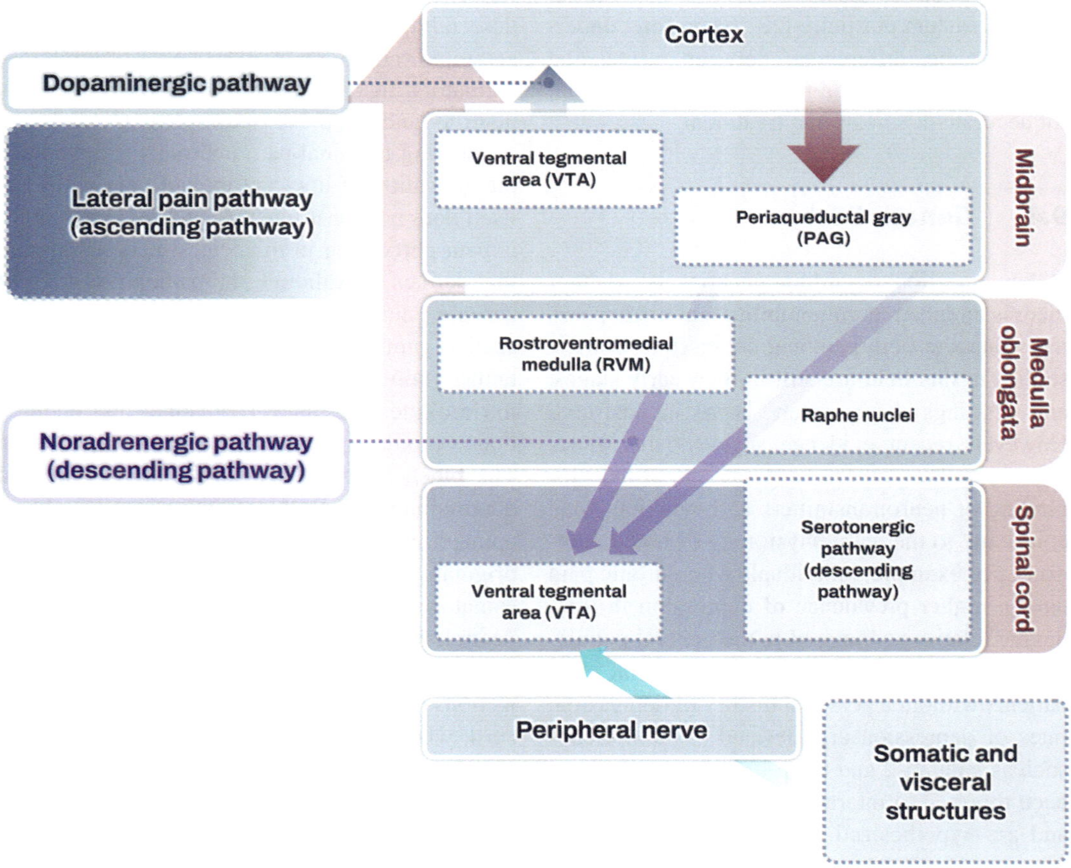

Fig. 9.1 Depression and pain perception

trophic factor (BDNF) have been reported and are associated with altered pain processing and central sensitization [16]. Heightened spinal cord sensitivity to pain has also been observed in patients with fibromyalgia [37]. Similar changes have been documented in patients with depression as well [38, 39].

9.6 Neuroimaging of Pain and Depression

Somatic pain is processed through a multidimensional system governed by several regions of the brain. It can largely be divided into the sensory-discriminative dimension (e.g., the location of pain) and the affective-emotional dimension (e.g., suffering). The primary somatosensory cortex and the posterior ventral insula are primarily involved in the sensory-discriminative aspect of somatic pain [40]. In contrast, psychological pain such as grief or sorrow is not directly triggered by physically harmful stimuli and is, thus, regulated by different brain regions. However, both types of pain activate neural mechanisms that assess and modulate threat. With recent advances in brain imaging techniques, it has become possible to identify the brain regions involved in both physical and psychological pain. Studies have revealed that the nociceptive pathways for psychological pain partially overlap with brain regions that process the emotional and affective components of physical pain [1]. Neuroimaging research has demonstrated that the insular cortex is involved in both physical pain and depression. However, it has also been proposed that different cortical areas are engaged in each condition. For example, one study found that patients with depression showed lower activation in the tegmental area and secondary somatosensory cortex compared to patients with pain [41]. Conversely, another study reported that patients with pain exhibited increased activation in the anterior insula and parietal operculum compared to patients with depression. Additionally, when patients became sensitized to pain, greater activation was observed in the thalamus, amygdala, mid-cingulate cortex, and sensorimotor areas. In contrast, depressed patients showed reduced activation in the midbrain and brainstem [42].

9.7 Psychosocial Factors

The frequent co-occurrence of pain and depression can be attributed to their overlapping psychosocial determinants. Cognitive and emotional factors that elevate the risk of developing depression or worsen its prognosis are commonly observed in patients with pain as well. According to the cognitive-behavioral model, thoughts evoke emotions, which in turn influence behavior. Applying this model to chronic pain, it is understood that patients tend to avoid activities and experiences that might bring them joy, receive less social reinforcement, and ultimately experience a diminished sense of life satisfaction, which may contribute to the development of depressive symptoms. However, the progression from pain to depression is not inevitable. Various psychosocial variables intervene in this relationship. A number of cognitive factors have been identified as mediators between pain and depression, including pessimism, perceived self-regulation, beliefs about fear-avoidance, self-efficacy, and perceived social support [1, 43]. Among these, one of the most influential cognitive patterns is catastrophizing, which refers to the tendency to interpret situations as far worse than they actually are. Pain-related catastrophizing involves a set of cognitive and emotional processes encompassing negative appraisals, feelings of helplessness, and a general tendency toward pessimism. Catastrophizing is associated with both pain and depression, and the two conditions often co-occur [1]. Catastrophizing is linked to greater pain intensity, decreased functioning, and a heightened sense of helplessness or worthlessness [1]. It has been shown to mediate the relationship between pain and depression [44] (see Fig. 9.2).

In the cognitive-behavioral model of pain, emotional responses are also critical. Negative affect can trigger the onset of depression in indi-

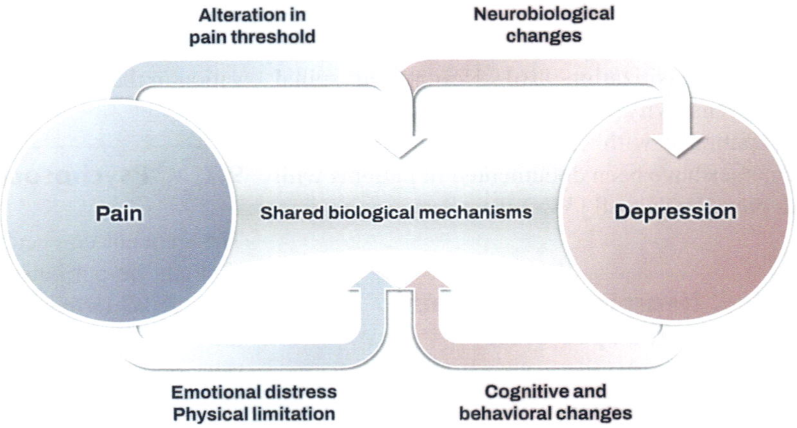

Fig. 9.2 Relationship between pain and depression

viduals suffering from chronic pain [1]. Conversely, positive emotions such as resilience, enthusiasm, perseverance, and grit have a beneficial impact by alleviating pain, reducing depressive symptoms, lowering fatigue, and mitigating catastrophizing tendencies [1]. Recent studies have confirmed that both negative and positive emotional states are closely related to clinical and experimentally induced pain. When pain is reduced, negative emotions tend to dissipate, and positive emotions are elicited, indicating that emotional regulation can significantly influence the pain-depression association [45]. From a behavioral perspective, two key factors in the pain-depression link are sleep hygiene and fear-avoidance. Sleep, pain, and depression form a triadic relationship—when one is improved or worsened, it influences the other two [1]. Thus, behaviors that impair sleep may contribute to the onset of depression in individuals with pain. Targeting sleep disturbances through therapeutic interventions can improve functioning in these patients [46]. Avoidance and withdrawal behaviors are common in both depression and chronic pain. Fear leads to activity restriction and limits social interaction [47]. Individuals who perceive chronic pain as a threat often exhibit fear-avoidance behaviors, which result in decreased function and increased disability [48]. These changes in daily functioning and social support can, in turn, contribute to depression. Accordingly, cognitive-behavioral therapy (CBT) incorporates behavioral activation strategies that help patients resume activity and overcome irrational fears through structured, systematic interventions.

9.8 Therapeutic Approaches to Pain and Depression

Before initiating treatment for pain and depression, it is essential to assess the underlying cause of the pain (see Fig. 9.3). In clinical practice, this evaluation begins with reviewing the patient's medical history, as conditions such as depression, diabetes, arthritis, and fibromyalgia are common causes of pain. When the cause cannot be clearly identified, consultation with specialists from other disciplines or referrals for further evaluation may be helpful. Gathering information about current medications is also beneficial, particularly with regard to which medications have been effective or ineffective in the past.

Pain assessment is especially important and should include various elements: the location of pain, functional impairment in daily life (both at rest and during activity), the quality and severity of the pain, the timing of onset, distribution, and precipitating or aggravating factors. It is important to ask patients about the character of the pain in detail. If the patient has difficulty articulating the nature of the pain, clinicians can ask specific questions such as: "Does it feel like a stabbing pain?," "Does it feel like being hit with a hammer?," or "Does it feel like squeezing or tightening?" The duration of pain is typically described

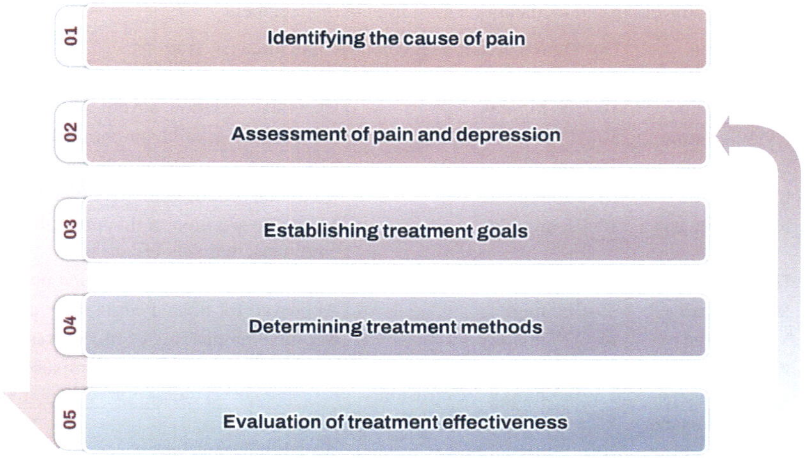

Fig. 9.3 Underlying cause of the pain

with terms such as frequent, occasional, or all day long. Pain episodes may also be inferred from the patient's emotional state, facial expressions, behaviors, or moaning. The severity of pain is usually assessed using the visual analogue scale (VAS), which asks patients to rate their pain on a scale from 0 (no pain) to 10 (worst pain imaginable). In children and adolescents, a faces pain scale, which is similar to the VAS, may be used.

To evaluate both physical pain and depressive symptoms, commonly used tools include the Hamilton Depression Rating Scale (HAM-D) and the Brief Inventory of Depressive Symptoms. A more recent and particularly useful tool in patients with depression accompanied by physical symptoms such as pain is the Depression and Somatic Symptoms Scale (DSSS), which has been validated in Korea. The DSSS consists of 5 items for somatic symptoms, 5 items for pain symptoms, and 12 items for depressive symptoms, with a cutoff score of 22 points [8].

9.9 Psychopharmacological Treatments

In managing chronic pain, psychotropic medications such as tricyclic antidepressants (TCAs) and anticonvulsants are frequently prescribed. Although there is no definitive evidence favoring one antidepressant over another for pain treatment, antidepressants that enhance serotonergic and noradrenergic activity such as TCAs, venlafaxine, duloxetine, and milnacipran are consistently reported to be effective for pain relief [49]. These medications are typically initiated at low doses and titrated upwards to minimize side effects.

TCAs act on multiple neurotransmitters including serotonin, norepinephrine, and dopamine. Some studies suggest that their analgesic effects may be independent of their antidepressant effects and can occur at doses lower than those used to treat depression [50]. Common side effects of TCAs include sedation, dry mouth, weight gain, blurred vision, urinary retention, constipation, and orthostatic hypotension. Amitriptyline and imipramine generally cause more severe side effects than nortriptyline and desipramine. Due to cardiotoxicity and potential arrhythmias, TCAs should be avoided in patients with ischemic heart disease, tachycardia, or conduction disorders, as well as in the elderly due to potential impacts on cognition and gait. Duloxetine has shown consistent efficacy for various pain conditions, including diabetic peripheral neuropathy, fibromyalgia, and osteoarthritis. It is typically titrated to 60 mg/day and maintained for at least 4 weeks, with possible increase up to 120 mg depending on the response. While venlafaxine is not officially indicated for pain, its mechanism of action is similar to duloxetine, and it is sometimes used off-label for pain.

Table 9.1 Psychotropic medications used in pain management

Medication	Dosage for pain management	Clinical considerations
Antidepressants		
Amitriptyline	10–100 mg/day	Excessive sedation, severe anticholinergic side effects
Clomipramine	50–100 mg/day	Mild sedation, mild anticholinergic side effects
Desipramine	25–100 mg/day	Mild sedation, mild anticholinergic side effects
Imipramine	25–100 mg/day	Moderate sedation, moderate anticholinergic side effects
Nortriptyline	10–75 mg/day	Moderate sedation, mild anticholinergic side effects, fewer cardiovascular side effects
Duloxetine	60–120 mg/day	Approved for fibromyalgia and neuropathic pain
Milnacipran	25–200 mg/day	Approved for fibromyalgia; may cause urinary dysfunction
Venlafaxine	75–225 mg/day	Requires monitoring of blood pressure, liver and renal function
Ketamine	0.75 mg/kg intranasal; 0.1–0.5 mg/kg IV infusion	Dissociation, hypertension, misuse
Anticonvulsants		
Carbamazepine	200–1200 mg/day	Anticholinergic side effects, hyponatremia, hematologic disorders, CYP450 inducer, elevated liver enzymes, electrocardiogram (ECG) changes
Gabapentin	100–3600 mg/day	Dizziness, sedation, weight gain, peripheral edema, renal function monitoring needed
Lamotrigine	200–400 mg/day	Sedation, headache, dizziness, ataxia, gastrointestinal symptoms, blurred vision, potentially fatal rash
Oxcarbazepine	300–1800 mg/day	Similar profile to carbamazepine
Pregabalin	150–600 mg/day	Dizziness, mild sedation, weight gain, peripheral edema, renal function monitoring needed
Topiramate	12.5–600 mg/day	Weight loss, decreased appetite, kidney stones, cognitive impairment

Milnacipran can be administered at 100–200 mg/day for fibromyalgia (see Table 9.1), Meta-analyses suggest that SSRIs are less effective for treating pain per se, but they are recommended when depressive symptoms coexist with pain [51, 52]. In one randomized controlled trial, patients with chronic pain and depression received 12 weeks of antidepressant treatment followed by six sessions of a pain self-management program. The study demonstrated improvement in both pain and depression, with effects lasting up to 12 months (see Table 9.1) [53].

Gabapentin and pregabalin bind to voltage-gated calcium channels and inhibit the release of excitatory neurotransmitters, thereby exerting analgesic effects. Gabapentin is indicated for neuropathic pain, and pregabalin is approved for both neuropathic pain and fibromyalgia. Topiramate acts on both GABA and NMDA receptors to suppress excitatory neurotransmission. It is effective for migraine prophylaxis and has also been reported to be useful for painful diabetic neuropathy [54]. Most psychotropic medications tend to cause weight gain, which can negatively impact pain management. In patients with metabolic syndrome or those at risk of weight gain, topiramate may be considered due to its weight-reducing properties. Carbamazepine and oxcarbazepine block sodium channels and inhibit pain transmission via various mechanisms, making them useful in treating neuropathic pain. Lamotrigine is sometimes used in clinical practice, especially in patients who are unresponsive to carbamazepine (see Table 9.1).

Ketamine, originally developed as a dissociative anesthetic and NMDA receptor antagonist, has long been used to manage acute pain from fractures, trauma, and postoperative conditions. Intravenous ketamine infusions have shown efficacy in managing chronic pain conditions such as complex regional pain syndrome, fibromyalgia, and chronic neuropathic pain [55]. However, optimal dosing, duration, and long-term analgesic effects in chronic pain remain to be fully elucidated. Ketamine has recently been approved for the treatment of depression and suicidal ideation at subanesthetic doses [56]. Given its shared efficacy for both depression and pain, ketamine may be a promising option in patients with comorbid conditions, although well-controlled studies are still lacking. Even at low doses, ketamine can cause dissociative symptoms and cardiovascular side effects, necessitating caution during administration [56].

Recent clinical studies also report that dopaminergic agents can be effective in treating both pain [57] and depression [58]. Activation of the endogenous dynorphin/κ-opioid system and subsequent suppression of mesolimbic dopamine release may underlie pain-related depressive symptoms. In preclinical studies, noxious acidic stimuli reduced extracellular dopamine levels in the septal area, supporting the notion that reduced mesolimbic dopamine contributes to the negative affective states of pain. Opioid analgesics blocked this dopamine reduction, indicating that their analgesic effects may influence affective components of pain [59]. Based on this, clinical attempts have been made to treat pain by enhancing dopamine activity. In a randomized controlled trial, the dopamine receptor agonist pramipexole significantly improved pain symptoms in patients with fibromyalgia compared to placebo [57]. Bupropion, a well-known antidepressant that modulates dopamine, has also demonstrated pain-relieving effects. In a 12-week double-blind trial, bupropion reduced pain scores and helped prevent quality of life impairment due to pain [60]. Interestingly, antipsychotics that typically reduce dopamine activity may also have analgesic effects. Although rarely used for this indication, medications like ziprasidone and olanzapine have been reported to produce analgesic benefits in some fibromyalgia patients [61, 62]. Their effects on pain may share mechanisms with their antidepressant action and could be considered in patients with prominent pain symptoms in the context of depressive disorders.

Collectively, these findings suggest that serotonin, norepinephrine, and dopamine are all involved in the pathophysiology of both pain and depression. They also represent potential pharmacological targets. Further research into the mechanisms of these medications will enhance our understanding of how they modulate pain pathways and expand the evidence base for psychopharmacological treatment of pain [63].

9.10 Cognitive-Behavioral Therapy (CBT)

For several decades, cognitive-behavioral therapy (CBT) has been used to treat chronic pain, and most studies show that both CBT and acceptance and commitment therapy (ACT) are effective across various types of pain. While CBT originated as a psychological treatment for depression, when applied to pain management, it typically does not directly address depressive symptoms. Instead, CBT for pain focuses on symptom relief and improving physical functioning. For example, patients learn how to challenge maladaptive beliefs, implement behavioral strategies to reduce pain, and increase activity levels [1]. Even when CBT does not directly target depression, it can alleviate depressive symptoms indirectly by reducing pain and increasing physical activity. Psychological interventions now play a central role in modern pain management and are considered essential components of care.

Numerous systematic reviews and meta-analyses have demonstrated the effectiveness of psychological interventions in clinical pain management. Among these, CBT—with its emphasis on cognitive coping strategies and behavioral rehearsal—has the strongest evidence base. However, most of the current evidence pertains to adults. There remains a lack of robust data for adolescents and older adults with chronic pain. Well-designed meta-analyses have shown that the overall effect size of CBT for adults is moderate, and combining CBT with pharmacotherapy consistently yields beneficial outcomes [64, 65].

9.11 Neurophysiological Treatments

Recently, neurophysiological or neuromodulatory interventions traditionally used for depression have been shown to be effective for pain management as well. These include electroconvulsive therapy (ECT), repetitive transcranial magnetic stimulation (rTMS), and transcranial direct current stimulation (tDCS). Approximately 79% of patients with major depressive disorder and co-occurring pain reported pain relief following ECT [66]. ECT has also been found to increase pain thresholds and tolerance in depressed patients [67]. Furthermore, studies have demonstrated ECT's effectiveness in managing complex regional pain syndrome [68] and fibromyalgia [69]. rTMS has strong evidence supporting its use for chronic neuropathic pain [70]. High-frequency stimulation of the motor cortex contralateral to the pain site is effective. In patients with major depressive disorder, high-frequency stimulation of the prefrontal cortex has improved both depression and pain [71–73]. rTMS has also shown benefit in fibromyalgia [74] and neuropathic pain following spinal cord injury [75]. Meta-analyses have demonstrated that tDCS provides comprehensive improvement in both pain and depressive symptoms in patients with chronic pain [76]. In fibromyalgia, tDCS was superior to sham treatment [77]. However, as these neurophysiological interventions are effective only in some patients, further well-controlled longitudinal studies are needed to establish their utility in treating comorbid pain and depression.

9.12 Conclusion

Depression and pain share numerous characteristics in terms of clinical presentation, neurobiological pathways, neurotransmitters, hormones, stress-related factors, neurotrophic factors, and inflammatory cytokines. These shared features have important implications for the pathogenesis and treatment of both conditions. Current research indicates that understanding brain mechanisms is essential for explaining how biological, psychological, and behavioral factors influence pain and depression, and for identifying optimal treatment strategies. Psychosocial and behavioral factors play a crucial role in initiating, maintaining, and exacerbating the experience of pain. Cognitive-behavioral therapy (CBT), whether delivered as a standalone treatment or as part of a multidisciplinary pain rehabilitation program, is strongly supported by empirical evidence. Since commonly prescribed medications are often insufficient to completely alleviate pain, it is increasingly clear that an individualized, multimodal approach that includes pharmacological, physical, and psychological components is necessary. Therefore, a comprehensive biopsychosocial model that integrates the pathogenesis, assessment, and management of both depression and pain is essential for effective treatment. Future advancements in theoretical, methodological, and technological domains will be crucial in clarifying the relationship between pain and depression and in developing more effective biological and psychological therapies for patients suffering from pain.

Declarations

Competing Interests The author(s) has no competing interests to declare that are relevant to the content of this manuscript.

Ethics Approval The author(s) declares that this manuscript does not include primary research with human participants.

The author(s) declares that this manuscript does not include primary studies involving animals.

References

1. Goesling J, Clauw DJ, Hassett AL. Pain and depression: an integrative review of neurobiological and psychological factors. Curr Psychiatry Rep. 2013;15:421.
2. Kupfer DJ, Frank E, Phillips ML. Major depressive disorder: new clinical, neurobiological, and treatment perspectives. Lancet. 2012;379:1045–55.
3. Lepine JP, Briley M. The epidemiology of pain in depression. Hum Psychopharmacol. 2004;19(Suppl 1):S3–7.
4. Pae CU, Luyten P, Marks DM, Han C, Park SH, Patkar AA, et al. The relationship between fibromyalgia and major depressive disorder: a comprehensive review. Curr Med Res Opin. 2008;24:2359–71.

5. Pae CU, Marks DM, Patkar AA, Masand PS, Luyten P, Serretti A. Pharmacological treatment of chronic fatigue syndrome: focusing on the role of antidepressants. Expert Opin Pharmacother. 2009;10:1561–70.
6. Sansone RA, Sansone LA. Pain, pain, go away: antidepressants and pain management. Psychiatry (Edgmont). 2008;5:16–9.
7. Bair MJ, Robinson RL, Katon W, Kroenke K. Depression and pain comorbidity: a literature review. Arch Intern Med. 2003;163:2433–45.
8. Jeon SW, Yoon SY, Ko YH, Joe SH, Kim YK, Han C, et al. Do somatic symptoms predict the severity of depression? A validation study of the Korean version of the depression and somatic symptoms scale. J Korean Med Sci. 2016;31:2002–9.
9. Leuchter AF, Husain MM, Cook IA, Trivedi MH, Wisniewski SR, Gilmer WS, et al. Painful physical symptoms and treatment outcome in major depressive disorder: a STAR*D (Sequenced Treatment Alternatives to Relieve Depression) report. Psychol Med. 2010;40:239–51.
10. Mathew RJ, Weinman ML, Mirabi M. Physical symptoms of depression. Br J Psychiatry. 1981;139:293–6.
11. Kroenke K, Spitzer RL, Williams JB, Linzer M, Hahn SR, de Gruy FV 3rd, et al. Physical symptoms in primary care. Predictors of psychiatric disorders and functional impairment. Arch Fam Med. 1994;3:774–9.
12. Croft PR, Papageorgiou AC, Ferry S, Thomas E, Jayson MI, Silman AJ. Psychologic distress and low back pain. Evidence from a prospective study in the general population. Spine (Phila Pa 1976). 1995;20:2731–7.
13. Von Korff M, Dworkin SF, Le Resche L, Kruger A. An epidemiologic comparison of pain complaints. Pain. 1988;32:173–83.
14. Li JX. Pain and depression comorbidity: a preclinical perspective. Behav Brain Res. 2015;276:92–8.
15. Kroenke K, Wu J, Bair MJ, Krebs EE, Damush TM, Tu W. Reciprocal relationship between pain and depression: a 12-month longitudinal analysis in primary care. J Pain. 2011;12:964–73.
16. Han C, Pae CU. Pain and depression: a neurobiological perspective of their relationship. Psychiatry Investig. 2015;12:1–8.
17. Ilgen MA, Kleinberg F, Ignacio RV, Bohnert AS, Valenstein M, McCarthy JF, et al. Noncancer pain conditions and risk of suicide. JAMA Psychiatry. 2013;70:692–7.
18. Leone M. Deep brain stimulation in headache. Lancet Neurol. 2006;5:873–7.
19. Bai YM, Chiou WF, Su TP, Li CT, Chen MH. Pro-inflammatory cytokine associated with somatic and pain symptoms in depression. J Affect Disord. 2014;155:28–34.
20. Burke NN, Geoghegan E, Kerr DM, Moriarty O, Finn DP, Roche M. Altered neuropathic pain behaviour in a rat model of depression is associated with changes in inflammatory gene expression in the amygdala. Genes Brain Behav. 2013;12:705–13.
21. Caumo W, Hidalgo MP, Souza A, Torres ILS, Antunes LC. Melatonin is a biomarker of circadian dysregulation and is correlated with major depression and fibromyalgia symptom severity. J Pain Res. 2019;31;12:545–56.
22. Magni G, Andreoli F, Arduino C, Arsie D, Ceccherelli F, Ambrosio F, et al. Modifications of [3H]imipramine binding sites in platelets of chronic pain patients treated with mianserin. Pain. 1987;30:311–20.
23. Nicolson SE, Caplan JP, Williams DE, Stern TA. Comorbid pain, depression, and anxiety: multifaceted pathology allows for multifaceted treatment. Harv Rev Psychiatry. 2009;17:407–20.
24. Sachs Ericsson N, Cromer K, Hemandez A, Kendall Tackett K. A review of childhood abuse, health, and pain-related problems; the role of psychiatric disorders and current life stress. J Trauma Dissociation. 2009;10:170–88.
25. Muhtz C, Rodriguez-Raecke R, Hinkelmann K, Moeller-Bertram T, Kiefer F, Wiedemann K, et al. Cortisol response to experimental pain in patients with chronic low back pain and patients with major depression. Pain Med. 2013;14:498–503.
26. Lee EJ, Wu MY, Lee GK, Cheing G, Chan F. Catastrophizing as a cognitive vulnerability factor related to depression in workers' compensation patients with chronic musculoskeletal pain. J Clin Psychol Med Settings. 2008;15:182–92.
27. Koh JS, Ko HJ, Wang SM, Cho KJ, Kim JC, Lee SJ, et al. Depression and somatic symptoms may influence on chronic prostatitis/chronic pelvic pain syndrome: a preliminary study. Psychiatry Investig. 2014;11:495–8.
28. Bonezzi C, Demartini L, Buonocore M. Chronic pain: not only a matter of time. Minerva Anestesiol. 2012;78:704–11.
29. Max MB, Wu T, Atlas SJ, Edwards RR, Haythornthwaite JA, Bollettino AF, et al. A clinical genetic method to identify mechanisms by which pain causes depression and anxiety. Mol Pain. 2006;2:14.
30. Lebe M, Hasenbring MI, Schmieder K, Jetschke K, Harders A, Epplen JT, et al. Association of serotonin-1A and -2A receptor promoter polymorphisms with depressive symptoms, functional recovery, and pain in patients 6 months after lumbar disc surgery. Pain. 2013;154:377–84.
31. Bras M, Dordevic V, Gregurck R, Bulajic M. Neurobiological and clinical relationship between psychiatric disorders and chronic pain. Pychiatr Danub. 2010;22:221–6.
32. Jann MW, Slade JH. Antidepressant agents for the treatment of chronic pain and depression. Pharmacotherapy. 2007;27:1571–87.
33. Sotres-Bayon F, Torres-Lopez E, Lopez-Avila A, del Angel R, Pellicer F. Lesion and electrical stimulation of the ventral tegmental area modify persistent nociceptive behavior in the rat. Brain Res. 2001;898:342–9.
34. Bendtsen L, Norregaard J, Jensen R, Olesen J. Evidence of qualitatively altered nociception

in patients with fibromyalgia. Arthritis Rheum. 1997;40:98–102.
35. Bennett RM. Emerging concepts in the neurobiology of chronic pain: evidence of abnormal sensory processing in fibromyalgia. Mayo Clin Proc. 1999;74:385–98.
36. Verne GN, Price DD, Callam CS, Zhang B, Peck J, Zhou Q. Viscerosomatic facilitation in a subset of IBS patients, an effect mediated by N-methyl-D-aspartate receptors. J Pain. 2012;13:901–9.
37. Staud R, Robinson ME, Price DD. Temporal summation of second pain and its maintenance are useful for characterizing widespread central sensitization of fibromyalgia patients. J Pain. 2007;8:893–901.
38. Blier P, Gobbi G, Haddjeri N, Santarelli L, Mathew G, Hen R. Impact of substance P receptor antagonism on the serotonin and norepinephrine systems: relevance to the antidepressant/anxiolytic response. J Psychiatry Neurosci. 2004;29:208–18.
39. Zelman DC, Howland EW, Nichols SN, Cleeland CS. The effects of induced mood on laboratory pain. Pain. 1991;46:105–11.
40. Jensen MP. A neuropsychological model of pain: research and clinical implications. J Pain. 2010;11:2–12.
41. Mutschler I, Ball T, Wankerl J, Strigo IA. Pain and emotion in the insular cortex: evidence for functional reorganization in major depression. Neurosci Lett. 2012;520:204–9.
42. Rodriguez-Raecke R, Ihle K, Ritter C, Muhrz C, Otte C, May A. Neuronal differences between chronic low back pain and depression regarding long-term habituation to pain. Eur J Pain (London, England). 2014;18:701–11.
43. Philips HC. Imagery and likelihood cognitive bias in pain. Behav Cogn Psychother. 2015;43:270–84.
44. Nicholas MK, Asghari A, Blyth FM, Wood BM, Murray R, McCabe R, et al. Self- management intervention for chronic pain in older adults: a randomised controlled trial. Pain. 2013;154:824–35.
45. Franklin JC, Lee KM, Hanra EK, Prinstein MJ. Feeling worse to feel better pain-offset relief simultaneously stimulates positive affect and reduces negative affect. Psychol Sci. 2013;24:521–9.
46. Tang NK, Goodchild CE, Salkovskis PM. Hybrid cognitive-behaviour therapy for individuals with insomnia and chronic pain: a pilot randomised controlled trial. Behav Res Ther. 2012;50:814–21.
47. Zale EL, Lange KL, Fields SA, Ditre JW. The relation between pain-related fear and disability: a meta-analysis. J Pain. 2013;14:1019–30.
48. Vlaeyen JW, Linton SJ. Fear-avoidance and its consequences in chronic musculoskeletal pain: a state of the art. Pain. 2000;85:317–32.
49. Hauser W, Wolfe F, Tolle T, Uceyler N, Sommer C. The role of antidepressants in the management of fibromyalgia syndrome: a systematic review and meta-analysis. CNS Drugs. 2012;26:297–307.
50. Guay DR. Adjunctive agents in the management of chronic pain. Pharmacotherapy. 2001;21:1070–81.
51. Mercier A, Auger-Aubin I, Lebeau JP, Schuers M, Boulet P, Hermil JL, et al. Evidence of prescription of antidepressants for non-psychiatric conditions in primary care: an analysis of guidelines and systematic reviews. BMC Fam Pract. 2013;14:55.
52. Kroenke K, Krebs EE, Bair MJ. Pharmacotherapy of chronic pain: a synthesis of recommendations from systematic reviews. Gen Hosp Psychiatry. 2009;31:206–19.
53. Kroenke K, Bair MJ, Damush TM, Wu J, Hoke S, Sutherland J, et al. Optimized antidepressant therapy and pain self-management in primary care patients with depression and musculoskeletal pain: a randomized controlled trial. JAMA. 2009;301:2099–110.
54. Raskin P, Donofrio PD, Rosenthal NR, Hewitt DJ, Jordan DM, Xiang J, et al. Topiramate vs placebo in painful diabetic neuropathy: analgesic and metabolic effect. Neurology. 2004;63:865–73.
55. Orhurhu V, Orhurhu MS, Bhatia A, Cohen SP. Ketamine infusions for chronic pain: a systematic review and meta-analysis of randomized controlled trials. Anesth Analg. 2019;129(1):241–54.
56. Subramanian S, Haroutounian S, Palanca BJA, Lenze EJ. Ketamine as a therapeutic agent for depression and pain: mechanisms and evidence. J Neurol Sci. 2022;434:120152. https://doi.org/10.1016/j.jns.2022.120152.
57. Holman AJ, Myers RR. A randomized, double-blind, placebo-controlled trial of pramipexole, dopamine agonist, in patients with fibromyalgia receiving concomitant medications. Arthritic Rheum. 2005;52:2495–505.
58. Corrigan MH, Denahan AQ, Wright CE, Ragual RJ, Evans DL. Comparison of pramipexole, fluoxetine, and placebo in patients with major depression. Depress Anxiety. 2000;11:58–65.
59. Leitl MD, Onvani S, Bowers MS, Cheng K, Rice KC, Carlezon WA Jr, et al. Pain-related depression of the mesolimbic dopamine system in rats: expression, blockade by analgesics, and role of endogenous kappa-opioids. Neuropsychopharmacology. 2014;39:614–24.
60. Semenchuk MR, Sherman 5, Davis B. Double-blind, randomized trial of bupropion SR for the treatment of neuropathic pain. Neurology. 2001;57:1583–8.
61. Rico-Villademoros F, Hidalgo J, Dominguez I, Garcia-Leiva JM, Calandre EP. Atypical antipsychotics in the treatment of fibromyalgia: a case series with olanzapine. Prog Neuro-Psychopharmacol Biol Psychiatry. 2005;29:161–4.
62. Calandre EP, Hidalgo J, Rico-Villademoros F. Use of ziprasidone in patients with fibromyalgia : a case series. Rheumatol Int. 2007;27:473–6.
63. Marks DM, Pae CU, Patkar AA. Triple reuptake inhibitors: a premise and promise. Psychiatry Investig. 2008;5:142–7.
64. Eccleston C, Morley SJ, Williams AC. Psychological approaches to chronic pain management: evidence and challenges. Br J Anaesth. 2013;111:59–63.

65. Turk DC, Swanson KS, Tunks ER. Psychological approaches in the treatment of chronic pain patients--when pills, scalpels, and needles are not enough. Can J Psychiatr. 2008;53:213–23.
66. Leong K, Tham JC, Scamvougeras A, Vila-Rodriguez F. Electroconvulsive therapy treatment in patients with somatic symptom and related disorders. Neuropsychiatr Dis Treat. 2015;11:2565–72.
67. Schreiber S, Shmueli D, Grunhaus L, Dolberg OT, Feldinger E, Magora F, et al. The influence of electroconvulsive therapy on pain threshold and pain tolerance in major depression patients before, during and after treatment. Eur J Pain (London, England). 2003;7:419–24.
68. McDaniel WW. Electroconvulsive therapy in complex regional pain syndromes. J CT. 2003;19:226–9.
69. Usui C, Doi N, Nishioka M, Komatsu H, Yamamoto R, Ohkubo T, et al. Electroconvulsive therapy improves severe pain associated with fibromyalgia. Pain. 2006;121:276–80.
70. Lefaucheur JP, Aleman A, Baeken C, Benninger DH, Brunelin J, Di Lazzaro V, et al. Evidence-based guidelines on the therapeutic use of repetitive transcranial magnetic stimulation (rTMS): an update (2014–2018). Clin Neurophysiol. 2020;131(2):474–528.
71. Avery DH, Holtzheimer PE 3rd, Fawaz W, Russo J, Neumaier J, Dunner DL, et al. Transcranial magnetic stimulation reduces pain in patients with major depression: a sham-controlled study. J Nerv Ment Dis. 2007;195:378–81.
72. Corlier J, Tadayonnejad R, Wilson AC, Lee JC, Marder KG, Ginder ND, et al. Repetitive transcranial magnetic stimulation treatment of major depressive disorder and comorbid chronic pain: response rates and neurophysiologic biomarkers. Psychol Med. 2021:1–10.
73. Phillips AL, Burr RL, Dunner DL. rTMS effects in patients with co-morbid somatic pain and depressive mood disorders. J Affect Disord. 2018;241:411–6.
74. Hou WH, Wang TY, Kang JH. The effects of add-on non-invasive brain stimulation in fibromyalgia: a meta-analysis and meta-regression of randomized controlled trials. Rheumatology (Oxford, England). 2016;55:1507–17.
75. Gao F, Chu H, Li J, Yang M, Du L, Li J, et al. Repetitive transcranial magnetic stimulation for pain after spinal cord injury: a systematic review and meta-analysis. J Neurosurg Sci. 2016;61(5):514–22.
76. Wen YR, Shi J, Hu ZY, Lin YY, Lin YT, Jiang X, et al. Is transcranial direct current stimulation beneficial for treating pain, depression, and anxiety symptoms in patients with chronic pain? A systematic review and meta-analysis. Front Mol Neurosci. 2022;15:1056966.
77. Kang JH, Choi SE, Park DJ, Xu H, Lee JK, Lee SS. Effects of add-on transcranial direct current stimulation on pain in Korean patients with fibromyalgia. Sci Rep. 2020;10(1):12114. https://doi.org/10.1038/s41598-020-69131-7.

Obesity and Depression

10

Young Sup Woo and Young Joon Kwon

10.1 Introduction

Recent studies have increasingly reported a significant association between depression and obesity. Although the relationship between these two conditions has long been suspected, early investigations failed to demonstrate a clear link between psychopathology of depression and obesity. Both depression and obesity are of major concern in public health. According to the World Health Organization (WHO), the lifetime prevalence of major depressive disorder (MDD) ranges from 6% to 21%. Obesity is also common, with international studies reporting prevalence rates of approximately 11% in men and 15% in women. Depression can lead to changes in appetite, weight, sleep, and physical activity, which may contribute to the development of overweight or obesity. Conversely, obesity can increase the risk of depression through factors such as negative body image, low self-esteem, and maladaptive cognitive schemas, thus supporting the notion of a relationship between the two conditions [1]. However, a study conducted in the 1960s involving 1660 residents of New York, which examined the relationship between obesity and mental health, reported that although obese individuals scored higher on traits such as "immaturity," "rigidity," and "suspiciousness," there were no significant differences in levels of depression or anxiety [2]. In fact, some researchers even found lower levels of psychopathology among obese individuals compared to those of normal weight [3]. This study formed the basis of the so-called "jolly fat" hypothesis, which posits that obesity or eating behaviors leading to obesity may serve as protective factors against negative emotions, including depression. In this study, obese men were found to have lower levels of depression than men of normal weight [3]. However, these early studies had methodological limitations, including inconsistent definitions of obesity and varied assessment tools for psychopathology and mood symptoms, which may account for their inconsistent findings [4].

More recent epidemiological studies, however, given the frequent co-occurrence of depression and obesity, have conceptualized their relationship as a bidirectional, reciprocal, and interconnected process [5]: that is, depression may increase the risk of future obesity, and obesity may elevate the risk of subsequent depression. Nevertheless, the mechanisms underlying this bidirectional relationship remain unclear. This chapter will review recent literature addressing the association between depression and obesity and will explore the biological mechanisms that may mediate this link.

Y. S. Woo (✉)
Woo and Bahk Psychiatry Clinic, Seoul, Republic of Korea
e-mail: woo.youngsup@hotmail.com

Y. J. Kwon
Department of Psychiatry, Soonchunhyang University Cheonan Hospital, College of Medicine, Soonchunhyang University, Cheonan, Republic of Korea

W.-M. Bahk et al. (eds.), *Depressive Disorder*, https://doi.org/10.1007/978-981-92-1331-3_10

10.2 Epidemiological Associations Between Depression and Obesity

Epidemiological studies exploring the relationship between depression and obesity can broadly be classified into cross-sectional and longitudinal studies. Cross-sectional studies examine the prevalence of obesity among individuals with depression, or the prevalence of depression among individuals with obesity, as well as the comorbidity rates between the two conditions in the general population. Longitudinal studies, in contrast, investigate the incidence of obesity in cohorts with depression, or the incidence of depression in cohorts with obesity. It is important to note that variations in study design can significantly affect the interpretation of findings. Some studies focus exclusively on obesity, while others include overweight populations. Similarly, the variables considered may include formal diagnoses of depression or the presence and severity of depressive symptoms.

To date, a substantial number of cross-sectional studies have been conducted, and findings from systematic reviews and meta-analyses have also been published. While many of these studies suggest an association between obesity and depression, the results are not always consistent. Differences by gender and geographic region have also been noted. A meta-analysis of 17 cross-sectional studies found a positive correlation between depression and obesity (odds ratio [OR] = 1.18) [6]. However, when results were stratified by gender, the correlation was statistically significant only in women, and not in men. A separate systematic review of 20 studies reported that studies conducted in the United States found a significant association between obesity and depression in women but not in men, while studies conducted outside the United States showed no consistent association in either gender [7].

Prospective studies on the impact of obesity on the future onset of depression have yielded similar findings. One early study reported that obese adults aged 50 or older with a body mass index (BMI) ≥30 were more than twice as likely to develop depression within 5 years compared to their non-obese counterparts [8]. Subsequent studies have also found increased risks. Kasen et al. reported that the risk was more than fivefold among women [9]. Another study conducted in elderly populations similarly found an increased risk [10]. One study showed that each standard deviation increase in BMI was associated with a 1.11-fold increase in the risk of developing depression [11]. A meta-analysis also confirmed that individuals with obesity had a significantly elevated risk of future depression [12].

However, some studies have highlighted the influence of potential confounding factors in the association between obesity and depression. For instance, Fowler-Brown et al. [13] found that obesity at baseline did not predict the future onset of depressive symptoms in the overall population. Yet, among individuals with high socioeconomic status, baseline obesity nearly doubled the risk. Physical activity has also been proposed as a mediating factor. In a study investigating BMI, physical activity, and depressive symptoms in young women, physical activity was found to be protective against depressive symptoms [14]. However, physical activity did not mitigate the increased risk of depressive symptoms associated with weight gain. More recently, studies have suggested that not only obesity itself but also the presence of comorbid metabolic conditions may contribute to the risk of depression. Compared to normal-weight individuals without metabolic abnormalities, those with obesity and two or more metabolic disorders, such as hypertension, glucose dysregulation, systemic inflammation, low HDL cholesterol, or elevated triglycerides-had a 1.5-fold increased risk of developing depressive symptoms. In contrast, obese individuals with fewer than two metabolic abnormalities had a 1.4-fold increase in risk, although this did not reach statistical significance [15]. Sociocultural factors may also play a role. According to the aforementioned meta-analysis [12], studies conducted in the United States found that obesity predicted future depression (OR = 2.12), while studies conducted in Europe did not find a significant effect (OR = 1.33). The authors of that meta-analysis speculated that, in addition to cultural differences, the generally higher rates of obesity in the United States might contribute to a greater psychological burden, thereby increasing the risk of depression.

Several studies have also investigated whether depression increases the risk of developing obesity, representing the reverse direction of the relationship. Research from the late 1990s primarily focused on whether depression or depressive symptoms during adolescence could predict obesity in adulthood. Pine et al. [16] reported that adolescent depression predicted obesity in early adulthood. Barefoot et al. [17] found that depressive symptoms negatively affected existing weight trajectories, resulting in further weight loss among underweight individuals and additional weight gain among those who were overweight. In contrast, Bardone et al. [18] found that adolescent depression had no significant effect on BMI in later life. Subsequent studies have continued to produce mixed findings. While some researchers reported that depression was associated with future obesity [5, 19] or abdominal obesity, [20] others found no such link [8]. It is also important to consider that the effect of depression on obesity risk may be more pronounced in women [13, 21, 22]. However, a meta-analysis published in 2008 found that individuals with depressive symptoms had a significantly higher risk of future obesity compared to those without such symptoms (OR = 1.19), with the risk particularly elevated in adolescent females (OR = 2.57) [23]. Another meta-analysis by Luppino et al. [12] reported that baseline depression or depressive symptoms increased the risk of developing obesity by 1.6 times, and this association was not significantly influenced by other covariates.

10.3 Genetic Associations between Depression and Obesity

The association of depression and obesity may be explained by shared genetic factors [24]. The heritability of major depressive disorder (MDD) is estimated to be approximately 0.35, while the heritability of body weight ranges between 0.7 and 0.8 [25, 26]. Although some forms of obesity may result from single-gene mutations, the majority of cases of both depression and obesity exhibit polygenic inheritance. Genome-wide association studies (GWAS) based on these heritable traits have not established a definitive genetic link between depression and obesity; however, certain genetic variants associated with obesity or type 2 diabetes may influence susceptibility to depression.

GWAS findings have suggested that genes such as NEGR1 (neuronal growth regulator 1), OLFM4 (olfactomedin 4), and KSR2 (kinase suppressor of ras 2) may be associated with both increased body mass index (BMI) and depression [27–29]. In case–control studies, approximately 20% of genetic variants related to obesity also showed associations with depression. Notably, certain alleles of the fat mass and obesity-associated (FTO) gene may be implicated in both conditions [30, 31]. A meta-analysis examining the impact of the FTO single nucleotide polymorphism (SNP) rs9939609 found a significant interaction among depression, FTO SNP status, and BMI—individuals who had both depression and the risk allele exhibited higher BMI levels [31].

In addition, a SNP located near the SIRT1 gene, a variant linked to depression, has been associated with metabolic regulation [32]. The SIRT1 gene encodes sirtuin 1, a key regulator of carbohydrate and lipid metabolism. Sirtuin 1 deacetylates various transcription factors, including FOXO1 and CREB, thereby inhibiting processes such as lipogenesis, cholesterol synthesis, and gluconeogenesis.

The association between genetic traits, depression, and metabolic disorders may also arise from gene–environment interactions. For instance, serotonin plays a crucial role in inducing satiety and is believed to influence both depressive states and eating behaviors. Polymorphisms in the promoter region of the serotonin transporter gene SLC6A4 have been shown to affect the risk of developing depression following exposure to stressful life events. These polymorphisms have also been linked to obesity and overweight status [33, 34]. Furthermore, SNPs in genes such as

FKBP5 and CRHR1 have been associated with the onset of adult depression following early life adversity. These genetic variants are also involved in the regulation of stress responses and eating behaviors through the hypothalamic–pituitary–adrenal (HPA) axis [35].

10.4 Mediating Factors in the Association Between Depression and Obesity

As discussed above, numerous epidemiological studies have reported a relationship between depression and obesity. However, the influence of mediating variables such as gender, sociocultural factors, and physical activity cannot be excluded. Among sociodemographic variables, gender and socioeconomic status are considered influential. In particular, being female and having a low income level may increase the risk of comorbid depression and obesity [36]. Psychosocial factors also appear to play a role. For women, emotions such as anger, sadness, and emotional reactivity have been reported as mediators, while for men, poor interpersonal competence, loneliness, and ineffective conflict resolution have been identified [37]. Additionally, negative body image, weight-related stigma, and lack of social or interpersonal relationships are common contributors to both depression and obesity [1, 36].

While it is well established that physical activity affects both obesity and depression, its influence may vary by gender [38–40]. One study [38] found that in women, depression led to decreased physical activity, which in turn contributed to increased BMI. Conversely, in men, depression also decreased physical activity but resulted in reduced BMI, possibly due to different patterns of eating behavior.

These findings may be related to the effects of dietary habits. It is well known that mood disturbances, such as stress and depression, alter eating behaviors. While stress and negative emotions may suppress appetite and lead to weight loss in some individuals, they may increase appetite and weight gain in others. Both animal models of stress [41] and clinical studies in individuals with depression [42] have shown a tendency to prefer palatable, high-calorie foods. Sweet and fatty foods may temporarily improve mood [43], and such eating behaviors are believed to regulate stress responses [44]. However, these effects are not sustained over the long term.

The relationship between stress, negative mood, and eating behavior is mediated by the activation of the hypothalamic–pituitary–adrenal (HPA) axis, as well as the opioid and dopaminergic reward systems [43, 44]. According to the reward-based stress eating model, repeated stimulation of these systems leads to adaptation and compulsive overeating of high-calorie foods, which in turn contributes to obesity [43, 44]. Moreover, stress promotes the secretion of glucocorticoids and insulin, increasing appetite and thereby facilitating weight gain [45]. In this way, stress and negative mood states modify eating behaviors, promoting obesity and fat accumulation, which subsequently increase vulnerability to depression.

The type of food consumed may also affect the risk of depression. Diets high in saturated and trans fats contribute to general or abdominal obesity, thereby elevating the risk of depression. In contrast, diets rich in unsaturated fatty acids or omega-3 fatty acids are associated with a reduced risk of depression and an improvement in depressive symptoms [46–48]. As will be discussed later, abdominal obesity not only worsens metabolic abnormalities but may also serve as a causal factor in psychiatric disorders, including depression. Saturated fatty acids disrupt leptin and insulin signaling in the hypothalamus, impairing metabolism and promoting weight gain [49, 50]. Increased circulating levels of saturated fatty acids have also been linked to greater severity of depressive symptoms [51]. In summary, depression can lead to unhealthy eating behaviors; when these patterns become chronic, they may result in abdominal obesity and elevated levels of circulating saturated fats, further exacerbating depressive symptoms.

Another factor that influences the association between depression and obesity is the severity of obesity. Studies on depression risk according to degree of obesity have shown that individuals with class III obesity (BMI $\geq$40.0) have more than three times the risk of developing depression compared to individuals with normal weight, even after controlling for other variables [52, 53]. Furthermore, when comparing overweight and obese individuals, the latter group shows a higher risk of experiencing depressive symptoms [54, 55]. These findings suggest that the risk of depression increases with the severity of obesity.

To explain the pathways by which obesity may lead to depression, Markowitz et al. [56] proposed two behavioral mechanisms: the health concern pathway and the appearance concern pathway. They also suggested that the influence of depression on the development of obesity may occur through two distinct pathways—direct physiological mechanisms and indirect psychosocial mechanisms. The health concern pathway refers to the influence of functional impairment and negative perceptions of one's health, which can lead to depression. The appearance concern pathway involves psychological and behavioral consequences of obesity, such as stigma, body dissatisfaction, and repeated dieting behaviors, which particularly increase the risk of depression in women. Indirect psychosocial mechanisms include difficulties in self-care experienced by individuals with depression—such as poor treatment adherence, binge eating, negative thinking patterns, and lack of social support. Direct physiological mechanisms, on the other hand, will be described in the following section on biological changes.

In conclusion, the association between depression and obesity is mediated by a range of factors, including the severity of obesity, gender, social stigma, psychological traits, and eating behaviors. A better understanding of these mediating variables may lead to more effective and tailored interventions for individuals suffering from both depression and obesity.

10.5 Neurobiological Mechanisms Underlying the Association Between Depression and Obesity

Depression and obesity share several neurobiological abnormalities. Key mediators of their interrelationship include dysregulation of the hypothalamic–pituitary–adrenal (HPA) axis, insulin and leptin resistance, inflammatory signaling pathways, oxidative stress, and orexin system dysfunction.

Dysfunction of the Hypothalamic–Pituitary–Adrenal (HPA) Axis

Dysregulation of the HPA axis and elevated cortisol levels contribute to the pathophysiology of both obesity and depression. Stress induces dysregulation of the hypothalamic–pituitary–adrenal (HPA) axis, resulting in elevated cortisol and corticotropin-releasing hormone (CRH) levels. CRH, a central regulator of the HPA axis, plays a crucial role in obesity by modulating metabolic processes, including fat accumulation, glucose homeostasis, and the development of insulin resistance. Notably, placental CRH secretion during pregnancy is essential for fetal development; however, excessive CRH exposure has been linked to an increased risk of metabolic disorders in offspring. Evidence from animal studies indicates that maternal stress and excessive glucocorticoid exposure can disrupt fetal CRH signaling, thereby influencing long-term metabolic outcomes in offspring. Furthermore, CRH-related peptides, including urocortins, have been shown to regulate food intake and glucose homeostasis, thereby contributing to metabolic regulation [57]. This cascade contributes to the overactivation of the mitogen-activated protein kinase pathway, which enhances serotonin transporter activity and exacerbates depressive symptoms [58, 59]. In cases of obesity—particularly abdominal obesity—the negative feedback mechanism that normally suppresses cortisol secretion becomes impaired. As a result, stress-induced cortisol secretion increases [60]. A recent meta-analysis reported that increased abdominal fat is associated with heightened activity of the HPA axis and increased secretion of corticotropin-releasing hormone (CRH) in response to stress [60]. Elevated cortisol levels promote the differentiation of preadipocytes into adipocytes, leading to adipocyte hyperplasia and subsequent fat accumulation and weight gain. Hypercortisolemia, in particular, is known to promote central (abdominal) fat accumulation. HPA axis dysfunction is also well established in the pathophysiology of depression. Glucocorticoids influence mood and behavior by regulating HPA axis activity and maintaining energy homeostasis via glucocorticoid receptors located in emotion-regulating regions of the brain, such as the midbrain and limbic system [61]. In animal models, chronic exposure to cortisol and the resultant overexpression of glucocorticoid receptors have been shown to produce depressive-like behaviors [62]. In humans, increased blood cortisol levels have been observed in individuals with depression, particularly those with melancholic features. Elevated cortisol levels in patients with depression have also been associated with increased abdominal fat, further supporting the link between depression, obesity, and HPA axis dysfunction [63]. Moreover, research has reported blunted cortisol responses in females with a history of sexual abuse, while polyvictimization has been associated with reduced cortisol reactivity and increased adult BMI. Collectively, these findings support a potential dose–response relationship between childhood maltreatment and adult BMI [64].

The relationship between excess glucocorticoids, abdominal obesity, and depression may also involve cortisol metabolism within adipose tissue, which is regulated by the enzymes 11β-hydroxysteroid dehydrogenases (11β-HSDs). These enzymes interconvert active cortisol and its inactive form, cortisone. 11β-HSD2 converts cortisol to cortisone, while 11β-HSD1 catalyzes the reverse reaction, generating active cortisol from cortisone. Overexpression of 11β-HSD1 has been shown to promote visceral fat accumulation and induce metabolic abnormalities such as insulin resistance. 11β-HSD1 is also widely distributed in brain regions involved in emotional regulation, including the hippocampus and hypothalamus, making it a key component in the glucocorticoid hypothesis of depression [65]. Polymorphisms in the gene encoding 11β-HSD1 have been linked to altered enzyme expression in central HPA feedback regions and are associated with increased vulnerability to depression [66]. In animal studies, genetic ablation of 11β-HSD1 resulted in an antidepressant-like phenotype [67].

In summary, dysregulation of the HPA axis appears to be a shared pathophysiological mechanism in both depression and obesity. In particular, the consumption of saturated fats and the accumulation of visceral fat may play a critical role in driving HPA axis dysfunction and the development of both conditions.

Leptin

Leptin is one of the hormones derived from adipocytes, and its concentration increases in proportion to body fat mass. While leptin plays a well-known role in suppressing appetite and reducing body weight, it also affects mood regulation. The antidepressant-like effects of leptin have been demonstrated in several animal models of depression. In models of chronic stress-induced depression, leptin levels were found to be decreased, which coincided with reduced sucrose preference-interpreted as a behavioral correlate of anhedonia [68]. In studies using genetically modified mice, ob/ob mice, which lack the gene for leptin, and db/db mice, which lack the leptin receptor, exhibited more depressive behaviors [69]. Conversely, leptin administration in wild-type mice elicited antidepressant effects, and depressive-like behaviors were alleviated in both chronic stress models and ob/ob mice [69]. These antidepressant effects were accompanied by increased neuronal activity in the hippocampus, a brain region closely associated with mood regulation [70].

However, studies in humans have yet to establish a clear association between leptin and depression. Several investigations have examined leptin concentrations in patients with depression, but findings have been inconsistent. Some studies have reported reduced leptin levels, whereas others have found elevated levels. Similarly, reports on the effects of antidepressant treatment on leptin levels have been mixed, with some showing increases and others showing no change. A recent meta-analysis further reflected this inconsistency [71]: peripheral leptin concentrations did not differ significantly between patients with depression and healthy controls, nor between those with severe major depressive disorder (MDD) and controls. However, leptin levels were elevated in patients with mild-to-moderate MDD compared to controls. Additionally, antidepressant treatment did not alter serum leptin levels [71]. The authors suggested that these discrepancies may be due to heterogeneity in study populations or diagnostic criteria. They also proposed that individuals with mild to moderate MDD may have less visceral adiposity and metabolic dysregulation than those with severe MDD, and that interactions between leptin and abdominal obesity may contribute to depression risk. Body mass index (BMI) differences between the MDD and control groups could have influenced the findings.

The "leptin hypothesis of depression" [72] emphasizes that in obese individuals with elevated leptin levels, the response to leptin is not straightforward. Similar to insulin resistance in type 2 diabetes, obesity induces leptin resistance, where peripheral leptin concentrations are high, but central leptin signaling is impaired [73]. Therefore, it is not the absolute level of leptin but rather impaired leptin signaling that may play a critical role in the pathophysiology of MDD. In obesity, leptin signaling may be attenuated by defects in transport of leptin across the blood–brain barrier (BBB), downregulation or dysfunction of leptin receptors, or impaired signaling through long isoform leptin receptors (LepRb), which are particularly important for central nervous system function [74]. Based on findings from animal studies demonstrating leptin's ability to suppress depressive-like behavior, it is plausible that leptin resistance in individuals with obesity contributes to an increased risk of depression.

One proposed mechanism for how leptin signaling dysfunction affects mood involves its modulation of the HPA axis. Serum leptin and cortisol concentrations are inversely correlated, and chronic stress-induced activation of the HPA axis reduces circulating leptin levels [75]. Leptin administration reduces elevated corticosterone levels in fasted ob/ob mice and suppresses CRH production in the paraventricular nucleus of the hypothalamus [76]. Moreover, leptin's effects are mediated via LepRb signaling, which has been implicated in depression pathophysiology. In mice with targeted deletion of LepRb in the hippocampus, leptin resistance and depressive-like behaviors were observed. Similarly, deletion of LepRb from glutamatergic neurons in the hippocampus and prefrontal cortex also induced depressive behaviors [77]. Leptin also modulates mood via its effects on dopamine and serotonin signaling pathways. Inhibitory neurons in the lateral hypothalamus that project to the ventral tegmental area (VTA) express leptin receptors. Leptin regulates these neurons, restoring expression of tyrosine hydroxylase (TH)—the rate-limiting enzyme in dopamine synthesis—in the VTA, thus modulating mesolimbic dopamine transmission [78]. Leptin also activates dopamine neurons in the VTA through the signal transducer and activator of transcription 3 (STAT3) pathway, [79] and influences dopamine transporter function and dopamine release in other brain regions [80]. Although leptin's regulation of serotonin signaling is less clearly understood than its effects on dopamine, some studies have suggested that leptin increases serotonin levels and metabolism in the forebrain [81, 82]. In ob/ob mice, expression of hypothalamic 5-HT_1A receptors is increased, while serotonin turnover in the hypothalamus and hippocampus is decreased compared to control mice [83]. However, other studies have found that while leptin administration increases serum serotonin levels, it may actually decrease serotonin concentrations in brain regions such as the hypothalamus and hippocampus [84]. In summary, although the relationship between leptin, obesity, and depression remains incompletely understood, impaired leptin signaling is considered to be a significant factor in the shared pathophysiology of both conditions.

Other Adipocyte-Derived Hormones

In addition to leptin, other adipocyte-derived hormones that influence energy metabolism and insulin sensitivity—and may consequently affect both obesity and depression—include adiponectin and resistin. Adiponectin enhances insulin sensitivity, but its circulating levels are reduced by obesity, increased waist circumference, visceral fat accumulation, and insulin resistance. Interestingly, in metabolically healthy obesity, adiponectin levels are not necessarily reduced, suggesting that this hormone is more closely related to metabolic disturbances associated with obesity than to obesity itself [63]. Adiponectin levels are also thought to be influenced by depressive symptoms, but studies have reported inconsistent findings, with some indicating a positive correlation, others a negative correlation, and still others reporting no association at all [63]. The relationship between resistin and obesity has also produced conflicting results. Early studies in both animals and humans showed elevated resistin levels in obesity, but subsequent studies suggested downregulation. In the context of depression, increased resistin levels have been observed in atypical depression but not in typical depression, and levels tend to be lower during remission [85, 86]. According to a meta-analysis [71], both adiponectin and resistin levels were lower in individuals with depression compared to healthy controls, and neither hormone appeared to be significantly altered by antidepressant treatment.

Insulin

Insulin resistance is closely linked to both obesity and depression [87]. The presence of insulin resistance in individuals with obesity significantly increases the risk of depression [15]. Additionally, a meta-analysis confirmed the presence of insulin resistance in patients with depression [87]. Mechanistically, alterations in insulin signaling—including insulin bioavailability and receptor sensitivity—are believed to play an important role in the pathophysiology of depression [88]. Insulin exerts its effects via receptors located in key brain regions such as the cerebral cortex, hippocampus, cerebellum, hypothalamus, and olfactory bulb. Upon ligand binding, insulin receptors activate intracellular signaling cascades via phosphorylation of insulin receptor substrate (IRS) docking proteins. Two major downstream pathways are the IRS–phosphatidylinositol 3-kinase (PI3K)–Akt pathway and the Ras–mitogen-activated protein kinase (MAPK)/MAPK kinase (MEK)–extracellular signal-regulated kinase (ERK) pathway, both of which are implicated in the neurobiology of depression [89]. Insulin also influences mood by regulating adult neurogenesis. Insulin receptors are highly expressed in the hippocampus and olfactory bulb, both regions characterized by robust neurogenesis during adulthood [90]. Insulin not only acts as a growth factor itself but also enhances levels of other neurotrophic and angiogenic factors—such as brain-derived neurotrophic factor (BDNF), vascular endothelial growth factor (VEGF), and insulin-like growth factor 1 (IGF-1)—that contribute to hippocampal neurogenesis. Thus, insulin resistance may impair neuroplasticity in brain regions critical for mood regulation by disrupting central insulin signaling [91]. Monoaminergic systems also mediate the relationship between insulin and mood. For instance, dopamine release in response to amphetamine is diminished under insulin-deficient conditions, suggesting that insulin signaling modulates dopaminergic neurotransmission [92]. Moreover, circulating insulin levels affect the activity of norepinephrine and serotonin transporters, thereby influencing extracellular concentrations of these monoamines [93].

Clinical studies have shown that insulin administration can improve depressive symptoms. Intravenous insulin infusions have been associated with increased hippocampal neuronal activity and mood enhancement [94]. Intranasal insulin administration has also been shown to improve mood and cognitive function in healthy controls, patients with obesity, and those with Alzheimer's disease [95]. Based on these findings, pharmacologic agents used for diabetes treatment—such as glucagon-like peptide-1 (GLP-1) receptor agonists and insulin sensitizers like pioglitazone—are being explored for use in patients with depression. Notably, the antidepressant effects of pioglitazone have been correlated with improvements in insulin resistance, and other studies have reported a relationship between the severity of insulin resistance and the intensity of depressive symptoms [93].

Therefore, insulin resistance appears to be a critical factor in the interplay between obesity and depression, and ongoing research into insulin-sensitizing medications may reveal novel therapeutic strategies for treating depressive disorders.

Orexin

Another potential mediator of the relationship between depression and obesity is orexin A. Orexin A is synthesized primarily in the hypothalamus and the perifornical area, and it exerts its effects by binding to two types of central nervous system receptors: OX1R and OX2R. Orexin plays a crucial role in regulating the sleep–wake cycle, feeding behavior, and energy homeostasis [96]. It helps maintain wakefulness during periods of fasting or caloric restriction. Evidence from animal models of depression has shown reduced levels of orexin A, suggesting that this neuropeptide may be involved in the link between depression and obesity. Decreased orexin A activity in depressive states may lead to dysregulation of arousal, feeding, and energy balance, thereby contributing to both mood disturbances and metabolic abnormalities [97].

Inflammatory Signaling

Obesity is widely recognized as a state of chronic low-grade systemic inflammation. Depression is highly prevalent among patients with comorbid chronic inflammatory conditions, such as obesity, diabetes, and autoimmune diseases. These patients frequently display elevated levels of inflammatory markers, including C-reactive protein (CRP) and interleukin-1β, which may contribute to the severity of depression and its clinical manifestations [98, 99].

Neuroinflammation is thought to play a pivotal role in stress-related conditions, including depression and obesity [100]; from a pathophysiological perspective, depression and obesity share a common proinflammatory cascade as well as structural and functional abnormalities in cortical and subcortical regions implicated in affective and cognitive functions [101]. In individuals with obesity, the levels of pro-inflammatory cytokines—such as interleukin-1β (IL-1β), tumor necrosis factor-α (TNF-α), interleukin-6 (IL-6), and C-reactive protein (CRP)—as well as inflammatory signaling activity are elevated. Emerging evidence suggests a potential link between affective neural circuits and inflammatory markers in patients with depression and obesity. This association between inflammatory biomarkers and neural targets may serve as a predictive factor for depression and anxiety in individuals with obesity, as well [102]. Multiple mechanisms contribute to the increase in inflammation associated with obesity.

White adipose tissue (WAT), particularly visceral fat, plays a central role in this process. A strong correlation exists between visceral fat accumulation and circulating cytokine levels. Adipocytes, along with infiltrating immune cells such as macrophages and T cells, accumulate in WAT and release pro-inflammatory mediators [103]. In diet-induced obesity, an increase in the number and size of adipocytes is accompanied by immunologic changes. Macrophages in adipose tissue polarize toward the pro-inflammatory M1 phenotype, leading to increased secretion of cytokines and reactive oxygen species (ROS). Obesity also skews T-cell responses toward a Th1-dominant state, further promoting inflammation [104]. Obesity activates the innate immune system through toll-like receptors (TLRs), especially TLR4. Free fatty acids can bind to TLR4 and activate transcription factors such as nuclear factor κB (NF-κB) and activator protein-1 (AP-1), which upregulate the expression of pro-inflammatory cytokines and chemokines [105]. Inflammation induced by obesity is not limited to adipose tissue—it also affects other organs such as the liver, pancreas, and skeletal muscle. For instance, hepatic inflammation alters metabolic function and promotes the polarization of Kupffer cells toward a pro-inflammatory phenotype. The combined effects of unhealthy dietary behaviors and liver metabolic disturbances lead to elevated circulating inflammatory mediators, contributing to obesity-related metabolic inflammation [106].

Emerging evidence also implicates alterations in the gut microbiota in the pathogenesis of obesity, particularly through inflammatory and metabolic pathways as well as effects on energy homeostasis [107, 108]. In animal models of depression, including chronic social defeat stress and maternal separation, alterations in the gut microbiota have been linked to depressive behaviors, decreased levels of serotonin (5-HT), and heightened neuroinflammation. Administration of probiotics, prebiotics, or specific gut microbiota strains has been shown to ameliorate these depressive behaviors, highlighting the therapeutic potential of targeting the gut–brain axis [109].

Obesity is associated with increased proportions of lipopolysaccharide (LPS)-bearing species such as Firmicutes and Enterobacteriaceae, along with reduced Bacteroidetes and overall microbial diversity. These changes compromise the integrity of the intestinal epithelial barrier, allowing translocation of bacterial components such as LPS, which then activate macrophages and elevate pro-inflammatory cytokine production. Elevated systemic LPS levels—termed "metabolic endotoxemia"—along with increased free fatty acids in organs such as the liver, adipose tissue, and muscle, stimulate pro-inflammatory M1 macrophages and exacerbate tissue inflammation [110]. Moreover, the NOD-like receptor protein 3 (NLRP3) inflammasome and other immune mechanisms have been associated with depression, particularly in response to chronic stressors. Inflammation-induced depressive behaviors may be modulated by caspase-1 inhibition and alterations in the gut microbiota [111, 112]. However, a pilot study of fecal microbiota transplantation in patients with obesity demonstrated changes in microbiome composition and bile acid profiles; however, no significant reduction in body mass index (BMI) was observed [113].

The central nervous system is also affected by this systemic inflammatory state. In obesity, both peripheral-to-central signaling and neuroimmune responses are altered. The protective function of the blood–brain barrier (BBB) against peripheral inflammation is compromised [114], and the blood–cerebrospinal fluid (CSF) barrier at the choroid plexus is also disrupted [115]. Changes in the concentrations of peripheral mediators—such as leptin, insulin, fatty acids, and cytokines—can influence the cellular phenotype within the brain. Microglia, the resident immune cells of the central nervous system, are activated by saturated and monounsaturated fatty acids through the TLR4/NF-κB signaling pathway, resulting in cytokine production and ROS generation [116]. Astrocytes, too, can be stimulated by saturated fatty acids to produce IL-6 and TNF-α [117].

The hypothalamus is particularly susceptible to these inflammatory changes in obesity [118]. The arcuate nucleus of the hypothalamus plays a critical role in energy homeostasis by integrating peripheral metabolic signals such as leptin, insulin, and ghrelin. However, this regulatory function is disrupted by obesity-induced neuroinflammation [118]. High-fat diets can increase gliosis within just 1 week, and even a single day of high-fat intake has been shown to increase microglial activation in the hypothalamus. Obesity also leads to increased expression of IL-6 and TNF-α in the hypothalamus and is associated with activation of the IKKβ/NF-κB pathway due to endoplasmic reticulum (ER) stress [118]. Importantly, the effects of obesity-induced neuroinflammation are not restricted to the hypothalamus. Similar neuroinflammatory processes—characterized by increased IKKβ/NF-κB signaling, upregulated pro-inflammatory cytokine expression, and increased microglial and astrocytic activation—have also been observed in the hippocampus and cerebral cortex of obese animal models [119].

Numerous studies have investigated changes in inflammatory biomarkers in individuals with depression. These studies suggest that elevated levels of pro-inflammatory cytokines may induce depressive symptoms. In patients with depression, increased levels of cytokines such as interleukin-1 (IL-1), IL-6, and tumor necrosis factor-α (TNF-α), as well as markers like C-reactive protein (CRP), chemokines, and adhesion molecules have been reported [120]. The depressogenic effects of cytokines are believed to be mediated through the disruption of monoaminergic neurotransmission, impairment of neuronal growth and survival, and alterations in hypothalamic–pituitary–adrenal (HPA) axis function. Cytokines influence mood by modulating the activity of key enzymes such as indoleamine 2,3-dioxygenase (IDO) and GTP-cyclohydrolase 1 (GTP-CH1), which regulate the synthesis, transport, and metabolism of monoamine neurotransmitters [121]. For example, the kynurenine pathway, modulated by proinflammatory cytokines, has been implicated in linking inflammation to serotonin dysregulation in depression [122]. Cytokine-induced stimulation of IDO accelerates the catabolism of tryptophan, leading to decreased serotonin production and increased levels of kynurenine—a neurotoxic metabolite within the glutamatergic pathway—thus contributing to the development of depressive symptoms [123]. Immune activation also affects the synthesis of tetrahydrobiopterin (BH4), an essential cofactor in the production of dopamine and serotonin, by altering GTP-CH1 activity. This shift favors the production of neopterin at the expense of BH4 [124]. As a result, cytokine-mediated activation of GTP-CH1 inhibits monoaminergic neurotransmission. Supporting this mechanism, studies have shown that patients with depression exhibit elevated levels of neurotoxic kynurenine metabolites [125], decreased concentrations of BH4 [126], and a positive correlation between neopterin levels and the frequency of depressive episodes (Fig. 10.1) [127]. In addition, high-density lipoprotein (HDL) and low-density lipoprotein (LDL) cholesterol have been shown to exert distinct and opposing effects on lipopolysaccharide-induced neuroinflammation. Furthermore, HDL cholesterol and cholesteryl ester, along with the tryptophan–kynurenine pathway, have been proposed as potential blood biomarkers in first-episode, drug-naïve patients with major depression [128, 129]. Recent findings also suggest that LDL cholesterol may serve

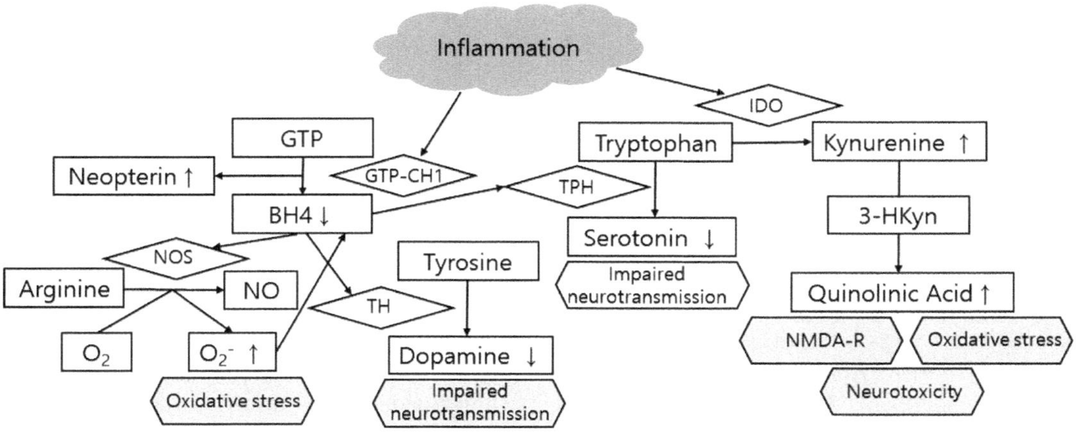

Fig. 10.1 Inflammation-induced alterations in monoamine neurotransmission. Inflammatory processes activate GTP-cyclohydrolase-1 (GTP-CH1), leading to reduced production of tetrahydrobiopterin (BH4), an essential cofactor for tyrosine hydroxylase (TH) and tryptophan hydroxylase (TPH). Consequently, diminished BH4 availability impairs dopamine and serotonin synthesis. Furthermore, reduced BH4 levels suppress nitric oxide synthase activity, thereby increasing oxidative stress, which in turn further depletes BH4. Inflammatory cytokines also activate indoleamine 2,3-dioxygenase (IDO) in macrophages, monocytes, and microglia, accelerating the catabolism of tryptophan into kynurenine. This process not only decreases serotonin availability but also generates neuroactive metabolites such as 3-hydroxykynurenine (3-HK) and quinolinic acid. These metabolites stimulate N-methyl-D-aspartate (NMDA) receptors and promote oxidative stress, thereby exacerbating neurotoxic effects and contributing to the pathophysiology of depression.

as a potential biomarker for pathological social withdrawal [130].

Neuroinflammation also negatively impacts neuronal growth and survival. Pro-inflammatory cytokines induce excitotoxicity by stimulating glutamate N-methyl-D-aspartate (NMDA) receptors, thereby suppressing the production of brain-derived neurotrophic factor (BDNF) [131]. Additionally, cytokine-induced oxidative stress damages glial cells in mood-regulating brain regions such as the prefrontal cortex and amygdala [132]. Beyond impairing neuroplasticity, cytokines also disrupt the functioning of the HPA axis, which is known to be central to depression. During inflammation, glucocorticoid resistance can develop due to the inhibition of glucocorticoid receptor (GR) activity at glucocorticoid response elements (GREs) [133]. Several molecular pathways mediate this cytokine-induced glucocorticoid resistance. Activation of IL-1 receptors leads to phosphorylation of mitogen-activated protein kinase kinases (MAPKK or MEK), which subsequently activate MAPKs and Jun N-terminal kinases (JNKs). These, in turn, activate the transcription factor c-JUN, a component of the AP-1 complex, which interferes with GR–GRE interactions [120]. Similarly, TNF receptor activation triggers a signaling cascade that activates IKKβ, resulting in phosphorylation and degradation of IκB from the IκB–NF-κB complex. The liberated NF-κB translocates to the nucleus, where it disrupts GR function [134]. Additionally, activation of interferon receptors phosphorylates Janus kinase-1 (Jak1), which then activates STAT5. Like NF-κB, STAT5 translocates to the nucleus and impairs GR–GRE interactions [135]. Collectively, these pathways demonstrate that cytokine signaling-via inflammatory mediators like NF-κB-interferes with GR expression and activity. This cytokine-induced glucocorticoid resistance contributes to the onset and persistence of depressive symptoms [136].

The impact of inflammation on depression may vary by individual susceptibility. In physiologically vulnerable individuals, even low-grade inflammation may be sufficient to trigger depressive symptoms. This phenomenon is referred to as "immune response element amplification" and is characterized by features such as diminished parasympathetic signaling, reduced BDNF production, impaired negative feedback regulation of the HPA axis, heightened anterior cingulate and amygdala reactivity to social threats, and reduced hippocampal volume—all of which are consistent with known biological markers of major depressive disorder [137].

Oxidative and Nitrosative Stress

Mitochondria are responsible for cellular energy production, and in this process, reactive oxygen species (ROS) and reactive nitrogen species (RNS) are generated. ROS and RNS play important roles in regulating various cellular functions. However, when there is an imbalance between their production and the antioxidant defense systems responsible for their elimination, these reactive species accumulate, resulting in damage to cellular components, excessive autoimmune responses, and ultimately cellular dysfunction [138]. In obesity, oxidative stress is increased, while antioxidant defenses are impaired. This imbalance is driven by multiple obesity-related factors, including high-fat and high-carbohydrate diets. Mechanisms such as endoplasmic reticulum (ER) stress in adipocytes and the activation of intracellular signaling systems such as nicotinamide adenine dinucleotide (NADH)/nicotinamide adenine dinucleotide phosphate (NADPH) oxidase contribute to enhanced oxidative stress. ROS-mediated oxidative signaling promotes adipogenesis, further contributing to the development of obesity. In turn, obesity exacerbates ROS generation through mechanisms such as chronic adipose tissue inflammation, fatty acid oxidation, cellular damage accumulation, and changes in mitochondrial activity and diet composition. As such, obesity and oxidative stress create a vicious cycle of mutual reinforcement [139]. Moreover, ROS modulate redox-sensitive transcription factors, including nuclear factor-κB (NF-κB) and activator protein-1 (AP-1), thereby stimulating the production of pro-inflammatory cytokines. This further amplifies ROS generation, sustaining a self-perpetuating cycle of oxidative and inflammatory damage [138–140]. Oxidative stress is also closely associated with depression [141]. Depression has been linked to reduced activity of enzymes involved in the mitochondrial respiratory chain, decreased ATP production, and other mitochondrial dysfunctions, which result in the accumulation of free radicals [142]. Mitochondrial impairments increase the production of ROS and RNS and disturb calcium homeostasis, all of which contribute to the pathophysiology of depression. In patients with depression, several biomarkers of oxidative and nitrosative stress are altered, including malondialdehyde, glutathione, NF-κB, and superoxide dismutase (SOD), while overall antioxidant capacity is reduced [142].

Taken together, these findings suggest that oxidative and nitrosative stress plays a significant role in both depression and obesity. By disrupting redox balance and inflammatory signaling pathways, these stress responses may provide a common biological ground for the co-occurrence and mutual reinforcement of both disorders.

10.6 Summary

The bidirectional relationship between obesity and depression is underpinned by a wide range of complex and multifaceted mechanisms. These include neurobiological factors such as leptin resistance, insulin dysregulation, inflammatory signaling pathways, and dysfunction of the hypothalamic–pituitary–adrenal (HPA) axis, which together contribute to the shared pathophysiology of both conditions (Fig. 10.2). It is also important to note that beyond these biological mechanisms, a variety of behavioral and psychosocial factors similarly contribute to both obesity and depression.

This chapter focused primarily on biological pathways that have been relatively well-studied in both disorders. However, other mechanisms not covered in this review may also mediate the association between obesity and depression [63]. Given the growing evidence of overlapping pathophysiological processes, some researchers have proposed the concept of a "metabolic subtype" or "obesity subtype" of depression [143]. This framework may offer valuable insights in clinical practice. For instance, individuals with comorbid obesity and depression often have poorer antidepressant treatment outcomes [144, 145], and improvements in depressive symptoms may promote weight loss, or vice versa [146].

Therefore, clinicians should assess for the presence of depression in patients with obesity, and similarly evaluate for obesity in patients with depression, incorporating these findings into treatment planning. In patients with comorbid

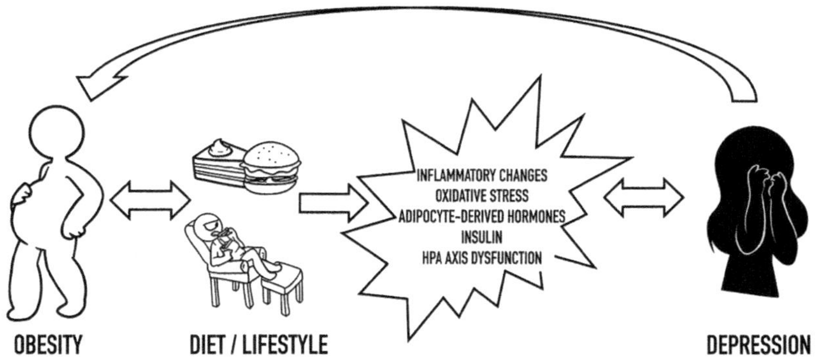

Fig. 10.2 Factors influencing obesity and depression. Obesity is associated with depression through multiple mechanisms, including inflammatory changes, oxidative stress, and dysfunction of the hypothalamic–pituitary–adrenal (HPA) axis. Through these mechanisms, obesity and depression bidirectionally increase the risk of developing one another

depression and obesity, additional risk factors—such as maladaptive eating behaviors that influence both disorders—should also be evaluated and addressed. Interventions aimed at preventing further weight gain should be considered an essential component of comprehensive care for these individuals.

Declarations

Competing Interests The author(s) has no competing interests to declare that are relevant to the content of this manuscript.

Ethics Approval The author(s) declares that this manuscript does not include primary research with human participants.

The author(s) declares that this manuscript does not include primary studies involving animals.

References

1. Gavin AR, Simon GE, Ludman EJ. The association between obesity, depression, and educational attainment in women: the mediating role of body image dissatisfaction. J Psychosom Res. 2010;69(6):573–81. https://doi.org/10.1016/j.jpsychores.2010.05.001.
2. Moore ME, Stunkard A, Srole L. Obesity, social class, and mental illness. JAMA. 1962;181:962–6.
3. Crisp AH, McGuiness B. Jolly fat: relation between obesity and psychoneurosis in general population. Br Med J. 1976;1(6000):7–9.
4. Friedman MA, Brownell KD. Psychological correlates of obesity: moving to the next research generation. Psychol Bull. 1995;117(1):3–20.
5. Vittengl JR. Mediation of the bidirectional relations between obesity and depression among women. Psychiatry Res. 2018;264:254–9. https://doi.org/10.1016/j.psychres.2018.03.023.
6. de Wit L, Luppino F, van Straten A, Penninx B, Zitman F, Cuijpers P. Depression and obesity: a meta-analysis of community-based studies. Psychiatry Res. 2010;178(2):230–5. https://doi.org/10.1016/j.psychres.2009.04.015.
7. Atlantis E, Baker M. Obesity effects on depression: systematic review of epidemiological studies. Int J Obes. 2008;32(6):881–91. https://doi.org/10.1038/ijo.2008.54.
8. Roberts RE, Deleger S, Strawbridge WJ, Kaplan GA. Prospective association between obesity and depression: evidence from the Alameda County study. Int J Obes Relat Metab Disord. 2003;27(4):514–21. https://doi.org/10.1038/sj.ijo.0802204.
9. Kasen S, Cohen P, Chen H, Must A. Obesity and psychopathology in women: a three decade prospective study. Int J Obes. 2008;32(3):558–66. https://doi.org/10.1038/sj.ijo.0803736.
10. Godin O, Elbejjani M, Kaufman JS. Body mass index, blood pressure, and risk of depression in the elderly: a marginal structural model. Am J Epidemiol. 2012;176(3):204–13. https://doi.org/10.1093/aje/kws003.
11. Bjerkeset O, Romundstad P, Evans J, Gunnell D. Association of adult body mass index and height with anxiety, depression, and suicide in the general population: the HUNT study. Am J Epidemiol. 2008;167(2):193–202. https://doi.org/10.1093/aje/kwm280.
12. Luppino FS, de Wit LM, Bouvy PF, Stijnen T, Cuijpers P, Penninx BW, et al. Overweight, obesity, and depression: a systematic review and meta-analysis of longitudinal studies. Arch Gen Psychiatry. 2010;67(3):220–9. https://doi.org/10.1001/archgenpsychiatry.2010.2.
13. Fowler-Brown AG, Ngo LH, Wee CC. The relationship between symptoms of depression and body weight in younger adults. Obesity (Silver Spring). 2012;20(9):1922–8. https://doi.org/10.1038/oby.2011.311.
14. Ball K, Burton NW, Brown WJ. A prospective study of overweight, physical activity, and depressive symptoms in young women. Obesity (Silver Spring). 2009;17(1):66–71. https://doi.org/10.1038/oby.2008.497.
15. Hamer M, Batty GD, Kivimaki M. Risk of future depression in people who are obese but metabolically healthy: the English longitudinal study of ageing. Mol Psychiatry. 2012;17(9):940–5. https://doi.org/10.1038/mp.2012.30.
16. Pine DS, Cohen P, Brook J, Coplan JD. Psychiatric symptoms in adolescence as predictors of obesity in early adulthood: a longitudinal study. Am J Public Health. 1997;87(8):1303–10.
17. Barefoot JC, Heitmann BL, Helms MJ, Williams RB, Surwit RS, Siegler IC. Symptoms of depression and changes in body weight from adolescence to mid-life. Int J Obes Relat Metab Disord. 1998;22(7):688–94.
18. Bardone AM, Moffitt TE, Caspi A, Dickson N, Stanton WR, Silva PA. Adult physical health outcomes of adolescent girls with conduct disorder, depression, and anxiety. J Am Acad Child Adolesc Psychiatry. 1998;37(6):594–601. https://doi.org/10.1097/00004583-199806000-00009.
19. Goodman E, Whitaker RC. A prospective study of the role of depression in the development and persistence of adolescent obesity. Pediatrics. 2002;110(3):497–504.
20. Vogelzangs N, Kritchevsky SB, Beekman AT, Newman AB, Satterfield S, Simonsick EM, et al. Depressive symptoms and change in abdominal obesity in older persons. Arch Gen

Psychiatry. 2008;65(12):1386–93. https://doi.org/10.1001/archpsyc.65.12.1386.
21. Richardson LP, Davis R, Poulton R, McCauley E, Moffitt TE, Caspi A, et al. A longitudinal evaluation of adolescent depression and adult obesity. Arch Pediatr Adolesc Med. 2003;157(8):739–45. https://doi.org/10.1001/archpedi.157.8.739.
22. Hasler G, Pine DS, Kleinbaum DG, Gamma A, Luckenbaugh D, Ajdacic V, et al. Depressive symptoms during childhood and adult obesity: the Zurich cohort study. Mol Psychiatry. 2005;10(9):842–50. https://doi.org/10.1038/sj.mp.4001671.
23. Blaine B. Does depression cause obesity?: a meta-analysis of longitudinal studies of depression and weight control. J Health Psychol. 2008;13(8):1190–7. https://doi.org/10.1177/1359105308095977.
24. Pistis G, Milaneschi Y, Vandeleur CL, Lasserre AM, Penninx B, Lamers F, et al. Obesity and atypical depression symptoms: findings from Mendelian randomization in two European cohorts. Transl Psychiatry. 2021;11(1):96. https://doi.org/10.1038/s41398-021-01236-7.
25. Geschwind DH, Flint J. Genetics and genomics of psychiatric disease. Science. 2015;349(6255):1489–94. https://doi.org/10.1126/science.aaa8954.
26. Stunkard AJ, Foch TT, Hrubec Z. A twin study of human obesity. JAMA. 1986;256(1):51–4.
27. Wheeler E, Huang N, Bochukova EG, Keogh JM, Lindsay S, Garg S, et al. Genome-wide SNP and CNV analysis identifies common and low-frequency variants associated with severe early-onset obesity. Nat Genet. 2013;45(5):513–7. https://doi.org/10.1038/ng.2607.
28. Pearce LR, Atanassova N, Banton MC, Bottomley B, van der Klaauw AA, Revelli JP, et al. KSR2 mutations are associated with obesity, insulin resistance, and impaired cellular fuel oxidation. Cell. 2013;155(4):765–77. https://doi.org/10.1016/j.cell.2013.09.058.
29. Locke AE, Kahali B, Berndt SI, Justice AE, Pers TH, Day FR, et al. Genetic studies of body mass index yield new insights for obesity biology. Nature. 2015;518(7538):197–206. https://doi.org/10.1038/nature14177.
30. Afari N, Noonan C, Goldberg J, Roy-Byrne P, Schur E, Golnari G, et al. Depression and obesity: do shared genes explain the relationship? Depress Anxiety. 2010;27(9):799–806. https://doi.org/10.1002/da.20704.
31. Rivera M, Locke AE, Corre T, Czamara D, Wolf C, Ching-Lopez A, et al. Interaction between the FTO gene, body mass index and depression: meta-analysis of 13701 individuals. Br J Psychiatry. 2017;211(2):70–6. https://doi.org/10.1192/bjp.bp.116.183475.
32. consortium C. Sparse whole-genome sequencing identifies two loci for major depressive disorder. Nature. 2015;523(7562):588–91. https://doi.org/10.1038/nature14659.
33. Sookoian S, Gemma C, Garcia SI, Gianotti TF, Dieuzeide G, Roussos A, et al. Short allele of serotonin transporter gene promoter is a risk factor for obesity in adolescents. Obesity (Silver Spring). 2007;15(2):271–6. https://doi.org/10.1038/oby.2007.519.
34. Fuemmeler BF, Agurs-Collins TD, McClernon FJ, Kollins SH, Kail ME, Bergen AW, et al. Genes implicated in serotonergic and dopaminergic functioning predict BMI categories. Obesity (Silver Spring). 2008;16(2):348–55. https://doi.org/10.1038/oby.2007.65.
35. Owens M, Harrison AJ, Burkhouse KL, McGeary JE, Knopik VS, Palmer RH, et al. Eye tracking indices of attentional bias in children of depressed mothers: polygenic influences help to clarify previous mixed findings. Dev Psychopathol. 2016;28(2):385–97. https://doi.org/10.1017/S0954579415000462.
36. Preiss K, Brennan L, Clarke D. A systematic review of variables associated with the relationship between obesity and depression. Obes Rev. 2013;14(11):906–18. https://doi.org/10.1111/obr.12052.
37. Musante GJ, Costanzo PR, Friedman KE. The comorbidity of depression and eating dysregulation processes in a diet-seeking obese population: a matter of gender specificity. Int J Eat Disord. 1998;23(1):65–75.
38. Beydoun MA, Wang Y. Pathways linking socioeconomic status to obesity through depression and lifestyle factors among young US adults. J Affect Disord. 2010;123(1–3):52–63. https://doi.org/10.1016/j.jad.2009.09.021.
39. Siegel JM, Yancey AK, McCarthy WJ. Overweight and depressive symptoms among African-American women. Prev Med. 2000;31(3):232–40. https://doi.org/10.1006/pmed.2000.0712.
40. Jorm AF, Korten AE, Christensen H, Jacomb PA, Rodgers B, Parslow RA. Association of obesity with anxiety, depression and emotional well-being: a community survey. Aust N Z J Public Health. 2003;27(4):434–40.
41. Cottone P, Sabino V, Roberto M, Bajo M, Pockros L, Frihauf JB, et al. CRF system recruitment mediates dark side of compulsive eating. Proc Natl Acad Sci USA. 2009;106(47):20016–20. https://doi.org/10.1073/pnas.0908789106.
42. Macht M. How emotions affect eating: a five-way model. Appetite. 2008;50(1):1–11. https://doi.org/10.1016/j.appet.2007.07.002.
43. Gibson EL. Emotional influences on food choice: sensory, physiological and psychological pathways. Physiol Behav. 2006;89(1):53–61. https://doi.org/10.1016/j.physbeh.2006.01.024.
44. Adam TC, Epel ES. Stress, eating and the reward system. Physiol Behav. 2007;91(4):449–58. https://doi.org/10.1016/j.physbeh.2007.04.011.
45. Dallman MF. Stress-induced obesity and the emotional nervous system. Trends Endocrinol Metab.

2010;21(3):159–65. https://doi.org/10.1016/j.tem.2009.10.004.
46. Sanchez-Villegas A, Martinez-Gonzalez MA. Diet, a new target to prevent depression? BMC Med. 2013;11:3. https://doi.org/10.1186/1741-7015-11-3.
47. Edwards R, Peet M, Shay J, Horrobin D. Omega-3 polyunsaturated fatty acid levels in the diet and in red blood cell membranes of depressed patients. J Affect Disord. 1998;48(2–3):149–55.
48. Lin PY, Su KP. A meta-analytic review of double-blind, placebo-controlled trials of antidepressant efficacy of omega-3 fatty acids. J Clin Psychiatry. 2007;68(7):1056–61.
49. Posey KA, Clegg DJ, Printz RL, Byun J, Morton GJ, Vivekanandan-Giri A, et al. Hypothalamic proinflammatory lipid accumulation, inflammation, and insulin resistance in rats fed a high-fat diet. Am J Physiol Endocrinol Metab. 2009;296(5):E1003–12. https://doi.org/10.1152/ajpendo.90377.2008.
50. Kleinridders A, Schenten D, Konner AC, Belgardt BF, Mauer J, Okamura T, et al. MyD88 signaling in the CNS is required for development of fatty acid-induced leptin resistance and diet-induced obesity. Cell Metab. 2009;10(4):249–59. https://doi.org/10.1016/j.cmet.2009.08.013.
51. Tsuboi H, Watanabe M, Kobayashi F, Kimura K, Kinae N. Associations of depressive symptoms with serum proportions of palmitic and arachidonic acids, and alpha-tocopherol effects among male population–a preliminary study. Clin Nutr. 2013;32(2):289–93. https://doi.org/10.1016/j.clnu.2012.07.011.
52. Keddie AM. Associations between severe obesity and depression: results from the National Health and nutrition examination survey, 2005–2006. Prev Chronic Dis. 2011;8(3):A57.
53. Ma J, Xiao L. Obesity and depression in US women: results from the 2005–2006 national health and nutritional examination survey. Obesity (Silver Spring). 2010;18(2):347–53. https://doi.org/10.1038/oby.2009.213.
54. Barry D, Pietrzak RH, Petry NM. Gender differences in associations between body mass index and DSM-IV mood and anxiety disorders: results from the National Epidemiologic Survey on alcohol and related conditions. Ann Epidemiol. 2008;18(6):458–66. https://doi.org/10.1016/j.annepidem.2007.12.009.
55. Johnston E, Johnson S, McLeod P, Johnston M. The relation of body mass index to depressive symptoms. Can J Public Health. 2004;95(3):179–83.
56. Markowitz S, Friedman MA, Arent SM. Understanding the relation between obesity and depression: causal mechanisms and implications for treatment. Clin Psychol Sci Pract. 2008;15(1):1–20.
57. Vasconcelos I, von Hafe M, Adao R, Leite-Moreira A, Bras-Silva C. Corticotropin-releasing hormone and obesity: from fetal life to adulthood. Obes Rev. 2024;25(8):e13763. https://doi.org/10.1111/obr.13763.
58. Dooley LN, Kuhlman KR, Robles TF, Eisenberger NI, Craske MG, Bower JE. The role of inflammation in core features of depression: insights from paradigms using exogenously-induced inflammation. Neurosci Biobehav Rev. 2018;94:219–37. https://doi.org/10.1016/j.neubiorev.2018.09.006.
59. Su KP, Lai HC, Peng CY, Su WP, Chang JP, Pariante CM. Interferon-alpha-induced depression: comparisons between early- and late-onset subgroups and with patients with major depressive disorder. Brain Behav Immun. 2019;80:512–8. https://doi.org/10.1016/j.bbi.2019.04.032.
60. Incollingo Rodriguez AC, Epel ES, White ML, Standen EC, Seckl JR, Tomiyama AJ. Hypothalamic-pituitary-adrenal axis dysregulation and cortisol activity in obesity: a systematic review. Psychoneuroendocrinology. 2015;62:301–18. https://doi.org/10.1016/j.psyneuen.2015.08.014.
61. Herman JP, Figueiredo H, Mueller NK, Ulrich-Lai Y, Ostrander MM, Choi DC, et al. Central mechanisms of stress integration: hierarchical circuitry controlling hypothalamo-pituitary-adrenocortical responsiveness. Front Neuroendocrinol. 2003;24(3):151–80.
62. Gregus A, Wintink AJ, Davis AC, Kalynchuk LE. Effect of repeated corticosterone injections and restraint stress on anxiety and depression-like behavior in male rats. Behav Brain Res. 2005;156(1):105–14. https://doi.org/10.1016/j.bbr.2004.05.013.
63. Hryhorczuk C, Sharma S, Fulton SE. Metabolic disturbances connecting obesity and depression. Front Neurosci. 2013;7:177. https://doi.org/10.3389/fnins.2013.00177.
64. Wallace C, Krugman R. More than what you eat: a review on the association between childhood maltreatment and elevated adult BMI. Curr Nutr Rep. 2024;13(3):377–81. https://doi.org/10.1007/s13668-024-00558-4.
65. Wyrwoll CS, Holmes MC, Seckl JR. 11beta-hydroxysteroid dehydrogenases and the brain: from zero to hero, a decade of progress. Front Neuroendocrinol. 2011;32(3):265–86. https://doi.org/10.1016/j.yfrne.2010.12.001.
66. Dekker MJ, Tiemeier H, Luijendijk HJ, Kuningas M, Hofman A, de Jong FH, et al. The effect of common genetic variation in 11beta-hydroxysteroid dehydrogenase type 1 on hypothalamic-pituitary-adrenal axis activity and incident depression. J Clin Endocrinol Metab. 2012;97(2):E233–7. https://doi.org/10.1210/jc.2011-0601.
67. Slattery DA, Uzunov DP, Cryan JF. 11-beta hydroxysteroid type 1 knockout mice display an antidepressant-like phenotype in the forced swim test. Acta Neuropsychiatr. 2016;28(1):55–60. https://doi.org/10.1017/neu.2015.50.
68. Willner P. Chronic mild stress (CMS) revisited: consistency and behavioural-neurobiological

concordance in the effects of CMS. Neuropsychobiology. 2005;52(2):90–110. https://doi.org/10.1159/000087097.
69. Yamada N, Katsuura G, Ochi Y, Ebihara K, Kusakabe T, Hosoda K, et al. Impaired CNS leptin action is implicated in depression associated with obesity. Endocrinology. 2011;152(7):2634–43. https://doi.org/10.1210/en.2011-0004.
70. Lu XY, Kim CS, Frazer A, Zhang W. Leptin: a potential novel antidepressant. Proc Natl Acad Sci USA. 2006;103(5):1593–8. https://doi.org/10.1073/pnas.0508901103.
71. Carvalho AF, Rocha DQ, McIntyre RS, Mesquita LM, Kohler CA, Hyphantis TN, et al. Adipokines as emerging depression biomarkers: a systematic review and meta-analysis. J Psychiatr Res. 2014;59:28–37. https://doi.org/10.1016/j.jpsychires.2014.08.002.
72. Lu XY. The leptin hypothesis of depression: a potential link between mood disorders and obesity? Curr Opin Pharmacol. 2007;7(6):648–52. https://doi.org/10.1016/j.coph.2007.10.010.
73. Munzberg H, Myers MG Jr. Molecular and anatomical determinants of central leptin resistance. Nat Neurosci. 2005;8(5):566–70. https://doi.org/10.1038/nn1454.
74. Myers MG Jr, Heymsfield SB, Haft C, Kahn BB, Laughlin M, Leibel RL, et al. Challenges and opportunities of defining clinical leptin resistance. Cell Metab. 2012;15(2):150–6. https://doi.org/10.1016/j.cmet.2012.01.002.
75. Ge JF, Qi CC, Zhou JN. Imbalance of leptin pathway and hypothalamus synaptic plasticity markers are associated with stress-induced depression in rats. Behav Brain Res. 2013;249:38–43. https://doi.org/10.1016/j.bbr.2013.04.020.
76. Huang Q, Rivest R, Richard D. Effects of leptin on corticotropin-releasing factor (CRF) synthesis and CRF neuron activation in the paraventricular hypothalamic nucleus of obese (ob/ob) mice. Endocrinology. 1998;139(4):1524–32. https://doi.org/10.1210/endo.139.4.5889.
77. Guo M, Huang TY, Garza JC, Chua SC, Lu XY. Selective deletion of leptin receptors in adult hippocampus induces depression-related behaviours. Int J Neuropsychopharmacol. 2013;16(4):857–67. https://doi.org/10.1017/S1461145712000703.
78. Leinninger GM, Jo YH, Leshan RL, Louis GW, Yang H, Barrera JG, et al. Leptin acts via leptin receptor-expressing lateral hypothalamic neurons to modulate the mesolimbic dopamine system and suppress feeding. Cell Metab. 2009;10(2):89–98. https://doi.org/10.1016/j.cmet.2009.06.011.
79. Fulton S, Pissios P, Manchon RP, Stiles L, Frank L, Pothos EN, et al. Leptin regulation of the mesoaccumbens dopamine pathway. Neuron. 2006;51(6):811–22. https://doi.org/10.1016/j.neuron.2006.09.006.
80. Liu J, Perez SM, Zhang W, Lodge DJ, Lu XY. Selective deletion of the leptin receptor in dopamine neurons produces anxiogenic-like behavior and increases dopaminergic activity in amygdala. Mol Psychiatry. 2011;16(10):1024–38. https://doi.org/10.1038/mp.2011.36.
81. Calapai G, Corica F, Corsonello A, Sautebin L, Di Rosa M, Campo GM, et al. Leptin increases serotonin turnover by inhibition of brain nitric oxide synthesis. J Clin Invest. 1999;104(7):975–82. https://doi.org/10.1172/JCI5867.
82. Harris RB, Zhou J, Redmann SM Jr, Smagin GN, Smith SR, Rodgers E, et al. A leptin dose-response study in obese (ob/ob) and lean (+/?) mice. Endocrinology. 1998;139(1):8–19. https://doi.org/10.1210/endo.139.1.5675.
83. Schellekens H, Clarke G, Jeffery IB, Dinan TG, Cryan JF. Dynamic 5-HT2C receptor editing in a mouse model of obesity. PLoS One. 2012;7(3):e32266. https://doi.org/10.1371/journal.pone.0032266.
84. Haleem DJ, Haque Z, Inam QU, Ikram H, Haleem MA. Behavioral, hormonal and central serotonin modulating effects of injected leptin. Peptides. 2015;74:1–8. https://doi.org/10.1016/j.peptides.2015.10.002.
85. Lehto SM, Huotari A, Niskanen L, Tolmunen T, Koivumaa-Honkanen H, Honkalampi K, et al. Serum adiponectin and resistin levels in major depressive disorder. Acta Psychiatr Scand. 2010;121(3):209–15. https://doi.org/10.1111/j.1600-0447.2009.01463.x.
86. Weber-Hamann B, Kratzsch J, Kopf D, Lederbogen F, Gilles M, Heuser I, et al. Resistin and adiponectin in major depression: the association with free cortisol and effects of antidepressant treatment. J Psychiatr Res. 2007;41(3–4, 344):–50. https://doi.org/10.1016/j.jpsychires.2006.01.002.
87. Kan C, Silva N, Golden SH, Rajala U, Timonen M, Stahl D, et al. A systematic review and meta-analysis of the association between depression and insulin resistance. Diabetes Care. 2013;36(2):480–9. https://doi.org/10.2337/dc12-1442.
88. Cha DS, Best MW, Bowie CR, Gallaugher LA, Woldeyohannes HO, Soczynska JK, et al. A randomized, double-blind, placebo-controlled, crossover trial evaluating the effect of intranasal insulin on cognition and mood in individuals with treatment-resistant major depressive disorder. J Affect Disord. 2017;210:57–65. https://doi.org/10.1016/j.jad.2016.12.006.
89. Chaudhury D, Liu H, Han MH. Neuronal correlates of depression. Cell Mol Life Sci. 2015;72(24):4825–48. https://doi.org/10.1007/s00018-015-2044-6.
90. McNay EC, Recknagel AK. Brain insulin signaling: a key component of cognitive processes and a potential basis for cognitive impairment in type 2 diabetes. Neurobiol Learn Mem. 2011;96(3):432–42. https://doi.org/10.1016/j.nlm.2011.08.005.
91. Rosenblat JD, McIntyre RS, Alves GS, Fountoulakis KN, Carvalho AF. Beyond monoamines-novel targets for treatment-resistant depression: a comprehensive review. Curr Neuropharmacol. 2015;13(5):636–55.
92. Williams JM, Owens WA, Turner GH, Saunders C, Dipace C, Blakely RD, et al. Hypoinsulinemia

regulates amphetamine-induced reverse transport of dopamine. PLoS Biol. 2007;5(10):e274. https://doi.org/10.1371/journal.pbio.0050274.
93. Kemp DE, Ismail-Beigi F, Ganocy SJ, Conroy C, Gao K, Obral S, et al. Use of insulin sensitizers for the treatment of major depressive disorder: a pilot study of pioglitazone for major depression accompanied by abdominal obesity. J Affect Disord. 2012;136(3):1164–73. https://doi.org/10.1016/j.jad.2011.06.033.
94. Rotte M, Baerecke C, Pottag G, Klose S, Kanneberg E, Heinze HJ, et al. Insulin affects the neuronal response in the medial temporal lobe in humans. Neuroendocrinology. 2005;81(1):49–55. https://doi.org/10.1159/000084874.
95. Shemesh E, Rudich A, Harman-Boehm I, Cukierman-Yaffe T. Effect of intranasal insulin on cognitive function: a systematic review. J Clin Endocrinol Metab. 2012;97(2):366–76. https://doi.org/10.1210/jc.2011-1802.
96. Chieffi S, Carotenuto M, Monda V, Valenzano A, Villano I, Precenzano F, et al. Orexin system: the key for a healthy life. Front Physiol. 2017;8:357. https://doi.org/10.3389/fphys.2017.00357.
97. Arendt DH, Ronan PJ, Oliver KD, Callahan LB, Summers TR, Summers CH. Depressive behavior and activation of the orexin/hypocretin system. Behav Neurosci. 2013;127(1):86–94. https://doi.org/10.1037/a0031442.
98. Draganov M, Arranz MJ, Salazar J, de Diego-Adelino J, Gallego-Fabrega C, Jubero M, et al. Association study of polymorphisms within inflammatory genes and methylation status in treatment response in major depression. Eur Psychiatry. 2019;60:7–13. https://doi.org/10.1016/j.eurpsy.2019.05.003.
99. Halaris A. Inflammation and depression but where does the inflammation come from? Curr Opin Psychiatry. 2019;32(5):422–8. https://doi.org/10.1097/YCO.0000000000000531.
100. Bauer ME, Teixeira AL. Inflammation in psychiatric disorders: what comes first? Ann NY Acad Sci. 2019;1437(1):57–67. https://doi.org/10.1111/nyas.13712.
101. Hallihan H, Tsai P, Lv N, Xiao L, Penalver Bernabe B, Wu Y, et al. Affective neural circuits and inflammatory markers linked to depression and anxiety symptoms in patients with comorbid obesity. J Psychiatr Res. 2023;160:9–18. https://doi.org/10.1016/j.jpsychires.2023.01.044.
102. Lv N, Hallihan H, Xiao L, Williams LM, Ajilore OA, Ma J. Association of changes in neural targets and dietary outcomes among patients with comorbid obesity and depression: post hoc analysis of ENGAGE-2 mechanistic clinical trial. J Nutr. 2023;153(3):880–96. https://doi.org/10.1016/j.tjnut.2023.01.022.
103. Langlet C, Tamoutounour S, Henri S, Luche H, Ardouin L, Gregoire C, et al. CD64 expression distinguishes monocyte-derived and conventional dendritic cells and reveals their distinct role during intramuscular immunization. J Immunol. 2012;188(4):1751–60. https://doi.org/10.4049/jimmunol.1102744.
104. Lee BC, Lee J. Cellular and molecular players in adipose tissue inflammation in the development of obesity-induced insulin resistance. Biochim Biophys Acta. 2014;1842(3):446–62. https://doi.org/10.1016/j.bbadis.2013.05.017.
105. Konner AC, Bruning JC. Toll-like receptors: linking inflammation to metabolism. Trends Endocrinol Metab. 2011;22(1):16–23. https://doi.org/10.1016/j.tem.2010.08.007.
106. Guillemot-Legris O, Muccioli GG. Obesity-induced Neuroinflammation: beyond the hypothalamus. Trends Neurosci. 2017; https://doi.org/10.1016/j.tins.2017.02.005.
107. Finelli C, Padula MC, Martelli G, Tarantino G. Could the improvement of obesity-related co-morbidities depend on modified gut hormones secretion? World J Gastroenterol. 2014;20(44):16649–64. https://doi.org/10.3748/wjg.v20.i44.16649.
108. Verdam FJ, Fuentes S, de Jonge C, Zoetendal EG, Erbil R, Greve JW, et al. Human intestinal microbiota composition is associated with local and systemic inflammation in obesity. Obesity (Silver Spring). 2013;21(12):E607–15. https://doi.org/10.1002/oby.20466.
109. Jianguo L, Xueyang J, Cui W, Changxin W, Xuemei Q. Altered gut metabolome contributes to depression-like behaviors in rats exposed to chronic unpredictable mild stress. Transl Psychiatry. 2019;9(1):40. https://doi.org/10.1038/s41398-019-0391-z.
110. Bleau C, Karelis AD, St-Pierre DH, Lamontagne L. Crosstalk between intestinal microbiota, adipose tissue and skeletal muscle as an early event in systemic low-grade inflammation and the development of obesity and diabetes. Diabetes Metab Res Rev. 2015;31(6):545–61. https://doi.org/10.1002/dmrr.2617.
111. Carlessi AS, Borba LA, Zugno AI, Quevedo J, Reus GZ. Gut microbiota-brain axis in depression: the role of neuroinflammation. Eur J Neurosci. 2021;53(1):222–35. https://doi.org/10.1111/ejn.14631.
112. Inserra A, Mastronardi CA, Rogers G, Licinio J, Wong ML. Neuroimmunomodulation in major depressive disorder: focus on caspase 1, inducible nitric oxide synthase, and interferon-Gamma. Mol Neurobiol. 2019;56(6):4288–305. https://doi.org/10.1007/s12035-018-1359-3.
113. Ribeiro FM, Silva MA, Lyssa V, Marques G, Lima HK, Franco OL, et al. The molecular signaling of exercise and obesity in the microbiota-gut-brain axis. Front Endocrinol (Lausanne). 2022;13:927170. https://doi.org/10.3389/fendo.2022.927170.
114. Stranahan AM, Hao S, Dey A, Yu X, Baban B. Blood-brain barrier breakdown promotes macrophage infiltration and cognitive impairment in leptin receptor-deficient mice. J Cereb Blood Flow Metab.

2016;36(12):2108–21. https://doi.org/10.1177/0271678X16642233.

115. Balusu S, Van Wonterghem E, De Rycke R, Raemdonck K, Stremersch S, Gevaert K, et al. Identification of a novel mechanism of blood-brain communication during peripheral inflammation via choroid plexus-derived extracellular vesicles. EMBO Mol Med. 2016;8(10):1162–83. https://doi.org/10.15252/emmm.201606271.
116. Button EB, Mitchell AS, Domingos MM, Chung JH, Bradley RM, Hashemi A, et al. Microglial cell activation increases saturated and decreases monounsaturated fatty acid content, but both lipid species are proinflammatory. Lipids. 2014;49(4):305–16. https://doi.org/10.1007/s11745-014-3882-y.
117. Gupta S, Knight AG, Gupta S, Keller JN, Bruce-Keller AJ. Saturated long-chain fatty acids activate inflammatory signaling in astrocytes. J Neurochem. 2012;120(6):1060–71. https://doi.org/10.1111/j.1471-4159.2012.07660.x.
118. Thaler JP, Yi CX, Schur EA, Guyenet SJ, Hwang BH, Dietrich MO, et al. Obesity is associated with hypothalamic injury in rodents and humans. J Clin Invest. 2012;122(1):153–62. https://doi.org/10.1172/JCI59660.
119. Carlin JL, Grissom N, Ying Z, Gomez-Pinilla F, Reyes TM. Voluntary exercise blocks Western diet-induced gene expression of the chemokines CXCL10 and CCL2 in the prefrontal cortex. Brain Behav Immun. 2016;58:82–90. https://doi.org/10.1016/j.bbi.2016.07.161.
120. Pace TW, Miller AH. Cytokines and glucocorticoid receptor signaling. Relevance to major depression. Ann NY Acad Sci. 2009;1179:86–105. https://doi.org/10.1111/j.1749-6632.2009.04984.x.
121. Capuron L, Miller AH. Immune system to brain signaling: neuropsychopharmacological implications. Pharmacol Ther. 2011;130(2):226–38. https://doi.org/10.1016/j.pharmthera.2011.01.014.
122. Davies KA, Cooper E, Voon V, Tibble J, Cercignani M, Harrison NA. Interferon and anti-TNF therapies differentially modulate amygdala reactivity which predicts associated bidirectional changes in depressive symptoms. Mol Psychiatry. 2021;26(9):5150–60. https://doi.org/10.1038/s41380-020-0790-9.
123. Dantzer R, O'Connor JC, Lawson MA, Kelley KW. Inflammation-associated depression: from serotonin to kynurenine. Psychoneuroendocrinology. 2011;36(3):426–36. https://doi.org/10.1016/j.psyneuen.2010.09.012.
124. Capuron L, Lasselin J, Castanon N. Role of adiposity-driven inflammation in depressive morbidity. Neuropsychopharmacology. 2017;42(1):115–28. https://doi.org/10.1038/npp.2016.123.
125. Savitz J, Drevets WC, Smith CM, Victor TA, Wurfel BE, Bellgowan PS, et al. Putative neuroprotective and neurotoxic kynurenine pathway metabolites are associated with hippocampal and amygdalar volumes in subjects with major depressive disorder. Neuropsychopharmacology. 2015;40(2):463–71. https://doi.org/10.1038/npp.2014.194.
126. Hashimoto R, Mizutani M, Ohta T, Nakazawa K, Nagatsu T. Changes in plasma tetrahydrobiopterin levels of depressives in depressive and remission phases: reconfirmed by measurement with an internal standard. Neuropsychobiology. 1994;29(2):57–60.
127. Celik C, Erdem M, Cayci T, Ozdemir B, Ozgur Akgul E, Kurt YG, et al. The association between serum levels of neopterin and number of depressive episodes of major depression. Prog Neuro-Psychopharmacol Biol Psychiatry. 2010;34(2):372–5. https://doi.org/10.1016/j.pnpbp.2010.01.002.
128. Jukema RA, Ahmed TAN, Tardif JC. Does low-density lipoprotein cholesterol induce inflammation? If so, does it matter? Current insights and future perspectives for novel therapies. BMC Med. 2019;17(1):197. https://doi.org/10.1186/s12916-019-1433-3.
129. Radford-Smith DE, Yates AG, Rizvi L, Anthony DC, Probert F. HDL and LDL have distinct, opposing effects on LPS-induced brain inflammation. Lipids Health Dis. 2023;22(1):54. https://doi.org/10.1186/s12944-023-01817-z.
130. Hayakawa K, Watabe M, Horikawa H, Sato-Kasai M, Shimokawa N, Nakao T, et al. Low-density lipoprotein cholesterol is a possible blood biomarker of schizoid personality traits among females. J Pers Med. 2022;12(2) https://doi.org/10.3390/jpm12020131.
131. Eyre H, Baune BT. Neuroplastic changes in depression: a role for the immune system. Psychoneuroendocrinology. 2012;37(9):1397–416. https://doi.org/10.1016/j.psyneuen.2012.03.019.
132. Leonard B, Maes M. Mechanistic explanations how cell-mediated immune activation, inflammation and oxidative and nitrosative stress pathways and their sequels and concomitants play a role in the pathophysiology of unipolar depression. Neurosci Biobehav Rev. 2012;36(2):764–85. https://doi.org/10.1016/j.neubiorev.2011.12.005.
133. Shelton RC, Miller AH. Eating ourselves to death (and despair): the contribution of adiposity and inflammation to depression. Prog Neurobiol. 2010;91(4):275–99. https://doi.org/10.1016/j.pneurobio.2010.04.004.
134. McKay LI, Cidlowski JA. Molecular control of immune/inflammatory responses: interactions between nuclear factor-kappa B and steroid receptor-signaling pathways. Endocr Rev. 1999;20(4):435–59. https://doi.org/10.1210/edrv.20.4.0375.
135. Hu F, Pace TW, Miller AH. Interferon-alpha inhibits glucocorticoid receptor-mediated gene transcription via STAT5 activation in mouse HT22 cells. Brain Behav Immun. 2009;23(4):455–63. https://doi.org/10.1016/j.bbi.2009.01.001.
136. Kiecolt-Glaser JK, Derry HM, Fagundes CP. Inflammation: depression fans the flames and feasts on the heat. Am J Psychiatry. 2015;172(11):1075–91. https://doi.org/10.1176/appi.ajp.2015.15020152.

137. Raison CL, Miller AH. Is depression an inflammatory disorder? Curr Psychiatry Rep. 2011;13(6):467–75. https://doi.org/10.1007/s11920-011-0232-0.
138. Moylan S, Berk M, Dean OM, Samuni Y, Williams LJ, O'Neil A, et al. Oxidative & nitrosative stress in depression: why so much stress? Neurosci Biobehav Rev. 2014;45:46–62. https://doi.org/10.1016/j.neubiorev.2014.05.007.
139. Rani V, Deep G, Singh RK, Palle K, Yadav UC. Oxidative stress and metabolic disorders: pathogenesis and therapeutic strategies. Life Sci. 2016;148:183–93. https://doi.org/10.1016/j.lfs.2016.02.002.
140. Bryan S, Baregzay B, Spicer D, Singal PK, Khaper N. Redox-inflammatory synergy in the metabolic syndrome. Can J Physiol Pharmacol. 2013;91(1):22–30. https://doi.org/10.1139/cjpp-2012-0295.
141. Berk M, Williams LJ, Jacka FN, O'Neil A, Pasco JA, Moylan S, et al. So depression is an inflammatory disease, but where does the inflammation come from? BMC Med. 2013;11:200. https://doi.org/10.1186/1741-7015-11-200.
142. Maurya PK, Noto C, Rizzo LB, Rios AC, Nunes SO, Barbosa DS, et al. The role of oxidative and nitrosative stress in accelerated aging and major depressive disorder. Prog Neuro-Psychopharmacol Biol Psychiatry. 2016;65:134–44. https://doi.org/10.1016/j.pnpbp.2015.08.016.
143. Mansur RB, Brietzke E, McIntyre RS. Is there a "metabolic-mood syndrome"? A review of the relationship between obesity and mood disorders. Neurosci Biobehav Rev. 2015;52:89–104. https://doi.org/10.1016/j.neubiorev.2014.12.017.
144. Woo YS, Seo HJ, McIntyre RS, Bahk WM. Obesity and its potential effects on antidepressant treatment outcomes in patients with depressive disorders: a literature review. Int J Mol Sci. 2016;17(1) https://doi.org/10.3390/ijms17010080.
145. Grigolon RB, Trevizol AP, Gerchman F, Bambokian AD, Magee T, McIntyre RS, et al. Is obesity a determinant of success with pharmacological treatment for depression? A systematic review, meta-analysis and meta-regression. J Affect Disord. 2021;287:54–68. https://doi.org/10.1016/j.jad.2021.03.032.
146. Jantaratnotai N, Mosikanon K, Lee Y, McIntyre RS. The interface of depression and obesity. Obes Res Clin Pract. 2017;11(1):1–10. https://doi.org/10.1016/j.orcp.2016.07.003.

Part III

Treatment

11 Novel Antidepressants

Lee Jung Goo and Young-Min Park

11.1 Introduction

Major depressive disorder (MDD) is a highly prevalent and debilitating psychiatric condition that affects more than 280 million people globally and is a leading cause of disability worldwide [1]. Despite the widespread use of conventional antidepressants—primarily selective serotonin reuptake inhibitors (SSRIs), serotonin-norepinephrine reuptake inhibitors (SNRIs), and tricyclic antidepressants (TCAs)—a significant proportion of patients fails to achieve remission. Approximately 30–50% of individuals with MDD exhibit partial or no response to initial treatments, leading to the classification of treatment-resistant depression (TRD) in nearly one-third of cases [2, 3].

One of the major limitations of existing antidepressants is their delayed onset of action, typically requiring several weeks to exert therapeutic effects. This latency can result in prolonged suffering and increased suicide risk during the initial treatment phase [4]. Furthermore, the current pharmacologic options largely target monoaminergic pathways, which may not sufficiently address the heterogeneous and complex pathophysiology of depression, including glutamatergic dysregulation, neuroinflammation, hypothalamic–pituitary–adrenal (HPA) axis abnormalities, and deficits in neuroplasticity [5, 6].

In response to these unmet clinical needs, the last two decades have witnessed growing interest and investment in the development of novel antidepressants with mechanisms beyond monoamine modulation. This includes agents acting on glutamate receptors (e.g., N-methyl-D-aspartate [NMDA] antagonists), GABAergic neurosteroids, trace amine-associated receptor 1 (TAAR1) agonists, melatonergic agents, and psychedelics such as psilocybin [7, 8]. The U.S. Food and Drug Administration (U.S. FDA) approval of esketamine in 2019 and brexanolone shortly thereafter marked a paradigm shift in antidepressant pharmacotherapy by introducing agents with rapid-onset and distinct mechanisms of action [9].

These novel treatments have shown promise, particularly in cases of TRD, postpartum depression (PPD), and acute suicidal ideation, where rapid symptom relief is critically needed. However, they also raise important considerations regarding safety, accessibility, long-term efficacy, and integration into existing treatment algorithms [10].

L. J. Goo
Department of Psychiatry, Haeundae Paik Hospital, College of Medicine, Inje University, Busan, Republic of Korea

Paik Institute for Clinical Research, Inje University, Busan, Republic of Korea

Y.-M. Park (✉)
Brain and Mind Mental Health Clinic, Goyang, Republic of Korea

Brain and Mind Institute, Goyang, Republic of Korea
e-mail: youngminpark007@naver.com

W.-M. Bahk et al. (eds.), *Depressive Disorder*, https://doi.org/10.1007/978-981-92-1331-3_11

This chapter aims to provide a comprehensive overview of novel antidepressants, detailing their mechanisms of action, clinical trial evidence, comparative efficacy, and emerging therapeutic roles. The discussion will emphasize how these agents are reshaping modern approaches to the pharmacologic management of depression.

11.2 Mechanisms of Action of Novel Antidepressants

The development of novel antidepressants has been driven by increasing recognition that major depressive disorder (MDD) is a heterogeneous condition, with complex and multifaceted pathophysiological mechanisms that extend beyond the monoaminergic hypothesis. While conventional antidepressants have largely focused on increasing synaptic concentrations of serotonin (5-HT), norepinephrine (NE), and dopamine (DA), these treatments fail to benefit a significant portion of patients and often require weeks to achieve clinical effects [11, 12].

In contrast, novel antidepressants target a broader range of systems involved in emotional regulation, stress response, neuroinflammation, synaptic plasticity, and neurocircuitry dysfunction [13]. These agents aim to provide faster, more robust, and more personalized relief from depressive symptoms, especially in patients with treatment-resistant depression (TRD), suicidal ideation, or comorbid conditions.

Glutamatergic Modulation

The glutamatergic system is the brain's principal excitatory neurotransmitter network and plays a critical role in synaptic plasticity, learning, and mood regulation. Dysregulation of glutamate signaling—particularly via N-methyl-D-aspartate (NMDA) receptors—has been implicated in MDD pathogenesis, with evidence of excitotoxicity, impaired neurogenesis, and disrupted cortico-limbic connectivity in depressed individuals [5, 14].

Esketamine, the S-enantiomer of ketamine, is a non-competitive NMDA receptor antagonist that has demonstrated rapid antidepressant effects within hours of administration [15]. These effects are believed to be mediated not by direct monoaminergic enhancement, but through a surge in glutamate release, activation of α-amino-3-hydroxy-5-methyl-4-isoxazolepropionic acid (AMPA) receptors, and brain-derived neurotrophic factor-mammalian target of rapamycin (BDNF-mTOR) signaling cascades, ultimately enhancing synaptogenesis in the prefrontal cortex [15].

Additional NMDA-modulating agents are under development:

- REL-1017 (esmethadone): a low-potency NMDA channel blocker with fewer dissociative effects than ketamine [15].
- AV-101 (4-chlorokynurenine): a prodrug of 7-chlorokynurenic acid, an NMDA glycine site antagonist, designed to minimize psychotomimetic effects [16].
- Rapastinel and Apimostinel: partial agonists at NMDA glycine modulatory sites with promising preclinical efficacy [17].

Despite their promise, glutamate-based therapies require careful monitoring due to potential for dissociation, hypertension, and abuse liability.

GABAergic Neurosteroids

Gamma-aminobutyric acid (GABA) is the primary inhibitory neurotransmitter in the central nervous system (CNS), balancing excitatory input and maintaining mood stability. Reduced GABAergic tone, especially in corticolimbic circuits, is associated with anxiety, anhedonia, and rumination, common features of depression [18]. Neurosteroids, such as allopregnanolone, enhance GABA A receptor activity, promoting anxiolytic and antidepressant effects.

Brexanolone, an intravenous formulation of allopregnanolone, was the first FDA-approved drug specifically for postpartum depression

(PPD), a condition thought to involve acute neurosteroid withdrawal [19]. Its administration leads to rapid symptom remission, typically within 60 h. However, limitations include its cost, need for continuous infusion, and sedation risk.

To overcome these limitations, zuranolone, an oral analog of brexanolone, has been developed. Zuranolone exhibits positive allosteric modulation of both synaptic and extrasynaptic GABA A receptors and demonstrates significant efficacy in MDD and PPD with better convenience [20]. Ongoing trials are also exploring its role in generalized anxiety disorder and bipolar depression.

Psychedelic Compounds and 5-HT2A Agonists

Psychedelic agents such as psilocybin, ayahuasca (DMT), and Lysergic acid diethylamide (LSD) have re-emerged in clinical research after decades of regulatory prohibition. Psilocybin, the most studied psychedelic in depression, acts as a 5-HT2A receptor partial agonist, modulating default mode network connectivity, emotional salience, and self-referential thinking [21].

Single-dose psilocybin-assisted psychotherapy has shown rapid and sustained antidepressant effects in both treatment-resistant and major depression, often lasting weeks to months after administration [22]. It also increases BDNF expression and may enhance psychological flexibility and meaning-based cognition.

However, these agents require careful set and setting, trained therapeutic support, and have regulatory barriers. They are currently undergoing Phase II and III clinical trials for MDD and other mood disorders.

TAAR1 Agonists

The trace amine-associated receptor 1 (TAAR1) is a G-protein-coupled receptor expressed in monoaminergic neurons and modulates dopamine and serotonin signaling. Unlike traditional antidepressants, TAAR1 agonists do not bind directly to dopamine or serotonin transporters, offering an alternative pathway for emotional regulation [23].

SEP-363856 (ulotaront), a TAAR1 and 5-HT1A receptor agonist, was originally developed for schizophrenia but has demonstrated antidepressant-like effects in preclinical and early clinical models [18]. The drug has a unique mechanism that avoids direct D2 antagonism, potentially reducing extrapyramidal symptoms and weight gain.

TAAR1 agonism also influences sleep-wake cycles, stress reactivity, and metabolic homeostasis, making it a promising target for broader psychiatric use.

Melatonergic Agents

Disturbances in circadian rhythm and sleep-wake cycles are core features of depression. Agomelatine, a melatonin receptor (MT 1/MT 2) agonist and 5-HT2C antagonist, enhances circadian entrainment and increases dopamine and norepinephrine release in the frontal cortex [24].

Agomelatine has shown similar efficacy to SSRIs in multiple trials, with fewer sexual side effects, improved sleep quality, and no discontinuation syndrome. Although not FDA-approved in the United States, it is widely used in Europe and offers an attractive profile for patients with prominent sleep or circadian disturbances [25].

Anti-inflammatory and Immunomodulatory Approaches

Growing evidence suggests that a subset of MDD patients exhibit low-grade systemic inflammation, elevated C-reactive protein (CRP), interleukin-6 (IL-6), and tumor necrosis factor-alpha (TNF-α), which may impair neurotransmission and neurogenesis [26]. This has led to trials of anti-inflammatory agents as novel antidepressants.

- Minocycline, a tetracycline antibiotic, crosses the blood–brain barrier and inhibits microglial activation and cytokine production [27].
- Infliximab, a TNF-α monoclonal antibody, has

shown modest efficacy in high-inflammation MDD subgroups [28].
- Celecoxib, a COX-2 inhibitor, has demonstrated additive benefits when combined with SSRIs in some studies [29].

Identifying patients with inflammatory biomarkers may allow for stratified or precision approaches in depression treatment.

Triple Reuptake Inhibitors (TRIs)

Triple reuptake inhibitors (TRIs) inhibit serotonin, norepinephrine, and dopamine transporters (serotonin transporter (SERT), norepinephrine transporter (NET), dopamine transporter(DAT)), offering a broader monoaminergic approach. Compounds like amitifadine and tesofensine have shown enhanced antidepressant efficacy with fewer side effects than conventional TCAs [30].

TRIs may be particularly effective in melancholic or anergic subtypes of depression. However, stimulant-like properties, abuse potential, and dose-limiting side effects have limited their clinical development so far.

11.3 Clinical Efficacy and Trials

The clinical efficacy of novel antidepressants has been the subject of intense research in recent years, especially in populations with treatment-resistant depression (TRD), postpartum depression (PPD), and acute suicidal ideation. Unlike traditional antidepressants, many of these agents demonstrate rapid onset, higher response rates, and sustained remission in difficult-to-treat cases. This section summarizes the evidence from randomized controlled trials (RCTs), meta-analyses, and real-world studies evaluating these novel compounds.

Esketamine

Esketamine, the S-enantiomer of ketamine, was the first novel antidepressant approved by the FDA in over 30 years for TRD. In a pivotal Phase III trial, patients receiving intranasal esketamine plus an oral antidepressant demonstrated significantly greater reductions in MADRS (Montgomery–Åsberg Depression Rating Scale) scores at 28 days compared to placebo plus antidepressant (least-squares mean difference − 4.0, $p = 0.01$) [9]. The onset of symptom relief was observed as early as 24 h after the first dose [31].

A separate relapse-prevention trial demonstrated that continuation of esketamine significantly delayed time to relapse compared to placebo in patients who had previously responded (hazard ratio 0.49, $p = 0.003$) [32]. Common adverse effects included transient dissociation, dizziness, and nausea, which generally resolved within 1–2 h post-administration.

Brexanolone

Brexanolone, an intravenous formulation of the neurosteroid allopregnanolone, was specifically approved for postpartum depression. In two large, double-blind, placebo-controlled trials, brexanolone produced rapid and significant improvements in Hamilton Depression Rating Scale (HAM-D) scores by hour 60 (−17.7 vs. −13.1; $p = 0.0075$), with sustained effects through day 30 [19].

Importantly, brexanolone was effective even in patients with severe baseline depression (HAM-D $\geq$ 26). Despite the efficacy, its use is limited by cost, requirement for a 60-h infusion, and risk of excessive sedation or loss of consciousness, necessitating continuous monitoring under a Risk Evaluation and Mitigation Strategy (REMS) program [33].

Zuranolone

Zuranolone is an oral neurosteroid with similar GABA A receptor activity to brexanolone. In the SKYLARK trial, zuranolone 50 mg daily for 14 days significantly improved depressive symptoms in women with PPD by day 15 compared to placebo (mean HAM-D reduction −15.6 vs.

−11.6; $p < 0.001$) [20]. Another trial in MDD also showed sustained improvements at 42 days post-treatment, indicating durability beyond the dosing period [34]. Advantages of zuranolone include oral administration, rapid action, and good tolerability. Ongoing Phase III trials will further define its role in both PPD and MDD [35].

Psilocybin

Psilocybin, a 5-HT2A receptor agonist and classical psychedelic, has shown promising antidepressant effects with rapid onset and long duration. In a randomized clinical trial involving adults with major depression, a single 25 mg dose of psilocybin combined with psychological support produced a 71% response rate and 54% remission rate at week 4 [22]. These outcomes significantly surpassed those of conventional antidepressants over similar timeframes.

A head-to-head trial comparing psilocybin (2 sessions) to daily escitalopram (for 6 weeks) in moderate-to-severe depression found that psilocybin produced non-inferior and numerically better outcomes in terms of Quick Inventory of Depressive Symptomatology–Self Report (QIDS-SR) scores, with fewer adverse effects and lower emotional blunting [36].

Agomelatine

Agomelatine has been evaluated in multiple trials and meta-analyses. A pooled analysis of 7 RCTs ($n = 1877$) found agomelatine to be significantly more effective than placebo and as effective as SSRIs in reducing depressive symptoms, with additional benefits on sleep quality and circadian rhythm restoration [25].

In contrast to SSRIs, agomelatine has a lower incidence of sexual dysfunction, withdrawal symptoms, and weight gain, making it a preferred option for certain subgroups [37]. Its efficacy is particularly notable in anxious depression and melancholic features.

Other Agents in Clinical Trials

REL-1017 (esmethadone), a low-affinity NMDA receptor antagonist, demonstrated rapid improvement in MADRS scores at day 7, with a favorable side effect profile [15]. Similarly, SEP-363856 (ulotaront), a TAAR1 agonist, has shown early signs of antidepressant activity in schizophrenia trials, warranting further investigation in mood disorders [18].

Anti-inflammatory agents such as minocycline and infliximab have yielded mixed results. A meta-analysis of minocycline adjunctive therapy showed small-to-moderate effect sizes in MDD, especially in individuals with elevated inflammatory markers [38]. In contrast, infliximab showed benefit only in patients with high baseline CRP, suggesting a role for biomarker-guided antidepressant therapy [28].

11.4 Safety and Side Effects

The evaluation of safety and tolerability is essential for integrating novel antidepressants into clinical practice. While these agents offer advantages in terms of faster onset and efficacy in treatment-resistant populations, they also present unique adverse effect profiles and regulatory considerations. This section reviews the safety and side effect data associated with major novel antidepressants based on clinical trials and post-marketing surveillance.

Esketamine

Esketamine's rapid onset of action is accompanied by a well-documented side effect profile, most notably transient dissociation, elevated blood pressure, and sedation [9]. In pooled clinical trial data, dissociation was reported in approximately 25% of patients, peaking within 40 min and resolving within 1–2 h [31]. Transient increases in systolic and diastolic blood pressure are common and usually resolve within 90 min post-dose [32].

Due to concerns about abuse potential and sedation-related adverse events, esketamine is available only through a REMS (Risk Evaluation and Mitigation Strategy) program requiring administration under medical supervision [39].

Brexanolone

Brexanolone is associated with a risk of profound sedation and loss of consciousness, necessitating continuous intravenous infusion over 60 h and monitoring in a certified healthcare setting [33]. In clinical trials, 4% of patients experienced syncope or excessive sedation [40]. Other side effects include dry mouth, dizziness, and flushing.

The need for hospital-based administration, high cost, and intensive monitoring limit its widespread use despite clinical efficacy.

Zuranolone

Zuranolone is generally well tolerated and can be taken orally, offering improved practicality over brexanolone. The most commonly reported adverse effects include somnolence (15–20%), dizziness, and headache [20].

Psilocybin

Psilocybin's side effect profile is unique, given its classification as a psychedelic. Acute adverse effects include transient anxiety, perceptual disturbances, nausea, and elevated blood pressure during the acute phase of intoxication [22]. These effects are typically self-limiting and resolve within 4–6 h.

Importantly, in controlled therapeutic settings, no serious adverse events or psychotic breaks have been reported in modern trials involving screened patients [18]. However, there is still concern about its use in individuals with psychotic disorders or a family history of schizophrenia. Because of its profound psychological effects, psilocybin must be administered under professional supervision in structured settings.

Agomelatine

Agomelatine is well tolerated, with minimal sexual side effects, no weight gain, and a low risk of discontinuation syndrome, distinguishing it from SSRIs and SNRIs [25]. However, a notable concern is the risk of liver enzyme elevation. In clinical trials, up to 1.3% of patients showed >3× upper limit of normal (ULN) transaminase levels, necessitating regular liver function monitoring, especially in the first 12 weeks of treatment [41].

Anti-inflammatory Agents

Agents such as minocycline and infliximab carry side effects typical of their primary indications. Minocycline may cause dizziness, nausea, and photosensitivity, while long-term use can lead to autoimmune syndromes [42]. Infliximab, as a TNF-α inhibitor, may increase the risk of infections, infusion reactions, and rebound inflammation [43]. Therefore, the use of these agents in depression requires careful risk–benefit assessment and may be limited to patients with elevated inflammatory markers.

General Considerations

Across novel antidepressants, personalized risk assessment is increasingly important.

11.5 Comparison with Conventional Antidepressants

Conventional antidepressants, including selective serotonin reuptake inhibitors (SSRIs), serotonin-norepinephrine reuptake inhibitors (SNRIs), tricyclic antidepressants (TCAs), and monoamine oxidase inhibitors (MAOIs), have long served as first-line treatments for major depressive disorder (MDD). While effective in many cases, these agents are limited by delayed onset, low remission rates, and undesirable side effects such as sexual dysfunction, weight gain, and withdrawal symptoms [2, 44]. The development of novel antidepressants has sought to overcome these limitations by targeting alternative neurobiological pathways. This section compares novel antidepressants to conventional agents across several key domains: efficacy, onset of action, side effect profiles, mechanism of action, and clinical utility.

Onset of Action

Conventional antidepressants typically require 2–6 weeks to demonstrate significant clinical benefit, a period that can be especially risky for individuals with severe or suicidal depression [4]. In contrast, novel agents such as esketamine, brexanolone, zuranolone, and psilocybin often show symptom improvement within hours to days [9, 19, 34]. For example, esketamine has demonstrated clinically meaningful effects within 24 h of administration [9], while zuranolone improved depressive symptoms by day 3 to 5 [34]. This rapid onset is particularly valuable in treatment-resistant depression (TRD) and acute depressive crises.

Efficacy and Remission Rates

While SSRIs and SNRIs achieve remission in approximately 30–40% of patients in controlled trials [45], novel agents have demonstrated higher remission rates in certain subgroups. Psilocybin, for instance, achieved 54% remission at 4 weeks in a recent trial [22], and brexanolone resulted in significant and sustained remission in postpartum depression [19]. However, head-to-head comparisons remain limited, and many novel agents have not yet been tested in large, long-term, comparative studies.

Mechanism of Action

Conventional antidepressants act by enhancing monoaminergic transmission through inhibition of serotonin and/or norepinephrine reuptake. This narrow mechanism may not address the full neurobiological complexity of depression, including dysfunction in glutamatergic, GABAergic, circadian, neuroimmune, and neurosteroid pathways [5, 6].

Novel agents offer mechanistic diversity:

- Esketamine modulates glutamatergic transmission via NMDA receptor antagonism [9].
- Zuranolone and brexanolone modulate GABA A receptors [19, 34].
- Psilocybin targets 5-HT2A receptors and alters network connectivity [22].
- Agomelatine acts on melatonin and 5-HT2C receptors to regulate circadian rhythms [24].

This broadened pharmacologic spectrum may explain improved efficacy in treatment-resistant populations and rapid symptom relief.

Side Effect Profiles

Conventional antidepressants are frequently associated with sexual dysfunction, weight gain, insomnia, emotional blunting, and discontinuation syndromes [46]. In contrast, several novel antidepressants offer improved tolerability in specific domains:

- Agomelatine is associated with minimal sexual dysfunction and no discontinuation syndrome [24].
- Zuranolone and brexanolone do not cause emotional blunting but may lead to sedation or somnolence [19, 34].
- Psilocybin does not produce chronic side effects but requires psychological supervision due to transient anxiety and perceptual disturbances [22].
- Esketamine is associated with dissociation and transient increases in blood pressure, necessitating in-clinic administration and monitoring [9].

Overall, the side effect burden is different rather than uniformly lower, and each novel agent carries unique risks that must be managed in clinical practice.

Practical Considerations

While novel agents provide clinical advantages, several practical barriers limit their widespread adoption:

- Cost: Both brexanolone and esketamine are associated with very high treatment costs, far exceeding those of conventional oral antidepressants [47, 48].
- Administration logistics: Esketamine and brexanolone require REMS programs and supervised administration, limiting accessibility [9, 19].
- Regulatory status: Many agents, including psilocybin, remain investigational or are only approved for specific indications (e.g., PPD for zuranolone).

Despite these limitations, novel agents represent a transformative advancement, especially in patients who have not responded to standard therapies.

11.6 Future Perspectives: Focusing on Novel Targets

The future of antidepressant development is increasingly centered on identifying and exploiting new biological targets that extend beyond the traditional monoaminergic systems. This approach aims to provide mechanism-specific, personalized interventions that can address the heterogeneity of major depressive disorder (MDD), improve response rates, and shorten the time to therapeutic effect.

Expanding Beyond Current Mechanisms

Currently approved novel antidepressants primarily act via glutamatergic modulation (e.g., NMDA receptor antagonists such as esketamine), GABA A receptor modulation (e.g., brexanolone, zuranolone), melatonergic receptor agonism (e.g., agomelatine), and 5-HT2A receptor agonism (e.g., psilocybin). While these mechanisms represent a major step forward, research is rapidly moving toward additional molecular pathways that may open entirely new therapeutic avenues.

Key Novel Targets in Development

- Neuroplasticity Enhancers—Agents that directly enhance synaptic connectivity and resilience, such as brain-derived neurotrophic factor (BDNF) agonists and mTOR pathway activators, aim to correct structural and functional deficits in mood-regulating circuits [5].
- Kynurenine Pathway Modulators—Compounds targeting this pathway influence glutamate metabolism and neuroinflammatory cascades, with potential benefits for inflammation-linked depression [49].
- Orexin Receptor Antagonists—Originally developed for insomnia, these agents are being explored for patients with comorbid sleep disturbance and depression, potentially improving both mood and circadian regulation [50].
- Vagal Tone Enhancers—Techniques such as digital neurostimulation and biofeedback-based interventions aim to modulate autonomic function and stress reactivity, indirectly influencing mood stability [51].
- Epigenetic Modifiers—Histone deacetylase (HDAC) inhibitors and other chromatin-modifying agents seek to reverse maladaptive gene expression patterns underlying depressive symptoms [52].

Psychedelic and Neurotechnology Integration

Psychedelic-assisted psychotherapy—currently in Phase III trials for psilocybin and MDMA—represents a treatment model that combines neurobiological effects (e.g., 5-HT2A receptor modulation, network connectivity reorganization) with guided therapeutic interventions for lasting remission [21, 53].

In parallel, digital biomarkers, mobile health platforms, and neuroimaging-based predictors could be used to identify patients most likely to benefit from specific novel targets. Noninvasive neuromodulation such as transcranial magnetic stimulation (TMS) and transcranial direct current stimulation (tDCS) may be combined with targeted pharmacotherapy for synergistic effects [54].

11.7 Conclusion

Over the past two decades, the field of antidepressant development has undergone a transformative shift. The emergence of novel antidepressants—ranging from glutamatergic modulators and neurosteroid agents to psychedelics and TAAR1 agonists—has expanded the therapeutic arsenal for major depressive disorder (MDD) beyond traditional monoaminergic approaches. These agents not only demonstrate more rapid onset and broader mechanisms of action, but they also offer clinical benefits for patients with treatment-resistant depression (TRD), postpartum depression (PPD), and acute suicidal ideation, populations often underserved by conventional treatments.

Despite these advances, the clinical application of novel antidepressants remains in a transitional phase. While promising in efficacy, many of these agents face practical limitations, including high cost, limited accessibility, need for supervised administration, and regulatory constraints. Moreover, long-term safety data and real-world effectiveness are still evolving.

The future of antidepressant therapy will likely be defined by a multidimensional, personalized approach—integrating biomarker-guided treatment, novel pharmacological targets, digital health tools, and psychotherapeutic frameworks. The success of this paradigm shift will depend not only on scientific innovation but also on thoughtful implementation, training, and patient engagement.

Ultimately, novel antidepressants represent more than just new drugs; they embody a new philosophy of care—one that seeks precision, speed, tolerability, and most importantly, hope for those affected by the burden of depression.

Declarations

Competing Interests The author(s) has no competing interests to declare that are relevant to the content of this manuscript.

Ethics Approval The author(s) declares that this manuscript does not include primary research with human participants.

The author(s) declares that this manuscript does not include primary studies involving animals.

References

1. World Health Organization. Depression. Updated June 2023. https://www.who.int/news-room/fact-sheets/detail/depression.
2. Rush AJ, Trivedi MH, Wisniewski SR, et al. Acute and longer-term outcomes in depressed outpatients requiring one or several treatment steps: a STARD report. Am J Psychiatry. 2006;163(11):1905–17. https://doi.org/10.1176/ajp.2006.163.11.1905.
3. Gaynes BN, Warden D, Trivedi MH, Wisniewski SR, Fava M, Rush AJ. What did STAR*D teach us? Results from a large-scale, practical, clinical trial for patients with depression. Psychiatr Serv. 2009;60(11):1439–45. https://doi.org/10.1176/ps.2009.60.11.1439.
4. Machado-Vieira R, Baumann J, Wheeler-Castillo C, et al. The timing of antidepressant effects: a comparison of diverse pharmacological and somatic treatments. Pharmaceuticals. 2010;3(1):19–41. https://doi.org/10.3390/ph3010019.
5. Duman RS, Aghajanian GK. Synaptic dysfunction in depression: potential therapeutic targets. Science. 2012;338(6103):68–72. https://doi.org/10.1126/science.1222939.
6. Haroon E, Raison CL, Miller AH. Psychoneuroimmunology meets Neuropsychopharmacology: translational implications of the impact of inflammation on behavior. Neuropsychopharmacology. 2012;37(1):137–62. https://doi.org/10.1038/npp.2011.205.
7. Hindmarch I. Beyond the monoamine hypothesis: mechanisms, molecules and methods. Eur Psychiatry. 2002;17(S3):294s–9s. https://doi.org/10.1016/s0924-9338(02)00653-3.
8. Newport DJ, Carpenter LL, McDonald WM, et al. Ketamine and other NMDA antagonists: early clinical trials and possible mechanisms in depression. Am J Psychiatry. 2015;172(10):950–66. https://doi.org/10.1176/appi.ajp.2015.15040465.

9. Daly EJ, Trivedi MH, Janik A, et al. Efficacy of Esketamine nasal spray plus Oral antidepressant treatment for relapse prevention in patients with treatment-resistant depression: a randomized clinical trial. JAMA Psychiatry. 2019;76(9):893–903. https://doi.org/10.1001/jamapsychiatry.2019.1189.
10. Wilkinson ST, Sanacora G. Considerations on the off-label use of ketamine as a treatment for mood disorders. JAMA. 2017;318(9):793–4. https://doi.org/10.1001/jama.2017.10697.
11. Krystal JH, Sanacora G, Duman RS. Rapid-acting glutamatergic antidepressants: the path to ketamine and beyond. Biol Psychiatry. 2013;73(12):1133–41. https://doi.org/10.1016/j.biopsych.2013.03.026.
12. Belmaker RH, Agam G. Major Depressive Disorder. N Engl J Med. 2008;358(1):55–68. https://doi.org/10.1056/nejmra073096.
13. Abdallah CG, Sanacora G, Duman RS, Krystal JH. Ketamine and rapid-acting antidepressants: a window into a new neurobiology for mood disorder therapeutics. Annu Rev Med. 2015;66(1):1–15. https://doi.org/10.1146/annurev-med-053013-062946.
14. Zanos P, Gould TD. Mechanisms of ketamine action as an antidepressant. Mol Psychiatry. 2018;23(4):801–11. https://doi.org/10.1038/mp.2017.255.
15. Fava M, Stahl S, Pani L, et al. REL-1017 (Esmethadone) as adjunctive treatment in patients with major depressive disorder: a phase 2a randomized double-blind trial. Am J Psychiatry. 2021;179(2):122–31. https://doi.org/10.1176/appi.ajp.2021.21020197.
16. Henter ID, Park LT, Zarate CA. Novel glutamatergic modulators for the treatment of mood disorders: current status. CNS Drugs. 2021;35(5):527–43. https://doi.org/10.1007/s40263-021-00816-x.
17. Wilkinson ST, Sanacora G. A new generation of antidepressants: an update on the pharmaceutical pipeline for novel and rapid-acting therapeutics in mood disorders based on glutamate/GABA neurotransmitter systems. Drug Discov Today. 2018;24(2):606–15. https://doi.org/10.1016/j.drudis.2018.11.007.
18. Koblan KS, Kent J, Hopkins SC, et al. A non–D2-receptor-binding drug for the treatment of schizophrenia. N Engl J Med. 2020;382(16):1497–506. https://doi.org/10.1056/nejmoa1911772.
19. Meltzer-Brody S, Colquhoun H, Riesenberg R, et al. Brexanolone injection in postpartum depression: two multicenter, double-blind, randomized, placebo-controlled, phase 3 trials. Obstet Gynecol Surv. 2019;74(4):219–20. https://doi.org/10.1097/01.ogx.0000554376.54568.64.
20. Deligiannidis KM, Meltzer-Brody S, Gunduz-Bruce H, et al. Effect of Zuranolone vs placebo in postpartum depression: a randomized clinical trial. JAMA Psychiatry. 2021;78(9):951. https://doi.org/10.1001/jamapsychiatry.2021.1559.
21. Vollenweider FX, Preller KH. Psychedelic drugs: neurobiology and potential for treatment of psychiatric disorders. Nat Rev Neurosci. 2020;21(11):611–24. https://doi.org/10.1038/s41583-020-0367-2.
22. Davis AK, Barrett FS, May DG, et al. Effects of psilocybin-assisted therapy on major depressive disorder: a randomized clinical trial. JAMA Psychiatry. 2021;78(5):481–9. https://doi.org/10.1001/jamapsychiatry.2020.3285.
23. Wu R, Liu J, Seaman R, Johnson B, Zhang Y, Li JX. The selective TAAR1 partial agonist RO5263397 promoted novelty recognition memory in mice. Psychopharmacology. 2021;238(11):3221–8. https://doi.org/10.1007/s00213-021-05937-1.
24. Kennedy SH, Rizvi SJ. Agomelatine in the treatment of major depressive disorder: potential for clinical effectiveness. CNS Drugs. 2010;24(6):479–99. https://doi.org/10.2165/11534420-000000000-00000.
25. Kennedy SH, Emsley R. Placebo-controlled trial of agomelatine in the treatment of major depressive disorder. Eur Neuropsychopharmacol. 2006;16(2):93–100. https://doi.org/10.1016/j.euroneuro.2005.09.002.
26. Miller AH, Raison CL. The role of inflammation in depression: from evolutionary imperative to modern treatment target. Nat Rev Immunol. 2016;16(1):22–34. https://doi.org/10.1038/nri.2015.5.
27. Zazula R, Husain MI, Mohebbi M, et al. Minocycline as adjunctive treatment for major depressive disorder: pooled data from two randomized controlled trials. Aust N Z J Psychiatry. 2021;55(8):784–98. https://doi.org/10.1177/0004867420965697.
28. Raison CL, Rutherford RE, Woolwine BJ, et al. A randomized controlled trial of the tumor necrosis factor antagonist infliximab for treatment-resistant depression: the role of baseline inflammatory biomarkers. JAMA Psychiatry. 2013;70(1):31–41. https://doi.org/10.1001/2013.jamapsychiatry.4.
29. Akhondzadeh S, Jafari S, Raisi F, et al. Clinical trial of adjunctive celecoxib treatment in patients with major depression: a double blind and placebo controlled trial. Dépress Anxiety. 2009;26(7):607–11. https://doi.org/10.1002/da.20589.
30. Prins J, Olivier B, Korte SM. Triple reuptake inhibitors for treating subtypes of major depressive disorder: the monoamine hypothesis revisited. Expert Opin Investig Drugs. 2011;20(8):1107–30. https://doi.org/10.1517/13543784.2011.594039.
31. Popova V, Daly EJ, Trivedi M, et al. Efficacy and safety of flexibly dosed Esketamine nasal spray combined with a newly initiated Oral antidepressant in treatment-resistant depression: a randomized double-blind active-controlled study. Am J Psychiatry. 2019;176(6):428–38. https://doi.org/10.1176/appi.ajp.2019.19020172.
32. Fedgchin M, Trivedi M, Daly EJ, et al. Efficacy and safety of fixed-dose Esketamine nasal spray combined with a new Oral antidepressant in treatment-resistant depression: results of a randomized, double-blind, active-controlled study (TRANSFORM-1). Int J Neuropsychopharmacol. 2019;22(10):616–30. https://doi.org/10.1093/ijnp/pyz039.

33. Kanes S, Colquhoun H, Gunduz-Bruce H, et al. Brexanolone (SAGE-547 injection) in post-partum depression: a randomised controlled trial. Lancet. 2017;390(10093):480–9. https://doi.org/10.1016/s0140-6736(17)31264-3.
34. Gunduz-Bruce H, Silber C, Kaul I, et al. Trial of SAGE-217 in patients with major depressive disorder. N Engl J Med. 2019;381(10):903–11. https://doi.org/10.1056/nejmoa1815981.
35. Clayton AH, Lasser R, Nandy I, Sankoh AJ, Jonas J, Kanes SJ. Zuranolone in major depressive disorder: results from MOUNTAIN-A phase 3, multicenter, double-blind, randomized, placebo-controlled trial. J Clin Psychiatry. 2023;84(2) https://doi.org/10.4088/jcp.22m14445.
36. Carhart-Harris R, Giribaldi B, Watts R, et al. Trial of psilocybin versus escitalopram for depression. N Engl J Med. 2021;384(15):1402–11. https://doi.org/10.1056/nejmoa2032994.
37. Chen Y, Li J, Liao M, et al. Efficacy and safety of agomelatine versus SSRIs/SNRIs for post-stroke depression: a systematic review and meta-analysis of randomized controlled trials. Int Clin Psychopharmacol. 2024;39(3):163–73. https://doi.org/10.1097/yic.0000000000000509.
38. Andrade C. Anti-inflammatory treatments for depression: perspectives on how to read a meta-analysis critically. J Clin Psychiatry. 2019;80(3) https://doi.org/10.4088/jcp.19f12907.
39. Yavi M, Lee H, Henter ID, Park LT, Zarate CA. Ketamine treatment for depression: a review. Discov Ment Health. 2022;2(1):9. https://doi.org/10.1007/s44192-022-00012-3.
40. Hutcherson TC, Cieri-Hutcherson NE, Gosciak MF. Brexanolone for postpartum depression. Am J Health-Syst Pharm. 2020;77(5):336–45. https://doi.org/10.1093/ajhp/zxz333.
41. Gahr M, Kratzer W, Fuchs M, Connemann B. Safety and tolerability of Agomelatine: focus on hepatotoxicity. Curr Drug Metab. 2015;15(7):694–702. https://doi.org/10.2174/1389200215666140926155041.
42. Rosenblat JD, McIntyre RS. Efficacy and tolerability of minocycline for depression: a systematic review and meta-analysis of clinical trials. J Affect Disord. 2017;227:219–25. https://doi.org/10.1016/j.jad.2017.10.042.
43. McIntyre RS, Subramaniapillai M, Lee Y, et al. Efficacy of adjunctive infliximab vs placebo in the treatment of adults with bipolar I/II depression. JAMA Psychiatry. 2019;76(8):783–90. https://doi.org/10.1001/jamapsychiatry.2019.0779.
44. Cipriani A, Furukawa TA, Salanti G, et al. Comparative efficacy and acceptability of 21 antidepressant drugs for the acute treatment of adults with major depressive disorder: a systematic review and network meta-analysis. Lancet (Lond, Engl). 2018;391(10128):1357–66. https://doi.org/10.1016/s0140-6736(17)32802-7.
45. Thase ME. Evaluating antidepressant therapies: remission as the optimal outcome. J Clin Psychiatry. 2003;64(Suppl 13):18–25.
46. Kennedy SH, Rizvi S. Sexual dysfunction, depression, and the impact of antidepressants. J Clin Psychopharmacol. 2009;29(2):157–64. https://doi.org/10.1097/jcp.0b013e31819c76e9.
47. Patatanian E, Nguyen DR. Brexanolone: a novel drug for the treatment of postpartum depression. J Pharm Pract. 2022;35(3):431–6. https://doi.org/10.1177/0897190020979627.
48. Ross EL, Soeteman DI. Cost-effectiveness of Esketamine nasal spray for patients with treatment-resistant depression in the United States. Psychiatr Serv. 2020;71(10):988–97. https://doi.org/10.1176/appi.ps.201900625.
49. Almulla AF, Maes M. The tryptophan catabolite or kynurenine pathway's role in major depression. Curr Top Med Chem. 2022;22(21):1731–5. https://doi.org/10.2174/1568026622666220428095250.
50. Fagan H, Jones E, Baldwin DS. Orexin receptor antagonists in the treatment of depression: a leading article Summarising pre-clinical and clinical studies. CNS Drugs. 2023;37(1):1–12. https://doi.org/10.1007/s40263-022-00974-6.
51. Petrocchi N, Piccirillo G, Fiorucci C, et al. Transcranial direct current stimulation enhances soothing positive affect and vagal tone. Neuropsychologia. 2017;96:256–61. https://doi.org/10.1016/j.neuropsychologia.2017.01.028.
52. Fuchikami M, Yamamoto S, Morinobu S, Okada S, Yamawaki Y, Yamawaki S. The potential use of histone deacetylase inhibitors in the treatment of depression. Prog Neuro-Psychopharmacol Biol Psychiatry. 2016;64:320–4. https://doi.org/10.1016/j.pnpbp.2015.03.010.
53. Sloshower J, Skosnik PD, Safi-Aghdam H, et al. Psilocybin-assisted therapy for major depressive disorder: an exploratory placebo-controlled, fixed-order trial. J Psychopharmacol. 2023;37(7):698–706. https://doi.org/10.1177/02698811231154852.
54. Lan Y. The effectiveness of tDCS and TMS for treatment of depression. Highlights Sci Eng Technol. 2024;102:394–400. https://doi.org/10.54097/7jm5w890.

12 Potential Role of Psychedelics in the Treatment of Depressive Disorder

Sheng-Min Wang and Won-Myong Bahk

12.1 Introduction

Depression, a pervasive and debilitating mental health disorder, affects millions of individuals worldwide, contributing to substantial suffering and reduced quality of life [1]. According to the World Health Organization (WHO), major depressive disorder (MDD) affects more than 300 million people, and it is projected to become the leading contributor to the global burden of disease in the coming decades. Despite advances in psychopharmacology and psychotherapy, a substantial proportion of patients continue to suffer from treatment-resistant depression (TRD) [2]. Conventional antidepressants, such as selective serotonin reuptake inhibitors (SSRIs) and serotonin-norepinephrine reuptake inhibitors (SNRIs), often require prolonged administration and show variable efficacy. This therapeutic gap has prompted a resurgence of interest in novel treatment modalities, among which psychedelics have emerged as a promising avenue.

S.-M. Wang
Department of Psychiatry, Yeouido St. Mary's Hospital, College of Medicine, The Catholic University of Korea, Seoul, Republic of Korea

W.-M. Bahk (✉)
Department of Psychiatry, College of Medicine, The Catholic University of Korea, Seoul, Republic of Korea

Woo and Bahk Psychiatry Clinic, Seoul, Republic of Korea
e-mail: wmbahk@catholic.ac.kr

Psychedelics, including psilocybin, lysergic acid diethylamide (LSD), ayahuasca, and 3,4-methylenedioxymethamphetamine (MDMA), are psychoactive substances that profoundly alter perception, cognition, and consciousness [3]. These compounds, once stigmatized and heavily restricted due to political and social pressures, are now at the forefront of psychiatric innovation. With the rapid growth of neuroscience and renewed interest in integrative mental health, psychedelics are being re-examined not only as pharmacological agents but as catalysts for profound psychological and emotional transformation [4]. Their ability to induce rapid, sustained antidepressant effects suggests they may represent a paradigm shift in psychiatric care.

In this chapter, the discussion will center primarily on four psychedelic compounds with the most clinical relevance for depressive disorders: psilocybin, LSD, ayahuasca, and MDMA. Each of these agents has been investigated in modern research for their potential antidepressant properties and unique mechanisms of action. Ketamine, although sometimes grouped with psychedelics, will not be a focus here, since its enantiomer, esketamine, has already been fully approved and integrated into clinical practice as an evidence-based antidepressant. By narrowing the scope to psilocybin, LSD, ayahuasca, and MDMA, this chapter aims to highlight the emerging data on substances that remain investigational but hold considerable promise for expanding the therapeutic landscape of depression.

W.-M. Bahk et al. (eds.), *Depressive Disorder*, https://doi.org/10.1007/978-981-92-1331-3_12

12.2 Historical Context

Early Psychiatric Research

Psychedelics were first introduced into Western medicine in the 1940s and 1950s, following Albert Hofmann's discovery of LSD in 1943 [3]. Early clinical research explored LSD and psilocybin for the treatment of depression, anxiety, alcoholism, and existential distress [5]. During this period, tens of thousands of patients received psychedelic therapy under medical supervision. While results were often promising, methodological rigor was limited by contemporary standards.

Decline and Prohibition

Although early studies showed promising outcomes, the non-medical use of psychedelics such as LSD and psilocybin rose sharply in the United States, fueling negative public opinion and increasing criticism in the media [5]. In response, the US government banned the production, distribution, and use of hallucinogenic substances in 1963 [6]. This was followed by the 1970 Controlled Substances Act, which classified LSD and psilocybin as Schedule I drugs—defined as compounds with high abuse potential and no accepted medical application—thereby imposing even stricter restrictions on their availability and research [7].

Revival of Psychedelic Science

The re-emergence of psychedelic research began cautiously in the 1990s, when a handful of small pilot studies sought to re-examine substances like psilocybin and LSD after decades of prohibition [8]. These early investigations were designed with strict safety protocols and ethical oversight, reflecting the lingering concerns from the previous era of unregulated experimentation. Findings from these initial trials suggested that, under controlled conditions, psychedelics could be administered safely and might provide meaningful therapeutic benefits [9]. Organizations such as Johns Hopkins University, Imperial College London, and MAPS (Multidisciplinary Association for Psychedelic Studies) have been instrumental in advancing this research [10, 11].

12.3 Neurobiological Mechanisms of Action

Psilocybin

Psilocybin is classified as a psychoplastogen, meaning it can induce rapid and enduring changes in neural plasticity [12]. Once ingested, it is quickly metabolized and exerts its effects mainly through serotonin (5-hydroxytryptamine, 5-HT) receptor agonism [13]. Among these receptors, it binds most strongly to the 5-HT2A subtype, which is thought to underpin its antidepressant and anxiolytic properties [14]. The mechanisms of action (Fig. 12.1) include several neurobiological pathways [15]. First, psilocybin stimulates glutamatergic transmission, which enhances the release of neurotrophic factors such as brain-derived neurotrophic factor (BDNF), thereby fostering neuronal repair and plasticity [16]. Activation of 5-HT2A receptors on immune cells has also been linked to a reduction in neuroinflammatory mediators such as tumor necrosis factor-alpha (TNF-α) and interleukin-6, contributing to an anti-inflammatory effect in the brain [13, 17, 18]. Beyond these processes, psilocybin may attenuate threat sensitivity in the visual cortex, which appears more closely tied to its anxiolytic rather than antidepressant effects [19]. Another important mechanism involves the downregulation of the default mode network, a brain system associated with rumination and self-focused negative thought patterns, the suppression of which is correlated with improvements in both depressive and anxiety symptoms [20]. Agonism of the 5-HT2A receptor also mediates the subjective psychedelic experience, including mystical-type states and visual hallucinations [21]. Because these receptors are densely distributed in the visual cortex, their activation likely plays a direct role in hallucinatory phenomena

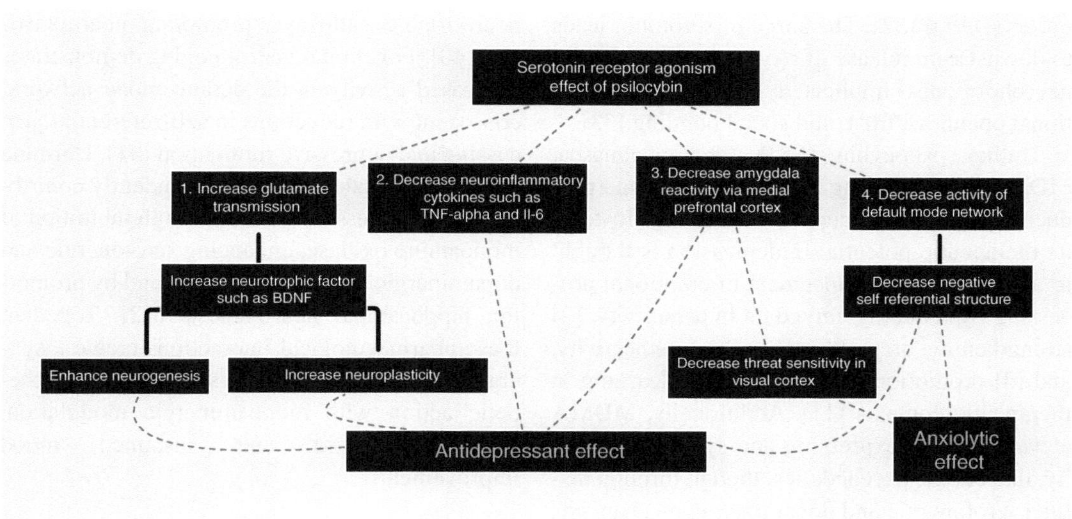

Fig. 12.1 Psilocybin exhibits antidepressant and anxiolytic effects through its agonistic action on serotonin receptors ($5HT_{2A}$). Reprinted with permission from Wang et al. [15]. BDNF brain-derived neurotrophic factor, IL-6 interleukin 6, TNF-alpha tumor necrosis factor-alpha

[22]. Additionally, 5-HT2A signaling increases dopamine release in the ventral striatum, contributing to altered states such as euphoria, depersonalization, and other hallucinogen-like experiences [23]. Finally, 5-HT2A receptor engagement in the thalamus and medial prefrontal cortex may reduce thalamic filtering capacity, leading to lowered arousal, diminished sensory gating, and alterations in consciousness [24].

Lysergic Acid Diethylamide (LSD)

LSD is a potent serotonergic psychedelic that, like psilocybin, exerts its primary effects through agonism at 5-HT2A receptors, although it also interacts with other serotonergic, dopaminergic, and adrenergic systems [25]. LSD shows high affinity not only for 5-HT2A but also for 5-HT1A, 5-HT2C, and dopamine D2 receptors, giving it a broader pharmacological profile [26]. Activation of 5-HT2A receptors leads to enhanced glutamatergic signaling in cortical pyramidal neurons, which in turn increases neurotrophic factors such as BDNF, supporting plasticity and synaptic remodeling [27]. Neuroimaging studies have shown that LSD decreases default mode network connectivity, facilitating greater global integration across brain networks, which is thought to underlie reductions in maladaptive rumination and depressive thinking [28]. Distinctively, LSD has prolonged receptor binding kinetics compared to psilocybin, leading to its longer duration of action [29]. LSD also increases dopaminergic signaling, especially in the striatum, contributing to its stimulant-like and euphoric properties [30]. The combination of serotonergic and dopaminergic effects, along with alterations in network-level connectivity, is believed to underlie both the hallucinogenic phenomena and potential antidepressant effects of LSD [31].

3,4-Methylenedioxymethamphetamine (MDMA)

MDMA differs mechanistically from the classic psychedelics, as it is primarily an entactogen rather than a hallucinogen. Its main action is as a monoamine releasing agent, markedly increasing extracellular levels of serotonin, norepinephrine, and dopamine through reversal of transporter function (serotonin transporter (SERT), norepinephrine transporter (NET), and dopamine transporter (DAT)) [32]. The surge of serotonin leads to downstream release of oxytocin and prolactin, neurohormones implicated in enhanced emotional openness, trust, and social bonding [33].

Unlike psilocybin, LSD, and ayahuasca, MDMA is not a strong 5-HT2A agonist and produces only mild perceptual alterations. Instead, its therapeutic potential in depression is thought to arise from [1] enhancement of emotional processing by reducing amygdala hyperactivity, [2] strengthening of prefrontal-limbic connectivity, and [3] promotion of fear extinction learning in therapeutic contexts [11]. Additionally, MDMA elevates BDNF expression and synaptic plasticity, like classic psychedelics, though through distinct serotonergic and dopaminergic mechanisms [34]. Functional imaging studies show decreased amygdala activity during negative emotional processing and increased connectivity between the amygdala and hippocampus, supporting improved regulation of traumatic or intrusive memories [35]. Adverse effects, such as mild cardiovascular stimulation (increased blood pressure and heart rate), are consistent with its sympathomimetic profile, but under clinical supervision, MDMA has shown a favorable safety profile [36].

Ayahuasca

Ayahuasca, a traditional Amazonian brew containing the psychedelic dimethyltryptamine (DMT) and monoamine oxidase inhibitors (MAOI) from Banisteriopsis caapi has attracted growing scientific interest for its potential antidepressant effects [37]. The MAOI components inhibit the breakdown of DMT, allowing for oral bioavailability. DMT itself is a 5-HT2A receptor agonist, similar to psilocybin and LSD, producing profound perceptual and cognitive alterations [38]. It also binds to sigma-1 receptors, which modulate calcium signaling, oxidative stress, and neuroinflammation, providing a potential mechanism for neuroprotective and antidepressant effects [39].

Preclinical and human studies indicate that ayahuasca acutely increases BDNF and other neurotrophic pathways, promoting neuroplasticity [40]. Functional neuroimaging demonstrates decreased activity in the default mode network, consistent with reductions in self-referential processing and depressive rumination [41]. Harmine and related alkaloids may independently contribute to antidepressant effects through inhibition of monoamine oxidase, enhancing serotonergic and dopaminergic neurotransmission, and by promoting hippocampal neurogenesis [42]. Together, these pharmacological interactions create a synergistic effect that combines serotonergic psychedelic action with monoaminergic modulation, supporting rapid and sustained mood improvements.

12.4 Clinical Evidence

Psilocybin

Psilocybin has received the most rigorous clinical evaluation. Twelve clinical trials that had investigated the effect of psilocybin in the treatment of depression were identified (Table 12.1). Among them, six were open-label studies and six were double-blind randomized controlled trials.

One open-label pilot study first demonstrated that psilocybin, when administered together with psychotherapy, could produce rapid and substantial reductions in depressive symptoms in patients with TRD [43]. In this study, patients who had failed to respond to multiple antidepressant trials received two psilocybin sessions (10 mg and 25 mg, 1 week apart), and the majority showed marked improvement within the first week, with many reaching remissions. These effects were maintained for several weeks, and the treatment was generally well tolerated, with adverse effects such as transient anxiety, nausea, or headache resolving quickly.

Other extension studies investigated the durability and predictors of therapeutic benefit. A 6-month follow-up of the Carhart-Harris [43] cohort showed that antidepressant effects persisted at 3 and 6 months, with large effect sizes still observed, although some patients relapsed over time [44]. Another open-label extension

Table 12.1 Clinical studies investigating psilocybin in the treatment of depression

Author (Year)	Subjects	Allocation	Size	Length	Intervention	1° outcome	Results
Carhart-Harris [43]	OL TRD	Psilocybin only	12	12 wk	Two oral psilocybin capsule (10 mg and 25 mg)	Subjective effect (0 ~ 1)	Low-dose session: 0·51 (SD 0·36) High-dose session: 0·75 (SD 0·27)
Carhart-Harris[a] [44]	OL TRD	Psilocybin only	20	6 mo	10 mg + 25 mg	QIDS-SR16	Improvement began 1 week after psilocybin and maintained at 6 mo
Roseman[a] [45]	OL TRD	Psilocybin only	20	6 mo	10 mg + 25 mg	ASC	High mystical experience + low anxiety predicted positive outcome
Lyons[a] [46]	OL TRD	Psilocybin CG	15 15	1 wk	10 mg + 25 mg Healthy subjects	BDI, POFLE	Depression and negative cognitive bias improved after psilocybin
Davis [47]	OL MDD	Psilocybin Waiting	15 12	4 wk	20 mg + 30 mg per 70 kg	GRID-HAMD	Significantly more improved in psilocybin group
Gukasyan [48]	OL MDD	Psilocybin only	27	12 mo	20 mg + 30 mg per 70 kg	GRID-HAMD	GRID-HAMD improved over 12 mo
Ross [49]	DB-RCT Cancer	Psilocybin 0.3 mg/kg Niacin 250 mg	14 15	7 wk + 5 mo	Cross over study, all in oral formulation	HADS-A, HADS-D	Psilocybin superior to niacin
Griffiths [50]	DB-RCT Cancer	Psilocybin 22 ~ 30 mg Psilocybin 1 ~ 3 mg	25 26	5 wk. + 5 mo	Cross over study, all in oral formulation	GRID-HAMD, HAM-A	High dose superior to low dose
Carhart-Harris [51]	DB-RCT MDD	Psilocybin 25 mg Escitalopram	30 29	6 wk	25 mg × 2 + PBO vs. 1 mg × 2 + Escitalopram	HADS-A, HADS-D	−8 points for psilocybin v − 6 points for escitalopram ($p > 0.05$)
von Rotz [52]	DB-RCT MDD	Psilocybin 0.215 mg/kg PBO	26 26	14 days	1 dose of gelatin capsules + psychological support	GRID-HAMD, HAM-A	0.215 mg/kg > PBO for MADRS and BDI
Goodwin [53]	DB-RCT TRD	Psilocybin 25 mg Psilocybin 10 mg Psilocybin 1 mg	79 75 79	12 wk	1 dose of synthetic formulation + psychological support	QIDS-SR-16	At wk. 3, 25 mg > 1 mg. 10 mg vs. 1 mg no difference
Raison [54]	DB-RCT MDD	Psilocybin 25 mg Niacin 100 mg	51 53	6 wk	1 dose + psychological support	MADRS	MADRS scores reduction more in psilocybin than niacin from day 8

[a]Extension of Carhart-Harris [43]; Extension of Davis [47]

1° Primary, *ASC* altered states of consciousness, *BDI* Beck's depression inventory, *CG* control group, *DB* double blinded, *GRID-HAMD* GRID Hamilton rating scale for depression, *HADS-A* hospital anxiety and depression scale-anxiety, *HADS-D* hospital anxiety and depression scale-depression, *HAM-D 17*, 17-item Hamilton depression rating scale, *MADRS* Montgomery–Åsberg depression rating scale, *MDD* major depressive disorder, *mo* Months, *POFLE* Prediction of future life events task, *QIDS-SR16* 16 item Quick inventory of depressive symptoms, *RCT* randomized clinical trial, *TRD* treatment-resistant depression, *wk* week focused on the role of the acute psychedelic experience in predicting outcomes [45]. Using validated questionnaires, it was shown that patients who experienced stronger mystical-type phenomena (such as oceanic boundlessness) and lower anxiety or ego dissolution during dosing tended to have better long-term results, emphasizing the therapeutic importance of the subjective experience itself. Building on this, a further extension study explored the cognitive mechanisms of benefit in TRD patients [46]. It found that cognitive bias, particularly pessimism about future life events, improved significantly 1 week after psilocybin treatment. Patients not only reported less pessimism but also demonstrated greater accuracy in predicting actual life events, while healthy controls showed no such improvement. These findings suggested that psilocybin may work partly by reshaping maladaptive cognitive patterns associated with chronic depression.

Two further open-label studies examined psilocybin in patients with MDD. A randomized waiting-list trial enrolled 27 patients and demonstrated rapid and robust reductions in depression severity, with significantly lower GRID-Hamilton Depression Rating Scale (GRID-HAMD) and Quick Inventory of Depressive Symptomatology (QIDS) scores in the immediate treatment group compared with the delayed treatment control group [47]. Psilocybin produced rapid symptom relief that was sustained for several weeks, and adverse events were generally mild, such as transient headaches or mild anxiety. A 12-month extension of this study confirmed the durability of antidepressant effects: at 1 year, 75% of participants maintained clinical response and 58% achieved remission, with no treatment-related serious adverse events reported [48].

Six double-blind randomized controlled trials have investigated psilocybin in the treatment of depression across cancer-related distress, MDD, and treatment-resistant depression (TRD). Two early trials were conducted in patients with life-threatening cancer and clinically significant symptoms of depression and anxiety [49, 50]. In a crossover study by Ross et al., patients who received a single high dose of psilocybin (0.3 mg/kg) showed significant reductions in depression and anxiety, as measured by Hospital Anxiety and Depression Scale (HADS), Beck's depression inventory (BDI), and State-Trait Anxiety Inventory (STAI), compared with the niacin control group [49]. These improvements were rapid, clinically meaningful, and sustained for more than 6 months, accompanied by improved quality of life and reduced fear of death. Similarly, Griffiths et al. randomized cancer patients to receive either a very low dose (1–3 mg/70 kg) or a high dose (22–30 mg/70 kg) of psilocybin in a counterbalanced sequence [50]. High-dose psilocybin produced markedly higher response and remission rates on GRID-HAMD and HAM-A at 5 weeks, and these benefits persisted at 6 months. Importantly, the therapeutic effect was mediated by the intensity of the mystical-type experience, and adverse events were mild and transient, including temporary increases in blood pressure, nausea, and anxiety.

Subsequent trials have investigated psilocybin in patients with MDD. A phase II trial by Carhart-Harris et al. compared psilocybin with escitalopram over 6 weeks in patients with moderate-to-severe depression [51]. Both groups demonstrated improvements in depression severity, but remission rates were significantly higher in the psilocybin group (57 vs. 28%) than in the escitalopram group. Secondary outcomes generally favored psilocybin, and both treatments were well tolerated, with the most common adverse effects being headache and transient anxiety. In another randomized controlled trials, von Rotz et al. randomized 52 patients with MDD to receive a single moderate dose of psilocybin (0.215 mg/kg) or placebo with psychological support [52]. Psilocybin produced rapid reductions in Montgomery–Åsberg depression rating scale (MADRS) and BDI scores within hours of administration, and these improvements remained significant at 14 days. Response and remission rates were also higher in the psilocybin group. Adverse events were mild and transient, including temporary increases in blood pressure, with no serious treatment-related events reported.

Larger multisite studies extended this evidence to TRD. Goodwin et al. randomized 233 adults with TRD to receive 25 mg, 10 mg, or 1 mg of psilocybin alongside psychological support [53]. At 3 weeks, the 25-mg group showed significantly greater reductions in MADRS scores and higher response and remission rates compared with the 1-mg control. The statistical analysis showed that the 25-mg group was superior to 1-mg group (−6.6; $p < 0.001$)). However, there were no statistical difference between 10-mg group and 1-mg group (−2.5; $p = 0.18$). In addition, the 25-mg group showed significantly higher rate of response (odds ratio [OR] = 2.9) and remission (OR = 4.8) at week 3, but not sustained response at week 12, than the 1-mg group. Notably, some participants receiving active doses experienced suicidal ideation or self-injurious behavior, underscoring the importance of careful monitoring. Most recently, a multisite phase II trial by Raison et al. randomized 104 adults with MDD to receive a single 25-mg dose of psilocybin or niacin placebo, both combined with psychotherapy [54]. Psilocybin treatment was associated with significantly greater reductions in MADRS scores compared with niacin from baseline to day 8 (mean difference, −12.0 [95% confidence interval [CI], −16.6 to −7.4]; $p < 0.001$) and from baseline to day 43 (mean difference, −12.3 [95% CI, −17.5 to −7.2]; $p < 0.001$). Functional outcomes also improved, with significantly greater reductions in Sheehan Disability Scale scores compared with niacin from baseline to day 43 (mean difference, −2.31 [95% CI, −3.50 to −1.11]; $p < 0.001$). Approximately 42% of participants receiving psilocybin achieved sustained response, although remission rates did not differ significantly between groups. No treatment-related serious adverse events were reported; however, psilocybin was associated with a higher rate of overall adverse events and more severe adverse events than placebo, most commonly transient headache, paranoia, panic, and perceptual disturbances, which resolved without sequelae.

A recent systematic review and meta-analysis synthesized evidence from nine randomized controlled trials including 436 participants with clinically significant depression [55]. Eligible studies included double-blind and open-label randomized trials with crossover or parallel designs, focusing exclusively on adults with clinically significant depressive symptoms. Trials were required to have a control condition (placebo, niacin, or very low-dose psychedelics), and if psychotherapy was provided, it had to be delivered equally in both groups to distinguish psilocybin's specific effects. Outcomes were included at all time points beyond 3 h post-administration. Psilocybin was found to produce a moderate-to-large antidepressant effect compared with placebo or non-psychoactive controls (Hedges' g = 0.66, 95% CI, 0.46–0.86). Importantly, psilocybin approximately doubled the likelihood of treatment response (relative risk [RR] = 2.17, 95% CI, 1.18–3.99) and nearly tripled remission rates (RR = 2.96, 95% CI, 1.69–5.17). Subgroup analyses suggested stronger effects in patients with secondary depression (e.g., cancer-related), in older adults, in those with previous psychedelic experience, and when outcomes were assessed using self-report scales. Adverse effects were generally mild and transient, most commonly headaches, short-lived anxiety, or slight increases in blood pressure, with no serious adverse events reported.

Complementing this, a recent 2025 meta-analysis of 17 randomized controlled trials ($n = 4960$) compared outcomes across psilocybin, esketamine, and SSRI trials for depression. Psilocybin trials ($n = 373$) showed large within-group improvements (standardized mean change (SMC) = 1.21), similar to SSRIs (1.28) and esketamine (1.43) [54]. However, control groups in psilocybin trials improved far less (SMC = 0.50) than controls in SSRI (1.00) or esketamine trials (1.12). This led to larger between-group effect sizes for psilocybin (standardized mean difference (SMD) = 0.70) compared with SSRIs (0.27) and esketamine (0.30). Yet the authors cautioned that this pattern may reflect unusually poor control group outcomes in psilocybin studies, possibly due to difficulties maintaining blinding or expectancy/nocebo effects. Response rates highlight this concern: only 19% of psilocybin control participants improved, versus 33% with SSRI controls and 42% with esketamine controls. Dropout rates were relatively low for psilocybin (5% active, 11% control) compared with SSRIs (~32–35%).

Taken together, the available evidence indicates that psilocybin, when administered with structured psychological support, produces rapid, clinically meaningful reductions in depressive symptoms across TRD, MDD, and cancer-related distress. Open-label studies demonstrate sustained benefits for up to a year in many patients, while double-blind randomized trials confirm efficacy over placebo and active comparators, though durability of effect beyond several weeks remains variable. Importantly, the quality and intensity of the acute psychedelic experience appear to mediate long-term therapeutic outcomes. Safety profiles are generally favorable, with most adverse events being mild and transient, but occasional reports of suicidality or self-injurious behavior highlight the need for careful monitoring. Recent meta-analyses reinforce psilocybin's robust antidepressant effects relative to placebo and standard treatments, while also underscoring methodological challenges such as expectancy effects and low control group response rates. Overall, psilocybin shows considerable promise as a novel, fast-acting intervention for depression, though larger and longer-term trials are needed to establish its durability, optimize therapeutic protocols, and ensure safe integration into clinical practice.

LSD

Evidence for LSD in depressive disorders is emerging but remains more limited than for psilocybin (Table 12.2). An initial mechanistic trial tested low-dose LSD (13 and 26 μg, sublingual) in 18 healthy adults using a randomized, within-subject, placebo-controlled design [56]. Neural responses were measured during a monetary incentive delay task with electroencephalography (EEG), focusing on reward-related event-related potentials. Compared with placebo, LSD—particularly the 13 μg dose—significantly increased neural markers of reward sensitivity (Reward Positivity, Feedback-P3, Late Positive Potential), which are typically blunted in depression. These changes occurred without strong psychedelic effects, suggesting that low doses may enhance reward processing independently of perceptual alterations and provide a rationale for future depression trials.

One of the earliest modern randomized controlled studies investigated LSD-assisted therapy in patients with anxiety associated with life-threatening illness but also assessed depressive symptoms as a secondary outcome [57]. In this double-blind, placebo-controlled phase II study, Holze and colleagues found that LSD (200 μg) significantly reduced both anxiety and depressive symptoms compared with placebo, and improvements were sustained at 16 weeks. One serious adverse event occurred (an acute delusional-anxious reaction during dosing, resolved with standard treatment), but otherwise adverse events were transient and mild, such as headache, nausea, and short-lived anxiety. These results provided preliminary support that LSD could alleviate depressive symptoms even when not the primary indication.

In a complementary study, Molla et al. examined the effects of low-dose LSD (26 μg) in 39 participants with mild depressive symptoms (BDI $\geq$ 17) compared with healthy controls [58]. Using a randomized, double-blind, placebo-controlled crossover design, participants received both LSD and placebo in counterbalanced sessions. In the depressed mood group, LSD produced greater acute increases in vigor, elation, and positively valenced altered states of consciousness, alongside significantly lower BDI scores 48 h post-dose. Adverse effects were mild and transient, including slight increases in blood pressure and perceptual changes. These findings suggest that even low doses of LSD may temporarily enhance mood in individuals with subclinical depression.

Most recently, Müller et al. performed the first modern randomized controlled trial of LSD-assisted therapy specifically in patients with MDD [59]. Sixty-one adults with moderate-to-severe MDD were randomized to high-dose LSD (100 μg at the first session, 200 μg at the second) or low-dose LSD (25 μg at both sessions) as an active control. All participants received structured psychotherapy, including preparation, dosing, and integration sessions. At

Table 12.2 Summary of clinical studies of LSD relevant to depression

Study (Year)	Population (*N*)	Design	Dose and intervention	Main depression-related outcomes	Safety
Glazer [56]	Healthy adults ($N = 18$)	DB, within-subject, PBO-controlled	13 μg & 26 μg LSD (sublingual, single dose)	Increased reward-related brain activity—relevant to anhedonia in depression	Well tolerated; no serious events
Holze [57]	Anxiety disorders ± life-threatening illness ($N = 42$)	Phase II, DB, PBO-controlled, crossover	200 μg LSD × 2 + psychotherapy	Significant reductions in HAM-D and BDI vs. placebo; sustained up to 16 weeks	1 SAE (acute anxiety/delusion, resolved); otherwise mild transient events (headache, nausea, anxiety)
Molla [58]	Mild depression (BDI ≥ 17) vs. controls ($N = 39$)	DB, PBO-controlled, crossover	26 μg LSD (single session)	Greater acute increases in positive mood and altered states in depressed group; BDI scores reduced 48 h post-dose	Mild, transient ↑BP, perceptual changes; no SAEs
Müller [59]	Major depressive disorder ($N = 61$)	Phase II, DB, randomized, parallel	High-dose: 100 μg + 200 μg vs. low-dose: 25 μg × 2; with psychotherapy	High-dose LSD significantly reduced IDS-C and IDS-SR vs. low-dose (effect sizes d = −0.63 to −0.73); benefits sustained to 6 weeks, partial at 12 weeks	Well tolerated; mild-to-moderate anxiety, nausea, transient ↑BP/HR; no SAEs

BDI Beck's depression inventory, *BP* blood pressure, *DB* double blinded, *HAM-D* 17-item Hamilton depression rating scale, *PBO* placebo, *SAE* serious adverse event

2 weeks after the second dosing, the high-dose group showed significantly greater reductions in depression severity: Inventory of Depressive Symptomatology - Clinican Rated (IDS-C) (−12.9 vs. –3.6; between-group difference −9.2; $p = 0.023$; d = −0.63) and Inventory of Depressive Symptomatology - Self Report (IDS-SR) (−11.8 vs. −1.6; between-group difference −10.2; $p = 0.004$; d = −0.73). Improvements remained significant at 6 weeks and were partially sustained at 12 weeks. Secondary measures, including BDI and symptom checklist-90-revised (SCL-90), also favored the high-dose group. LSD was well tolerated overall, with no treatment-related serious adverse events. The most common side effects were mild and transient, such as acute anxiety, headache, nausea, and moderate increases in blood pressure or heart rate. Importantly, no cases of psychosis or suicidality attributable to LSD were reported.

While evidence remains limited, emerging data from controlled studies indicate that LSD, like psilocybin, has antidepressant potential. Early work in anxiety with comorbid depression suggested efficacy, subsequent experimental studies demonstrated transient mood improvements even at low doses, and the first dedicated randomized controlled trial in MDD confirmed significant antidepressant effects of higher-dose LSD-assisted therapy. Larger trials with longer follow-up are now needed to establish the durability and safety of these effects in clinical populations.

MDMA

Unlike psilocybin and LSD, which have been studied primarily for MDD and TRD, MDMA research has largely focused on posttraumatic stress disorder (PTSD) [60]. Nevertheless, depressive symptoms are frequently measured as secondary outcomes in these trials, and emerging evidence suggests that MDMA-assisted therapy may also exert antidepressant effects. The first modern pilot studies of MDMA-assisted psychotherapy in patients with chronic PTSD reported substantial reductions in both PTSD severity and depressive symptoms [11]. In early randomized, placebo-controlled trials, patients who received two to three sessions of MDMA-assisted psychotherapy showed marked HAM-D and BDI scores compared with controls, with many patients no longer meeting criteria for comorbid depression after treatment. These improvements were durable, with follow-up studies showing sustained benefits up to 12 months.

More rigorous evidence comes from phase III, multisite randomized controlled trials. In 2021, a large study of 90 participants with severe, chronic PTSD demonstrated that MDMA-assisted therapy not only produced large reductions in PTSD symptoms but also led to significant improvements in comorbid depression, as measured by the MADRS [61]. Effect sizes for depression were in the moderate-to-large range, and benefits were sustained at follow-up. Importantly, these effects appeared to be mediated by both direct pharmacological action and the facilitation of emotional processing within psychotherapy sessions.

Beyond PTSD, there is growing interest in applying MDMA-assisted therapy directly to primary depression. The first open-label proof-of-principle study in MDD was published in 2025 and included 12 participants with moderate-to-severe depression [62]. All participants received two MDMA-assisted therapy sessions combined with preparatory and integration psychotherapy. Significant reductions in depressive symptoms were observed, with large decreases in MADRS and Sheehan Disability Scale scores that persisted up to 8 weeks post-treatment. The intervention was generally well tolerated, with common side effects including mild transient increases in blood pressure and heart rate, jaw tension, and temporary anxiety. No treatment-related serious adverse events were reported.

Overall, although the evidence base for MDMA in depression is smaller than for psilocybin or ayahuasca, available data suggest promising antidepressant effects. Secondary analyses of PTSD trials consistently demonstrate significant reductions in depressive symptoms, and the first proof-of-principle study in MDD shows feasibility, safety, and encouraging efficacy. Larger randomized controlled trials targeting MDD and TRD are now warranted to determine whether MDMA-assisted therapy can play a definitive role in the treatment of depressive disorders.

Ayahuasca

Compared with psilocybin and LSD, the clinical evidence base is smaller, but several controlled trials have now evaluated its efficacy in patients with MDD and TRD. The modern clinical study of ayahuasca in depression began with small open-label investigations in Brazil. In 2015, a pilot trial administered a single ayahuasca session to six patients with recurrent MDD [63]. Rapid reductions in depressive symptoms were observed within hours, with significant improvements maintained for up to 21 days on the HAM-D and MADRS. The treatment was generally well tolerated, with nausea, vomiting, and transient anxiety as the most common adverse effects, but no serious adverse events were reported.

In 2016, an open-label neuroimaging study extended these findings in 17 patients with recurrent depression [64]. A single ayahuasca dose produced significant reductions in MADRS scores at both 1 day and 7 days post-treatment. Single-photon emission computed tomography (SPECT) demonstrated increased blood flow in brain regions implicated in mood regulation, including the nucleus accumbens, insula, and subgenual anterior cingulate cortex, providing neurobiological support for the observed antidepressant effects. Ayahuasca was well tolerated. Vomiting was the only adverse effect recorded, being reported by 47% of the volunteers.

The first randomized, placebo-controlled trial was published in 2019 and included 35 adults with TRD [65]. This was a parallel-group, double-blind design conducted in a hospital setting, where participants were randomized to receive either a single oral dose of ayahuasca or a placebo beverage that was carefully designed to mimic its taste, color, and consistency. All participants had moderate-to-severe depression and had failed to respond to at least two prior antidepressant trials, making this a particularly difficult-to-treat population. Patients were monitored in a controlled environment and provided with psychological support throughout the dosing session and follow-up period. Both groups showed some initial improvement at day 1, likely reflecting expectancy and nonspecific care effects. However, by day 7 the ayahuasca group demonstrated significantly greater reductions in MADRS scores (mean difference ≈ −9.8; $p < 0.01$), corresponding to a large effect size. Response rates (≥50% reduction in MADRS) were 64% in the ayahuasca group compared with 27% in placebo, while remission rates (MADRS ≤10) were 36 versus 7%, respectively. Notably, antidepressant effects were already apparent within 24 h of administration, highlighting the rapid onset of benefit, and remained significant for at least a week after a single dose. The treatment was well tolerated overall. Common side effects included nausea, vomiting, and transient anxiety or emotional distress during the session, but these resolved spontaneously. Importantly, no cases of psychosis, mania, or suicidality were reported, and no treatment-related serious adverse events occurred. The presence of the traditional "purge" (nausea and vomiting) was frequent but not medically concerning in the supervised setting.

Overall, clinical studies conducted between 2015 and 2019 consistently demonstrate that ayahuasca produces rapid and robust antidepressant effects in patients with recurrent or treatment-resistant depression, with benefits lasting up to several weeks after a single administration. Neuroimaging findings provide biological plausibility, and placebo-controlled data confirm efficacy beyond expectancy effects. While nausea, vomiting, and transient anxiety are common, safety in controlled clinical settings has been favorable, with no treatment-related serious adverse events observed. Larger and longer-term randomized trials are now required to confirm efficacy, evaluate durability, and optimize therapeutic protocols.

Comparative Evidence Across Psychedelics

A recent systematic review and Bayesian network meta-analysis synthesized evidence from 19 randomized controlled trials, including 15 psychedelic trials ($n = 811$) and 5 escitalopram trials ($n = 1968$), to directly compare the antidepressant efficacy and safety of psilocybin, LSD, ayahuasca, and MDMA with escitalopram [66]. The study addressed a key methodological limitation of prior meta-analyses: the potential overestimation of psychedelic efficacy due to poor blinding and unusually low placebo responses. To mitigate this, control conditions were categorized as: (i) placebo in antidepressant trials (adequately blinded inert controls); (ii) placebo in psychedelic trials (e.g., niacin or inactive gelatin capsules, often compromised by unblinding); and (iii) extremely low-dose psychedelics (e.g., psilocybin 1–3 mg, MDMA ≤40 mg) functioning as "active placebos."

The results showed that placebo responses were consistently lower in psychedelic trials than in antidepressant trials (≈3.8 HAM-D points difference), confirming that earlier studies likely inflated effect sizes. High-dose psilocybin (≥20 mg) was the only psychedelic that demonstrated superiority over placebo when benchmarked against antidepressant trial placebo response, with a small but clinically relevant effect size (SMD = 0.31). Compared with escitalopram, high-dose psilocybin was associated with significantly greater reductions in depressive symptoms (≈4.7 HAM-D points), while LSD, ayahuasca, and MDMA showed more limited or inconsistent benefits in this comparative framework. In patients with MDD, high-dose psilocybin, ayahuasca, and escitalopram all outperformed antidepressant-trial placebo, though only psilocybin exceeded the threshold for minimal clinically important difference across all control comparisons. Safety outcomes were generally favorable: no higher risk of all-cause discontinuation or severe adverse events was found for psychedelics compared with placebo. Adverse events were mostly mild and transient (e.g., nausea, headache, anxiety, transient increases in blood pressure/heart rate).

This analysis provides the most rigorous comparative evidence to date. While earlier reports suggested very large antidepressant effects of psychedelics, much of this appears to have been driven by methodological artifacts, particularly weak placebo performance. When benchmarked against adequately blinded antidepressant trials, high-dose psilocybin emerges as the only psychedelic with reproducible superiority over placebo and escitalopram, though its effect size is small and comparable to conventional SSRIs. Evidence for LSD, MDMA, and ayahuasca remains promising but less consistent, warranting further high-quality trials with larger samples, longer follow-up, and improved blinding methods.

12.5 Conclusion

The modern reappraisal of psychedelics has revitalized psychiatric research and highlighted their therapeutic potential in depressive disorders. Across psilocybin, LSD, ayahuasca, and MDMA, converging lines of evidence suggest that these compounds engage both biological and psychological processes that extend beyond those of conventional antidepressants. Neurobiological data point to overlapping mechanisms such as 5-HT2A receptor agonism, modulation of glutamatergic and monoaminergic transmission, enhancement of neurotrophic signaling, and large-scale network reorganization, including suppression of default mode network hyperactivity. These changes appear to translate into rapid symptom relief, improvements in emotional processing, and sustained functional recovery in at least a subset of patients.

Clinically, psilocybin is the most extensively studied, with randomized controlled trials consistently showing substantial antidepressant effects, including superiority to placebo and comparability to established antidepressants such as escitalopram. LSD has re-emerged after decades of prohibition, with recent mechanistic and clinical trials demonstrating meaningful reductions in depressive symptoms, particularly at higher doses combined with psychotherapy. Ayahuasca, though studied primarily in South America, has yielded robust antidepressant signals in both open-label and placebo-controlled trials, with neuroimaging data providing biological plausibility for its effects. MDMA, traditionally categorized as an entactogen, has primarily been investigated for PTSD, yet evidence consistently shows secondary benefits on depression severity, and early trials in primary MDD indicate feasibility and promising efficacy. Across all four compounds, safety profiles in controlled research environments have been reassuring. Adverse effects are typically mild and transient—such as anxiety, nausea, vomiting, or modest cardiovascular changes—with very few reports of serious treatment-emergent events. Nonetheless, the potential for acute psychological distress, suicidality in vulnerable individuals, and cardiovascular risks underscores the need for careful screening, professional supervision, and integration of psychotherapy into treatment protocols.

Despite these encouraging developments, limitations must be acknowledged. Many trials remain small, heterogeneous, and of relatively short duration. The durability of antidepressant effects beyond several weeks is uncertain, with some evidence of relapse over time. Challenges in maintaining blinding due to the distinctive psychoactive effects of these drugs raise concerns about expectancy bias and inflated effect sizes. Furthermore, the heterogeneity of psychotherapeutic support across studies makes it difficult to disentangle pharmacological from psychological contributions to treatment outcomes.

Looking forward, rigorous, large-scale randomized controlled trials with extended follow-up are required to confirm efficacy and clarify long-term safety. Comparative effectiveness studies with standard antidepressants, exploration of biomarkers predictive of treatment response, and refinement of therapeutic frameworks will be essential to optimize clinical utility. Equally important are considerations of scalability, equity of access, training of therapists, and integration into existing health systems should these treatments achieve regulatory approval.

In summary, psychedelics represent a promising and potentially transformative class of interventions for depression. While psilocybin currently leads the field in terms of evidence, LSD, ayahuasca, and MDMA all show antidepressant potential that warrants further investigation. These agents may ultimately expand therapeutic options for patients who fail to respond to conventional treatments, offering rapid relief, novel mechanisms, and the possibility of durable recovery when combined with structured psychological support. Continued research will determine whether the promise of psychedelic-assisted therapy can be translated into safe, effective, and widely accessible treatments for depressive disorders.

Declarations

Competing Interests The author(s) has no competing interests to declare that are relevant to the content of this manuscript.

Ethics Approval The author(s) declares that this manuscript does not include primary research with human participants.

The author(s) declares that this manuscript does not include primary studies involving animals.

References

1. Serretti A. Anhedonia and depressive disorders. Clin Psychopharmacol Neurosci. 2023;21(3):401–9.
2. Fava M. The challenges of defining and managing treatment-resistant depression in research and practice. World Psychiatry. 2023;22(3):350–1.
3. Raj P, Rauniyar S, Sapkale B. Psychedelic drugs or hallucinogens: exploring their medicinal potential. Cureus. 2023;15(11):e48719.
4. Carhart-Harris RL, Goodwin GM. The therapeutic potential of psychedelic drugs: past, present, and future. Neuropsychopharmacology. 2017;42(11):2105–13.
5. Redden WM, Paracha SU, Sheheryar Q. Hallucinogen use and misuse in older adults. Clin Geriatr Med. 2022;38(1):55–66.
6. Sharma P, Nguyen QA, Matthews SJ, Carpenter E, Mathews DB, Patten CA, et al. Psilocybin history, action and reaction: a narrative clinical review. J Psychopharmacol. 2023;37(9):849–65.
7. Drug Enforcement Administration DoJ. Definition of "positional isomer" as it pertains to the control of schedule I controlled substances. Final Rule Fed Regist. 2007;72(231):67850–2.
8. Rucker JJH, Iliff J, Nutt DJ. Psychiatry & the psychedelic drugs. Past, present & future. Neuropharmacology. 2018;142:200–18.
9. Petranker R, Anderson T, Farb N. Psychedelic research and the need for transparency: polishing Alice's looking glass. Front Psychol. 2020;11:1681.
10. Johnson MW, Garcia-Romeu A, Griffiths RR. Long-term follow-up of psilocybin-facilitated smoking cessation. Am J Drug Alcohol Abuse. 2017;43(1):55–60.
11. Mithoefer MC, Wagner MT, Mithoefer AT, Jerome L, Doblin R. The safety and efficacy of +/-3,4-methylenedioxymethamphetamine-assisted psychotherapy in subjects with chronic, treatment-resistant posttraumatic stress disorder: the first randomized controlled pilot study. J Psychopharmacol. 2011;25(4):439–52.
12. Vargas MV, Meyer R, Avanes AA, Rus M, Olson DE. Psychedelics and other psychoplastogens for treating mental illness. Front Psych. 2021;12:727117.
13. Nau F Jr, Yu B, Martin D, Nichols CD. Serotonin 5-HT2A receptor activation blocks TNF-alpha mediated inflammation in vivo. PLoS One. 2013;8(10):e75426.
14. Muttoni S, Ardissino M, John C. Classical psychedelics for the treatment of depression and anxiety: a systematic review. J Affect Disord. 2019;258:11–24.
15. Wang SM, Kim S, Choi WS, Lim HK, Woo YS, Pae CU, et al. Current understanding on psilocybin for major depressive disorder: a review focusing on clinical trials. Clin Psychopharmacol Neurosci. 2024;22(2):222–31.
16. Mason NL, Kuypers KPC, Muller F, Reckweg J, Tse DHY, Toennes SW, et al. Me, myself, bye: regional alterations in glutamate and the experience of ego dissolution with psilocybin. Neuropsychopharmacology. 2020;45(12):2003–11.
17. Raval NR, Johansen A, Donovan LL, Ros NF, Ozenne B, Hansen HD, et al. A single dose of psilocybin increases synaptic density and decreases 5-HT(2A) receptor density in the pig brain. Int J Mol Sci. 2021;22(2):835.
18. Nkadimeng SM, Steinmann CML, Eloff JN. Anti-inflammatory effects of four psilocybin-containing magic mushroom water extracts in vitro on 15-lipoxygenase activity and on lipopolysaccharide-

induced Cyclooxygenase-2 and inflammatory cytokines in human U937 macrophage cells. J Inflamm Res. 2021;14:3729–38.
19. Mertens LJ, Wall MB, Roseman L, Demetriou L, Nutt DJ, Carhart-Harris RL. Therapeutic mechanisms of psilocybin: changes in amygdala and prefrontal functional connectivity during emotional processing after psilocybin for treatment-resistant depression. J Psychopharmacol. 2020;34(2):167–80.
20. Carhart-Harris RL, Roseman L, Bolstridge M, Demetriou L, Pannekoek JN, Wall MB, et al. Psilocybin for treatment-resistant depression: fMRI-measured brain mechanisms. Sci Rep. 2017;7(1):13187.
21. Ling S, Ceban F, Lui LMW, Lee Y, Teopiz KM, Rodrigues NB, et al. Molecular mechanisms of psilocybin and implications for the treatment of depression. CNS Drugs. 2022;36(1):17–30.
22. Mahapatra A, Gupta R. Role of psilocybin in the treatment of depression. Ther Adv Psychopharmacol. 2017;7(1):54–6.
23. Vollenweider FX, Vontobel P, Hell D, Leenders KL. 5-HT modulation of dopamine release in basal ganglia in psilocybin-induced psychosis in man–a PET study with [11C]raclopride. Neuropsychopharmacology. 1999;20(5):424–33.
24. Daniel J, Haberman M. Clinical potential of psilocybin as a treatment for mental health conditions. Ment Health Clin. 2017;7(1):24–8.
25. Nichols DE. Psychedelics. Pharmacol Rev. 2016;68(2):264–355.
26. Rickli A, Moning OD, Hoener MC, Liechti ME. Receptor interaction profiles of novel psychoactive tryptamines compared with classic hallucinogens. Eur Neuropsychopharmacol. 2016;26(8):1327–37.
27. Vollenweider FX, Preller KH. Psychedelic drugs: neurobiology and potential for treatment of psychiatric disorders. Nat Rev Neurosci. 2020;21(11):611–24.
28. Carhart-Harris RL, Muthukumaraswamy S, Roseman L, Kaelen M, Droog W, Murphy K, et al. Neural correlates of the LSD experience revealed by multimodal neuroimaging. Proc Natl Acad Sci USA. 2016;113(17):4853–8.
29. Wacker D, Wang S, McCorvy JD, Betz RM, Venkatakrishnan AJ, Levit A, et al. Crystal structure of an LSD-bound human serotonin receptor. Cell. 2017;168(3):377–89 e12.
30. Marona-Lewicka D, Chemel BR, Nichols DE. Dopamine D4 receptor involvement in the discriminative stimulus effects in rats of LSD, but not the phenethylamine hallucinogen DOI. Psychopharmacology. 2009;203(2):265–77.
31. Preller KH, Burt JB, Ji JL, Schleifer CH, Adkinson BD, Stampfli P, et al. Changes in global and thalamic brain connectivity in LSD-induced altered states of consciousness are attributable to the 5-HT2A receptor. elife. 2018;7:7.
32. Liechti M. Novel psychoactive substances (designer drugs): overview and pharmacology of modulators of monoamine signaling. Swiss Med Wkly. 2015;145:w14043.
33. Dumont GJ, Sweep FC, van der Steen R, Hermsen R, Donders AR, Touw DJ, et al. Increased oxytocin concentrations and prosocial feelings in humans after ecstasy (3,4-methylenedioxymethamphetamine) administration. Soc Neurosci. 2009;4(4):359–66.
34. Nardou R, Lewis EM, Rothhaas R, Xu R, Yang A, Boyden E, et al. Oxytocin-dependent reopening of a social reward learning critical period with MDMA. Nature. 2019;569(7754):116–20.
35. Carhart-Harris RL, Wall MB, Erritzoe D, Kaelen M, Ferguson B, De Meer I, et al. The effect of acutely administered MDMA on subjective and BOLD-fMRI responses to favourite and worst autobiographical memories. Int J Neuropsychopharmacol. 2014;17(4):527–40.
36. Sessa B. MDMA and PTSD treatment: "PTSD: from novel pathophysiology to innovative therapeutics". Neurosci Lett. 2017;649:176–80.
37. Palhano-Fontes F, Soares BL, Galvao-Coelho NL, Arcoverde E, Araujo DB. Ayahuasca for the treatment of depression. Curr Top Behav Neurosci. 2022;56:113–24.
38. Riba J, Valle M, Urbano G, Yritia M, Morte A, Barbanoj MJ. Human pharmacology of ayahuasca: subjective and cardiovascular effects, monoamine metabolite excretion, and pharmacokinetics. J Pharmacol Exp Ther. 2003;306(1):73–83.
39. Szabo A, Kovacs A, Frecska E, Rajnavolgyi E. Psychedelic N,N-dimethyltryptamine and 5-methoxy-N,N-dimethyltryptamine modulate innate and adaptive inflammatory responses through the sigma-1 receptor of human monocyte-derived dendritic cells. PLoS One. 2014;9(8):e106533.
40. de Almeida RN, Galvao ACM, da Silva FS, Silva E, Palhano-Fontes F, Maia-de-Oliveira JP, et al. Modulation of serum brain-derived neurotrophic factor by a single dose of Ayahuasca: observation from a randomized controlled trial. Front Psychol. 2019;10:1234.
41. Palhano-Fontes F, Andrade KC, Tofoli LF, Santos AC, Crippa JA, Hallak JE, et al. The psychedelic state induced by ayahuasca modulates the activity and connectivity of the default mode network. PLoS One. 2015;10(2):e0118143.
42. Morales-Garcia JA, de la Fuente Revenga M, Alonso-Gil S, Rodriguez-Franco MI, Feilding A, Perez-Castillo A, et al. The alkaloids of Banisteriopsis caapi, the plant source of the Amazonian hallucinogen Ayahuasca, stimulate adult neurogenesis in vitro. Sci Rep. 2017;7(1):5309.
43. Carhart-Harris RL, Bolstridge M, Rucker J, Day CM, Erritzoe D, Kaelen M, et al. Psilocybin with psychological support for treatment-resistant depression: an open-label feasibility study. Lancet Psychiatry. 2016;3(7):619–27.
44. Carhart-Harris RL, Bolstridge M, Day CMJ, Rucker J, Watts R, Erritzoe DE, et al. Psilocybin with psychological support for treatment-resistant depression: six-month follow-up. Psychopharmacology. 2018;235(2):399–408.

45. Roseman L, Nutt DJ, Carhart-Harris RL. Quality of acute psychedelic experience predicts therapeutic efficacy of psilocybin for treatment-resistant depression. Front Pharmacol. 2017;8:974.
46. Lyons T, Carhart-Harris RL. More realistic forecasting of future life events after psilocybin for treatment-resistant depression. Front Psychol. 2018;9:1721.
47. Davis AK, Barrett FS, May DG, Cosimano MP, Sepeda ND, Johnson MW, et al. Effects of psilocybin-assisted therapy on major depressive disorder: a randomized clinical trial. JAMA Psychiatry. 2021;78(5):481–9.
48. Gukasyan N, Davis AK, Barrett FS, Cosimano MP, Sepeda ND, Johnson MW, et al. Efficacy and safety of psilocybin-assisted treatment for major depressive disorder: prospective 12-month follow-up. J Psychopharmacol. 2022;36(2):151–8.
49. Ross S, Bossis A, Guss J, Agin-Liebes G, Malone T, Cohen B, et al. Rapid and sustained symptom reduction following psilocybin treatment for anxiety and depression in patients with life-threatening cancer: a randomized controlled trial. J Psychopharmacol. 2016;30(12):1165–80.
50. Griffiths RR, Johnson MW, Carducci MA, Umbricht A, Richards WA, Richards BD, et al. Psilocybin produces substantial and sustained decreases in depression and anxiety in patients with life-threatening cancer: a randomized double-blind trial. J Psychopharmacol. 2016;30(12):1181–97.
51. Carhart-Harris R, Giribaldi B, Watts R, Baker-Jones M, Murphy-Beiner A, Murphy R, et al. Trial of psilocybin versus Escitalopram for depression. N Engl J Med. 2021;384(15):1402–11.
52. von Rotz R, Schindowski EM, Jungwirth J, Schuldt A, Rieser NM, Zahoranszky K, et al. Single-dose psilocybin-assisted therapy in major depressive disorder: a placebo-controlled, double-blind, randomised clinical trial. EClinicalMedicine. 2023;56:101809.
53. Goodwin GM, Aaronson ST, Alvarez O, Arden PC, Baker A, Bennett JC, et al. Single-dose psilocybin for a treatment-resistant episode of major depression. N Engl J Med. 2022;387(18):1637–48.
54. Raison CL, Sanacora G, Woolley J, Heinzerling K, Dunlop BW, Brown RT, et al. Single-dose psilocybin treatment for major depressive disorder: a randomized clinical trial. JAMA. 2023;330(9):843–53.
55. Metaxa AM, Clarke M. Efficacy of psilocybin for treating symptoms of depression: systematic review and meta-analysis. BMJ. 2024;385:e078084.
56. Glazer J, Murray CH, Nusslock R, Lee R, de Wit H. Low doses of lysergic acid diethylamide (LSD) increase reward-related brain activity. Neuropsychopharmacology. 2023;48(2):418–26.
57. Holze F, Gasser P, Muller F, Dolder PC, Liechti ME. Lysergic acid diethylamide-assisted therapy in patients with anxiety with and without a life-threatening illness: a randomized, double-blind, Placebo-Controlled Phase II Study. Biol Psychiatry. 2023;93(3):215–23.
58. Molla H, Lee R, Tare I, de Wit H. Greater subjective effects of a low dose of LSD in participants with depressed mood. Neuropsychopharmacology. 2024;49(5):774–81.
59. Muller F, Zaczek H, Becker AM, Ley L, Borgwardt S, Santos de Jesus J, et al. Efficacy and safety of low-versus high-dose-LSD-assisted therapy in patients with major depression: a randomized trial. Med. 2025;6:100725.
60. Bahji A, Lunsky I, Gutierrez G, Vazquez G. Efficacy and safety of four Psychedelic-assisted therapies for adults with symptoms of depression, anxiety, and posttraumatic stress disorder: a systematic review and meta-analysis. J Psychoactive Drugs. 2025;57(1):1–16.
61. Mitchell JM, Ot'alora GM, van der Kolk B, Shannon S, Bogenschutz M, Gelfand Y, et al. MDMA-assisted therapy for moderate to severe PTSD: a randomized, placebo-controlled phase 3 trial. Nat Med. 2023;29(10):2473–80.
62. Kvam TM, Goksoyr IW, Rog J, van de Vooren IJ, Stewart LH, Autran I, et al. MDMA-assisted therapy as a treatment for major depressive disorder: proof of principle study. Br J Psychiatry. 2025;227:1–7.
63. Osorio FL, Sanches RF, Macedo LR, Santos RG, Maia-de-Oliveira JP, Wichert-Ana L, et al. Antidepressant effects of a single dose of ayahuasca in patients with recurrent depression: a preliminary report. Braz J Psychiatry. 2015;37(1):13–20.
64. Sanches RF, de Lima Osorio F, Dos Santos RG, Macedo LR, Maia-de-Oliveira JP, Wichert-Ana L, et al. Antidepressant effects of a single dose of Ayahuasca in patients with recurrent depression: a SPECT study. J Clin Psychopharmacol. 2016;36(1):77–81.
65. Palhano-Fontes F, Barreto D, Onias H, Andrade KC, Novaes MM, Pessoa JA, et al. Rapid antidepressant effects of the psychedelic ayahuasca in treatment-resistant depression: a randomized placebo-controlled trial. Psychol Med. 2019;49(4):655–63.
66. Hsu TW, Tsai CK, Kao YC, Thompson T, Carvalho AF, Yang FC, et al. Comparative oral monotherapy of psilocybin, lysergic acid diethylamide, 3,4-me thylenedioxymethamphetamine, ayahuasca, and escitalopram for depressive symptoms: systematic review and Bayesian network meta-analysis. BMJ. 2024;386:e078607.

13 Depression and Microbiome: Concepts and Therapeutic Applications

Seung-Ho Jang, Sang-Yeol Lee, and Won-Myong Bahk

13.1 Introduction

In Korea, a well-known verb states, "When a cousin buys land, your stomach aches," illustrating the close connection between psychological and gastrointestinal symptoms. Such a functional connection between the brain and the gastrointestinal tract can be understood from an embryological perspective. The enteric nervous system (ENS), like the central nervous system (CNS), originates from the neural crest and contains a similar number of neurons as the spinal cord. For this reason, the ENS is often referred to as the "second brain" or the "little brain" [1]. In ancient times, the concept of holism, which viewed the mind and body as one, dominated our understanding of disease. However, in the seventeenth century, the separation of mind and body gave rise to dualism. Technological advances have led to the discovery of various microorganisms. By the nineteenth century, the germ theory, which posits that microorganisms can cause disease, had shifted medical perspectives. Symptoms were expected to be linked to organic or pathological causes deemed medically valid [2]. Therefore, even when patients present with various physical symptoms, their symptoms are often dismissed as psychological in origin if pathological evidence cannot be identified through testing. In the early twentieth century, cumulative research confirmed the connection between the brain and gastrointestinal tract, leading to the development of the "brain–gut axis" concept. With an increasing number of studies on gut microbiota, this has evolved into the "brain–gut–microbiota axis" (Fig. 13.1). In this chapter, we explored the brain–gut–microbiota axis and its role in depression.

S.-H. Jang
Jeil Psychiatry Clinic, Gimje, Republic of Korea

S.-Y. Lee
Department of Psychiatry, Wonkwang University Hospital, College of Medicine, Wonkwang University, Iksan, Republic of Korea

W.-M. Bahk (✉)
Department of Psychiatry, College of Medicine, The Catholic University of Korea, Seoul, Republic of Korea

Woo and Bahk Psychiatry Clinic, Seoul, Republic of Korea
e-mail: wmbahk@catholic.ac.kr

W.-M. Bahk et al. (eds.), *Depressive Disorder*, https://doi.org/10.1007/978-981-92-1331-3_13

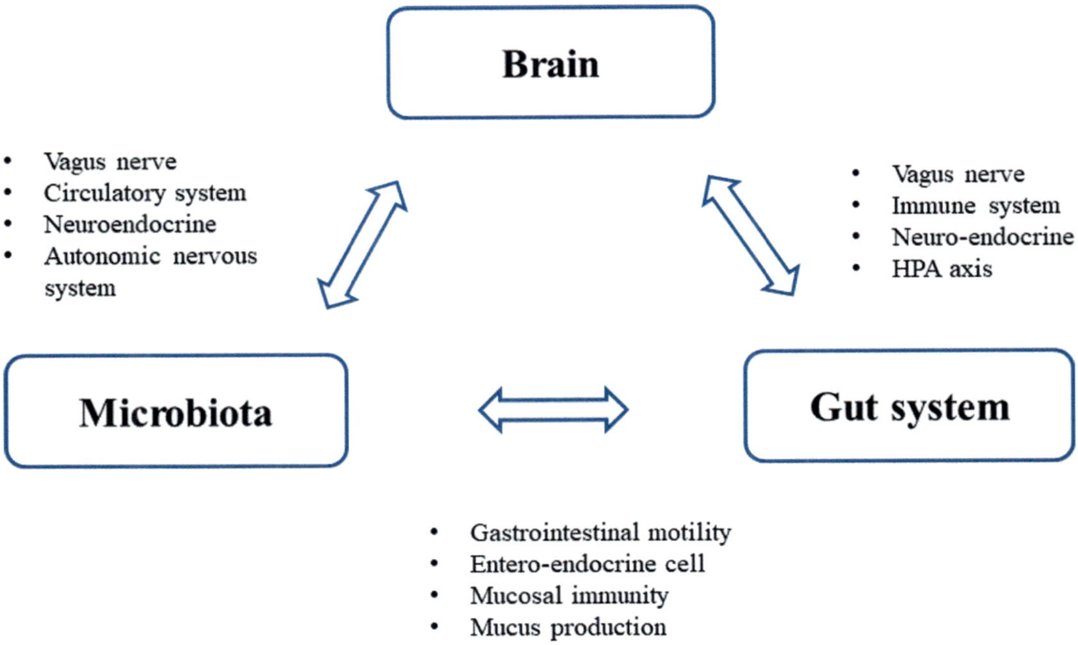

Fig. 13.1 Brain–gut–microbiota axis

13.2 Development of the Brain–Gut–Microbiota Axis Concept

The notion that gastrointestinal function is influenced by the brain began with observations in patients with gastric fistulas, in whom researchers noted changes in motility and metabolic secretions. In 1833, William Beaumont studied a sailor named Alexis St. Martin and found that emotional states such as stress, anxiety, and fear could affect gastric mucosal secretion and surface conditions [3]. This is the first documented evidence that psychological symptoms influence gastrointestinal function. Subsequent studies have demonstrated that emotions such as anger, pleasure, and aggression can cause mucosal hyperemia, altered motility, and secretory changes, whereas fear, depression, and anxiety are associated with mucosal pallor and reduced endocrine and motor functions [4]. Mental symptoms also affect colonic motility and secretion. In 1951, Dr. Thomas Almy experimented with a 22-year-old male medical student during sigmoidoscopy, leading the participant to believe that the tumor had been discovered. This unexpected diagnosis induced extreme fear and anxiety, resulting in rapid rectal contractions and mucosal congestion. Once the researchers explained that the situation had been fabricated, the rectum relaxed, demonstrating that anxiety alone could cause direct changes in colon motility without any underlying pathology. Similar findings were later confirmed in studies on patients with irritable bowel syndrome (IBS), in whom emotional changes such as grief, aggression, and self-blame directly influenced colonic motility. Physiological and scientific experimental designs have confirmed that stress decreases gastric motility and increases colonic motility [5]. The key mechanism involves corticotropin-releasing factor (CRF), a stress mediator secreted by the hypothalamus. CRF binds to CRF1 receptors, stimulating sacral parasympathetic nerves and increasing colonic motility, whereas binding to CRF2 receptors reduces gastric motility via the vagus nerve [6]. Stress enhances inflammation in the gastric mucosa. In rodent models exposed to water avoidance stress, CRF increases centrally, leading to elevated mast cell and protease-activated receptor-2 expression in the colonic mucosa, which, in turn, triggers an inflammatory cytokine surge [7]. CRF and other peptides influence the sensory, sympathetic, immune, and endocrine cells in the gastrointestinal tract, thereby affecting gut sensation and inflammation [8]. By the late twentieth century, extensive preclinical, translational, and fMRI studies established that stress and other mental symptoms influenced gastrointestinal motility, endocrine responses, and immune function. In the twenty-first century, it has become apparent that the gut microbiota not only contributes to disease but also plays essential roles in maintaining normal physiological functions and health. With an increase in research, concepts such as dysbiosis, imbalanced microbial communities, and their associations with specific diseases and psychiatric conditions have led to the continued development of the brain–gut axis. Studies have revealed that stress and other mental states can alter gastrointestinal motility and endocrine function, as well as the distribution and environment of the gut microbiota [9]. For example, a previous study showed that the levels of *Bacteroides* were reduced in stressed mice, whereas those of *Clostridium* were increased [10]. Another study reported that the *Lactobacillus* levels in university students decreased significantly during stressful examination periods [11]. These preclinical and clinical findings continue to improve our understanding of the brain–gut–microbiota axis.

13.3 Gut Microbiome

The microbiome refers to the ecological community of microorganisms, including bacteria, archaea, eukaryotes, fungi, viruses, and their genetic material, that inhabit the human body [12]. In an average adult, these microorganisms weigh approximately 1 kg, which is equivalent to the weight of the brain. It is estimated that the human gastrointestinal tract hosts between 10^{13} and 10^{14} microorganisms, a number that exceeds the total number of human cells. Furthermore, the microbiome contains more than 100 times the number of genes as the human genome [13]. Although the distribution of the gut microbiota varies among individuals, the relative abundance of specific microbial phylotypes within the intestinal tract tends to be similar in healthy individuals. Among these, Firmicutes and Bacteroidetes are predominant, accounting for over 75% of the total gut microbial population [14]. The gut microbiome has recently been shown to play a critical role not only in gastrointestinal function but also in brain health. Dysbiosis, defined as an imbalance in the gut microbiota from infancy to old age, is linked to alterations in brain function and is influenced by factors such as mode of delivery, diet, and exposure to antibiotics. With the advancement of sequencing techniques, the potential of utilizing the gut microbiome to maintain health and treat diseases is gaining increasing attention [15]. Notably, the gut microbiome holds promise as an efficient biomarker and is essential for shaping and developing the human immune system, thereby supporting key physiological functions. An imbalance in the gut microbiome can lead to systemic physiological dysfunction, which is associated with increased inflammatory responses and oxidative stress, both of which are recognized contributors to mental illnesses [16]. Therefore, research on the gut microbiome has significant implications for treating psychiatric disorders and understanding their pathophysiology.

13.4 Mechanisms by Which the Brain Influences the Gut Microbiota

The brain, particularly the autonomic nervous system, plays a crucial regulatory role in the gut. The autonomic nervous system governs gastrointestinal motility, secretion, permeability, and immune and inflammatory responses. Consequently, changes in activity in this system can impact gut microbiota composition [17]. For example, stress-induced alterations in intestinal motility or secretion can influence the rate of material transport through the gut, resulting in changes in microbial colonization. Changes in water and electrolyte secretion and stimulated immune responses also reshape the microbial community within the gut. Various gut hormones secreted in response to brain signals play important roles in these processes. Serotonin, cholecystokinin, and dynorphin are released from enteroendocrine cells in the intestinal mucosa and help regulate microbial ecosystems. Circadian rhythms regulated in the brain influence daily fluctuations in the gut microbiota [18]. Stress and other psychological stimuli can also affect gut function via the autonomic nervous system by altering bowel habits, gastric acid secretion, and intestinal permeability. Thus, these brain-derived signals exert broad effects on gut microbiome structure and function [19].

13.5 Influence of the Gut Microbiome on Brain and ENS Development

While past research on the brain–gut–microbiota axis has primarily focused on gastrointestinal disorders such as IBS, recent studies have increasingly investigated the influence of the gut microbiome on brain development. Notably, the period during which the gut microbiome matures after birth overlaps, at least in part, with the developmental windows of the brain and gastrointestinal tract. The gut microbiome plays a central role in neurogenesis, myelination, microglial activation, and blood–brain barrier (BBB) formation [20]. The critical role of the gut microbiota in brain development has been demonstrated by studies involving germ-free (GF) mice (i.e., mice raised in sterile environments without exposure to microorganisms). Compared with conventionally raised mice, GF mice exhibit significant differences in brain function and behavior, including heightened anxiety responses, abnormal locomotion, exaggerated reactions to stress, memory impairment, and hyperactivation of the hypothalamic–pituitary–adrenal (HPA) axis [21]. Interestingly, the abnormalities observed in GF mice can be reversed by colonizing them with normal gut microbiota. However, the timing of microbiota colonization is crucial, and the restoration of normal brain function and behavior is only possible if the microbiota is introduced early in development. Delayed colonization may result in irreversible deficits, underscoring the importance of critical periods and specific beneficial microbes in neurodevelopment. Further supporting evidence comes from human cohort studies in which antibiotic exposure during infancy has been associated with a negative impact on cognitive development. These findings highlight the essential role of the gut microbiome in shaping the developing nervous system and suggest that microbial balance during early life is a key determinant of lifelong brain health [22].

13.6 Mechanisms by Which the Gut Microbiome Affects the Brain

Although the precise mechanisms through which the gut microbiome influences the distant brain are not fully understood, current evidence suggests that these effects are mediated by the nervous, immune, and endocrine systems. The vagus nerve, the longest cranial nerve in vertebrates, plays a central role in bidirectional signaling between the gastrointestinal tract and brain [23]. Gut microbes exert their effects on the nervous system through several mechanisms. They produce metabolites such as short-chain fatty acids that can modulate neural activity. Additionally, microbial-associated molecular patterns, such as peptidoglycans and lipopolysaccharides (LPS), can translocate across the intestinal mucosa and interact with toll-like receptors expressed in the neural tissue. An indirect pathway has also been proposed in which gut microbes stimulate enteroendocrine cells to secrete serotonin, which, in turn, activates neural pathways [24]. Recent findings also suggest that modulation of the peripheral immune system can significantly influence brain function and behavior. The gut microbiome can act as an immune stimulant, and activated immune cells produce pro-inflammatory cytokines such as interleukin-1α (IL-1α), IL-1β, tumor necrosis factor-α (TNF-α), and IL-6, which may cross the BBB and bind to receptors on neurons, glial cells, and microglia, thereby altering brain activity. Notably, LPS itself is capable of penetrating the BBB. Animal studies demonstrated that intraperitoneal LPS injection in mice reduced their attention and exploratory behavior toward novel objects [25]. Enteroendocrine cells offer another route through which gut microbes influence the brain. At least 12 different types of enteroendocrine cells in the gastrointestinal tract collectively secrete over 20 signaling molecules in response to chemical and mechanical stimuli. These molecules can affect feeding behavior via the CNS or signals through vagal afferents, ultimately influencing brain function. Gastrointestinal hormones not only regulate digestion, but may also modulate emotion and mood. For example, ghrelin reduces anxiety- and depression-like symptoms during chronic stress, whereas peptide YY can enhance reward-related behaviors by modulating its plasma concentration. [26] Serotonin is a particularly important neurotransmitter in the gut–brain–microbiota axis is serotonin, which is also influenced by gut microbes. Although serotonin is widely known as a neurotransmitter, 95% of the body's serotonin is found in the gastrointestinal tract, and only 5% resides in the CNS. Moreover, 90% of gut-derived serotonin is produced by enterochromaffin cells, but not by neurons. When stimulated by gut signals, these cells release serotonin, which affects gut motility and secretion, and transmits signals to submucosal nerve endings [27]. The remaining 10% of gut serotonin acts as a neurotransmitter in the ENS. Nevertheless, because serotonin molecules are too large to cross the BBB, they cannot directly affect the CNS. Instead, precursors to neurotransmitters, such as tryptophan, can cross this barrier. The gut microbiota may regulate the metabolism and availability of these precursors, thereby indirectly influencing neurotransmission and brain function.

13.7 Studies on the Gut Microbiota in Depression

A growing body of research has investigated the role of the gut microbiota in the pathophysiology and modulation of depression. Gareau et al. studied 4–9-day-old neonatal mice that were separated from their mothers for 3 h daily and compared them with control groups. Two strains of *Lactobacillus* were administered, and serum corticosterone levels were measured 20 days later. The probiotic-treated group showed a significant reduction in corticosterone levels, which were elevated due to maternal separation [28]. Bharwani et al. administered *Lactobacillus rhamnosus* (strain JB-1) in C57BL/6 mice daily for 28 days. Behavioral assessments and immune profiling via 16S rRNA sequencing revealed a marked reduction in stress-induced anxiety-like behaviors and the prevention of social avoidance tendencies in the JB-1 group [29]. Burokas et al. demonstrated that the administration of fructo-oligosaccharides and galacto-oligosaccharides in C57BL/6J mice effectively reduced depressive and anxiety-related behaviors [30]. Desbonnet et al. used a maternal separation model and administered *Bifidobacterium* to mice. Behavioral analysis using the forced swim test showed reduced behavioral despair, normalized norepinephrine levels in the brainstem, and stabilization of immune responses in the probiotic-treated groups [31]. Bravo et al. reported that chronic administration of *L. rhamnosus* led to increased expression of GABA B1b mRNA in the cortex as well as reductions in stress-induced corticosterone levels, anxiety, and depressive-like behaviors [32]. Ait-Belgnaoui et al. administered *Lactobacillus farciminis* for 2 weeks while subjecting mice to partial restraint stress. The results indicated decreased levels of adrenocorticotropic hormone (≫ACTH), corticosterone, corticotropin-releasing hormone (CRH), proinflammatory cytokines, and circulating LPS. The probiotic also suppressed stress-induced increases in intestinal permeability and endotoxemia, thereby preventing HPA axis activation and neuroinflammation [33]. Liang et al. subjected mice to 21 days of restraint stress and compared the effects of *Lactobacillus helveticus* with those of the antidepressant citalopram. The *L. helveticus*-treated group exhibited reductions in depressive and anxiety-like behaviors comparable to the citalopram-treated group, along with improvements in cognitive function [34]. In a separate study, Bharwani et al. used a mouse

Table 13.1 Characteristics of prior studies investigating the relation between microbiome and depression

Authors (Years)	Subject	Method	Result
Gareau et al. [28]	Pups (n = 12)	Separated from the mother model, probiotics (two strains of Lactobacillus species)	Probiotic administration reduced the elevated corticosterone levels
Bharwani et al. [29]	Male C57BL/6 mice	*Lactobacillus rhamnosus* (JB-1)	Stress-induced anxiety behavior was reduced. Lack of social interaction was prevented
Burokas et al. [30]	Male C57BL/6 J mice	Probiotics (fructo-oligosaccharides (Fos) and galacto-oligosaccharides (Gos))	Antidepressant and anxiolytic effects. Reduced stress-induced corticosterone release
Desbonnet et al. [31]	Rats	Maternal separation model Bifidobacterium / citalopram Forced swimming test	Immune response, behavioral deficit, and basal noradrenaline concentration were normalized
Bravo et al. [32]	Male BALB/c mice (n = 36)	*Lactobacillus rhamnosus* (JB-1)	Increased expression of GABA B1bmRNA. Reduction in stress-induced corticosterone and anxiety and depression-related behavior
Ait-Belgnaoui et al. [33]	Female rats	Partial restraint stress *Lactobacillus farciminis* for 2 weeks	Induced hyperpermeability and endotoxemia Prevention of neuroinflammation and stress response in the HPA axis
Liang et al. [34]	Adult specific pathogen-free rats	*Lactobacillus helveticus* N58 or citalopram Behavioral test (Sucrose preference test, elevated-plus maze test, open-field test, object recognition test, object placement test)	Decreased anxiety and depressive behaviors. Cognitive dysfunctions were improved at a level similar to citalopram group
Bharwani et al. [35]	Male C57BL/6 mice	Chronic social defeat 16S rRNA marker gene Sequencing	The degree of social deficit was correlated with microbial community profile Functional diversity was reduced in chronic social defeat group
Kato-Kataoka et al. [36]	Double blind placebo-controlled trial (n = 24 vs. 23)	*Lactobacillus casei* Shirota (LcS)	Improving physical symptoms in stressful situations Significant increase in fecal serotonin level

Source: Cited from Jang et al. [44]
n number, *LPS* lipopolysaccharide, *GABA* gamma-aminobutyric acid

model of chronic social defeat stress and found a significant correlation between the degree of social impairment and the gut microbiota composition. Reduced microbial diversity is associated with decreased synthesis of neurotransmitter precursors and short-chain fatty acids [35]. Kato et al. administered *Lactobacillus casei* strain Shirota (LcS) five times in a human trial. After 2 weeks, the LcS group exhibited increased fecal serotonin concentrations, improved psychiatric symptoms, and alleviated somatic symptoms, even under stressful conditions [36] (Table 13.1).

13.8 Therapeutic Applications of Gut Microbiota

Modulation of the gut microbiota has emerged as a promising therapeutic strategy for the treatment of psychiatric symptoms and brain disorders. One of the earliest and most widely studied approaches involves the use of probiotics. Probiotics used to alleviate psychiatric symptoms are often referred to as "psychobiotics." Among the psychobiotic formulations, the combination of *L. helveticus* R0052 and *Bifidobacterium longum* R0175 was particularly noteworthy. In one clinical study, participants with mild depressive and anxiety symptoms received the combination for 1 month, resulting in improvements in depression, anxiety, somatization, anger, and hostility, along with a reduction in 24-h urinary cortisol levels [37]. These beneficial effects on psychiatric symptoms have also been observed in patients with major depressive disorders and individuals experiencing stress-related gastrointestinal symptoms, with additional improvements in sleep quality [38]. Other probiotic strains, including *Lactobacillus casei Shrota* and *Bifidobacterium animalis*, have positive effects on anxiety and cognitive function [39]. A recent meta-analysis of nine double-blind, randomized, placebo-controlled trials involving 1901 participants found that probiotics significantly reduced depressive symptoms compared with placebo [40]. Notably, probiotics had a significant effect in individuals with major depressive disorder but not in those with other clinical conditions. Multi-strain formulations were more effective than single-strain products in reducing depressive symptoms. These findings suggest that modifying the gut–brain axis using probiotics may be a viable approach for alleviating depression. However, large-scale clinical trials are required to confirm the efficacy of these specific strains and their combinations [40].

Recently, fecal microbiota transplantation (FMT) has recently gained attention as a microbiota-based therapeutic intervention. Initially established as a treatment for refractory *Clostridioides difficile* infection, FMT is currently being explored for neurological and psychiatric conditions based on growing evidence supporting the influence of the gut microbiota on brain function. For autism spectrum disorder (ASD), in which gastrointestinal symptoms and microbial dysbiosis are common, FMT has led to improvements in both core ASD symptoms and gastrointestinal issues, with effects lasting for up to 2 years after treatment [41]. Moreover, FMT is being investigated in clinical settings because of its potential benefits in Parkinson's disease, dementia, depression, epilepsy, amyotrophic lateral sclerosis, chronic fatigue syndrome, and multiple sclerosis [42]. In patients with IBS who also experience depression and anxiety, FMT has been associated with improvements in gastrointestinal symptoms, depressive symptoms, fatigue, and overall quality of life [43].

13.9 Summary

Advances in technologies for analyzing and evaluating gut microbiota have highlighted their potential utility in assessing both physical and mental health. The brain–gut–microbiota axis is a complex bidirectional communication system. Psychosocial stress activates the HPA axis, triggering the release of CRF, which in turn alters intestinal permeability and the ecological balance of the gut microbiota. Simultaneously, the autonomic nervous system influences gut motility and the secretion of neurotransmitters such as serotonin. Conversely, increased gut permeability allows microbial metabolites and inflammatory mediators to enter the bloodstream and reach the CNS, potentially contributing to psychiatric symptoms such as depression, anxiety, cognitive or social dysfunction, and neurodegenerative disorders. Thus, the connection between the brain, gut, and microbiota should be viewed as a bidirectional pathway rather than a unidirectional one. To date, most studies on the gut microbiota remain in the preclinical stage. While some human clinical trials have demonstrated improvements in depressive, anxiety, somatic, and stress-related symptoms, their sample sizes have been relatively small. Therefore, large-scale multicenter clinical studies are necessary to validate these findings. Despite the current limitations, microbiota-based therapies such as probiotics and FMT show potential as adjunctive treatments for patients with depression or anxiety who do not respond sufficiently to conventional psychotherapy or pharmacotherapy.

Declarations

Competing Interests The author(s) has no competing interests to declare that are relevant to the content of this manuscript.

Ethics Approval The author(s) declares that this manuscript does not include primary research with human participants.

The author(s) declares that this manuscript does not include primary studies involving animals.

References

1. Goldstein AM, Hofstra RM, Burns AJ. Building a brain in the gut: development of the enteric nervous system. Clin Genet. 2013;83:307–16.
2. Lucas G. Gut thinking: the gut microbiome and mental health beyond the head. Microb Ecol Health Dis. 2018;29:1548250.
3. Beaumont W. Experiments and observations on the gastric juice and the physiology of digestion. Nutr Rev. 1977;35:144–5.
4. Drossman DA. Functional gastrointestinal disorders: history, pathophysiology, clinical features and Rome IV. Gastroenterology. 2016;150:1262–79.
5. Monnikes H, Tebbe JJ, Hildebrandt M, et al. Role of stress in functional gastrointestinal disorders. Evidence for stress–induced alterations in gastrointestinal motility and sensitivity. Dig Dis. 2001;19:201–11.
6. Tache Y, Bonaz B. Corticotropin–releasing factor receptors and stress–related alterations of gut motor function. J Clin Invest. 2007;117:33–40.
7. Kim YS, Lee MY, Ryu HS, et al. Regional differences in chronic stress–induced alterations in mast cell and protease–activated receptor–2–positive cell numbers in the colon of Ws/Ws rats. J Neurogastroenterol Motil. 2014;20:54–63.
8. Buckinx R, Adriaensen D, Nassauw LV, et al. Corticotrophin–releasing factor, related peptides, and receptors in the normal and inflamed gastrointestinal tract. Front Neurosci. 2011;5:54.
9. Carabotti M, Scirocco A, Maselli MA, et al. The gut–brain axis: interactions between enteric microbiota, central and enteric nervous systems. Ann Gastroenterol. 2015;28:203–9.
10. Bailey MT, Dowd SE, Galley JD, et al. Exposure to a social stressor alters the structure of the intestinal microbiota: implications for stressor–induced immunomodulation. Brain Behav Immun. 2011;25:397–407.
11. Knowles SR, Nelson EA, Palombo EA. Investigating the role of perceived stress on bacterial flora activity and salivary cortisol secretion: a possible mechanism underlying susceptibility to illness. Biol Psychol. 2008;77:132–7.
12. Qin J, MetaHIT Consortium, Li R, Raes J, Arumugam M, et al. A human gut microbial gene catalogue established by metagenomic sequencing. Nature. 2010;464:59–65.
13. Dinan TG, Stilling RM, Stanton C, Cryan JF. Collective unconscious: how gut microbes shape human behavior. J Psychiatr Res. 2015;63:1–9.
14. Eckburg PB, Bik EM, Bernstein CN, Purdom E, Dethlefsen L, et al. Diversity of the human intestinal microbial flora. Science. 2005;308:1635–8.
15. Knight R, Callewaert C, Marotz C, Hyde ER, et al. The microbiome and human biology. Annu Rev Genom Hum Genet. 2017;18:65–86.
16. Rea K, Dinan TG, Cryan JF. Gut microbiota: a perspective for psychiatrists. Neuropsychobiology. 2019;79:50–62.
17. Martin CR, Osadchiy V, Kalani A, et al. The brain–gut–microbiome Axis. Cell Mol Gastroenterol Hepatol. 2018;6:133–48.
18. Paulose JK, Wright JM, Patel AG, et al. Human gut bacteria are sensitive to melatonin and express endogenous circadian rhythmicity. PLoS One. 2016;11:e0146643.
19. Quigley EMM. Gut microbiome as a clinical tool in gastrointestinal disease management: are we there yet? Nat Rev Gastroenterol Hepatol. 2017;14:315–20.
20. Sharon G, Sampson TR, Geschwind DH, et al. The central nervous system and the gut microbiome. Cell. 2016;167:915–32.
21. Spichak S, Guzzetta KE, O'Leary OF, et al. Without a bug's life: germ–free rodents to interrogate microbiota–gut–neuroimmune interactions. Disease model. 2018;28:79–93.
22. Slykerman R, Hood K, Wickens K, et al. Effect of Lactobacillus rhamnosus HN001 in pregnancy on postpartum symptoms of depression and anxiety: a randomised double–blind placebo–controlled trial. EBioMedicine. 2017;24:159–65.
23. Bonaz B, Bazin T, Pellissier S. The vagus nerve at the interface of the microbiota–gut–brain axis. Front Neurosci. 2018;12:49.
24. Sampson TR, Mazmanian SK. Control of brain development, function, and behavior by the microbiome. Cell Host Microbe. 2015;17:565–76.
25. Haba R, Shintani N, Onaka Y, et al. Lipopolysaccharide affects exploratory behaviors toward novel objects by impairing cognition and/or motivation in mice: possible role of activation of the central amygdala. Behav Brain Res. 2012;228:423–31.
26. Lutter M, Sakata I, Osborne–Lawrence S, et al. The orexigenic hormone ghrelin defends against depressive symptoms of chronic stress. Nat Neurosci. 2008;11:752–3.
27. Camilleri M. Serotonin in the gastrointestinal tract. Curr Opin Endocrinol Diabetes Obes. 2009;16:53–9.
28. Gareau MG, Jury J, MacQueen G, Sherman PM. Probiotic treatment of rat pups normalises corticosterone release and ameliorates colonic dysfunction induced by maternal separation. Gut. 2007;56:1522–8.
29. Bharwani A, Mian MF, Surette MG, Bienenstock J, et al. Oral treatment with Lactobacillus rhamnosus attenuates behavioral deficits and immune changes in chronic social stress. BMC Med. 2017;15:7.
30. Burokas A, Arboleya S, Moloney RD, Peterson V, Murphy K, et al. Targeting the microbiota–gut–brain axis: probiotics have anxiolytic and antidepressant–

like effects and reverse the impact of chronic stress in mice. Biol Psychiatry. 2017;82:472–87.
31. Desbonnet L, Garrett L, Clarke G, Kiely B, Cryan JF, et al. Effects of the probiotic Bifidobacterium infantis in the maternal separation model of depression. Neuroscience. 2010;170:1179–88.
32. Bravo JA, Forsythe P, Chew MV, Escaravage E, Savignac HM, et al. Ingestion of Lactobacillus strain regulates emotional behavior and central GABA receptor expression in a mouse via the vagus nerve. Proc Natl Acad Sci USA. 2011;108:16050–5.
33. Ait–Belgnaoui A, Durand H, Cartier C, Chaumaz G, et al. Prevention of gut leakiness by a probiotic treatment leads to attenuated HPA response to an acute psychological stress in rats. Psychoneuroendocrinology. 2012;37:1885–95.
34. Liang S, Wang T, Hu X, Luo J, Li W, et al. Administration of Lactobacillus helveticus NS8 improves behavioral, cognitive, and biochemical aberrations caused by chronic restraint stress. Neuroscience. 2015;310:561–77.
35. Bharwani A, Mian MF, Foster JA, Surette MG, et al. Structural & functional consequences of chronic psychosocial stress on the microbiome & host. Psychoneuroendocrinology. 2016;63:217–27.
36. Kato–Kataoka A, Nishida K, Takada M, Suda K, Kawai M, et al. Fermented milk containing Lactobacillus casei strain shirota prevents the onset of physical symptoms in medical students under academic examination stress. Benef Microbes. 2016;7:153–6.
37. Messaoudi M, Lalonde R, Violle N, et al. Assessment of psychotropic–like properties of a probiotic formulation (Lactobacillus helveticus R0052 and Bifidobacterium longum R0175) in rats and human subjects. Br J Nutr. 2011;105:755–64.
38. Kazemi A, Noorbalal AA, Azam K, et al. Effect of probiotic and prebiotic vs placebo on psychological outcomes in patients with major depressive disorder: a randomized clinical trial. Clin Nutr. 2019;38:522–8.
39. Tillisch K, Labus J, Kilpatrick L, et al. Consumption of fermented milk product with probiotic modulates brain activity. Gastroenterology. 2013;144:1394–401, 1401.e1–4.
40. Goh KK, Liu YW, Kuo PH, et al. Effect of probiotics on depressive symptoms: a meta–analysis of human studies. Psychiatry Res. 2019;282:112568.
41. Kang DW, Adams JB, Gregory AC, et al. Microbiota transfer therapy alters gut ecosystem and improves gastrointestinal and autism symptoms: an open–label study. Microbiome. 2017;5:10.
42. Wortelboer K, Nieuwdorp M, Herrema H. Fecal microbiota transplantation beyond Clostridioides difficile infections. EBioMedicine. 2019;44:716–29.
43. Lahtinen P, Jalanka J, Hartikainen A, et al. Randomised clinical trial: faecal microbiota transplantation versus autologous placebo administered via colonoscopy in irritable bowel syndrome. Aliment Pharmacol Ther. 2020;51:1321–31.
44. Jang SH, Woo YS, Lee SY, Bahk WM. The brain–gut–microbiome axis in psychiatry. Int J Mol Sci. 2020;21:7122.

Personalized Medicine for the Treatment of Depression

14

Daeyoung Roh and Moon-Doo Kim

14.1 Introduction

Psychiatry has witnessed substantial advancements in evidence-based pharmacotherapy and psychotherapies, yet treatment selection often relies on clinical interviews and symptom-based diagnoses. Depression is biologically heterogeneous and manifests diverse symptom profiles. Consequently, only about one-third of patients exhibit a substantial response to first-line therapy and even fewer achieve full remission. Trial-and-error switching due to lack of efficacy or adverse effects prolongs recovery and diminishes quality of life [1]. The goal of personalized medicine is to integrate clinical and biological factors—such as genetic variants, neural circuitry, cognitive traits and environmental exposures—to identify optimal treatment and prevention strategies for each patient. At the same time, personalized approach in psychiatry must also incorporate ecosocial determinants and the patient's context.

This chapter synthesizes recent advances in personalized medicine for depression. Evidence from genetics, immune markers, neuroimaging, digital technologies, and multi-omics is integrated with clinical experience to guide patient-centered care. Rather than exhaustively reviewing every study, the emphasis is on clinically meaningful findings, overarching concepts and practical implications. The chapter reviews core concepts, summarizes key biomarker domains, discusses emerging interventions and neuromodulation, and outlines challenges and future directions.

14.2 Core Concepts

Personalized medicine refers to tailoring treatment to the clinical features and preferences of an individual patient. This concept has a long history—from Hippocrates' emphasis on individualized care to the modern P4 medicine paradigm (predictive, preventive, personalized and participatory) [2]. Precision medicine is sometimes used interchangeably but more specifically denotes decisions informed by measurable biological markers. Precision psychiatry applies these principles to mental disorders by identifying clinically meaningful subtypes, linking them to differential treatment response, and improving prevention and diagnosis [3].

Psychiatry has long personalized care using demographic and clinical features, yet syndrome-based subtyping has not yielded reliable predictors of antidepressant response [4]. The National Institute of Mental Health's Research Domain

D. Roh
Department of Psychiatry, Ilsanpaik Hospital, Inje University, College of Medicine, Goyang, Republic of Korea

M.-D. Kim (✉)
Department of Psychiatry, Jeju National University Hospital, School of Medicine, Jeju National University, Jeju, Republic of Korea
e-mail: mdkim66@jejunu.ac.kr

W.-M. Bahk et al. (eds.), *Depressive Disorder*, https://doi.org/10.1007/978-981-92-1331-3_14

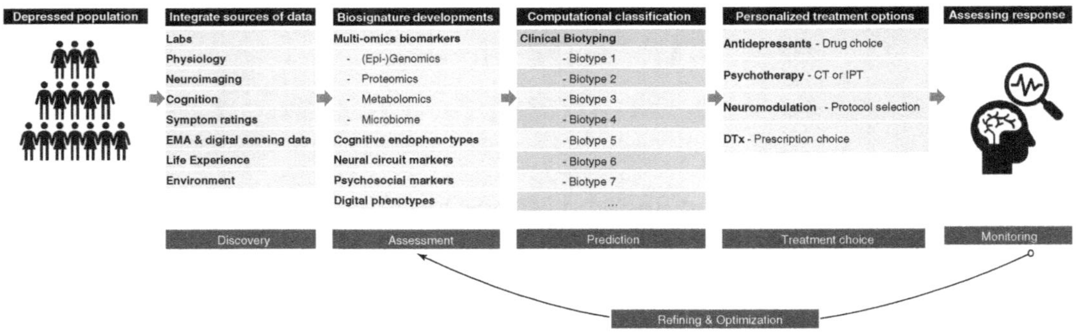

Fig. 14.1 An illustration of a precision psychiatry approach in the treatment of major depressive disorder. DTx digital therapeutics; EMA ecological momentary assessment

Criteria (RDoC)-aligned biological measures (genomics, proteomics, neuroimaging, and physiology) are intended to overcome this limitation [5], but current biomarkers show modest individual-level predictive value, and biomarkers alone are insufficient; assessment and treatment must also incorporate ecosocial determinants and the patient's context. Advances in artificial intelligence (AI) enable integration of heterogeneous, multimodal data (symptoms, genetics, imaging, inflammatory and digital measures) to build decision-support tools. Because model performance and generalizability remain variable, such tools should augment—rather than replace—clinical judgment and be externally validated. *Throughout this chapter, we differentiate findings that can be applied in routine clinical practice from those that remain investigational, and we calibrate all statements to the strength of the available evidence*. Figure 14.1 summarizes how integrating laboratory, physiological, neuroimaging, cognitive, and environmental data can support biosignatures, clinical biotypes, and treatment matching (medications, psychotherapies, neuromodulation).

14.3 Genetic Biomarkers

Genetic variation influences brain circuits and modulates mood, cognition, and behavior. Specifically, gene expression impacts the hypothalamic–pituitary–adrenal axis and contributes to depressive symptoms. While genetics may account for up to 42% of the variance in antidepressant response, *individual-level effects remain modest and context-dependent*. Pharmacogenomics (PGx) studies how gene variants alter drug targets, transporters, and metabolizing enzymes. Polymorphisms in serotonin receptors (HTR2A/HTR2C), dopamine receptor DRD2, transporters (ABCB1, OCT1), and drug-metabolizing enzymes *have been associated with* antidepressant pharmacokinetics and dosing [6]. Among the latter, CYP2D6 and CYP2C19 are the principal determinants of selective serotonin reuptake inhibitor (SSRI) exposure and dose requirements, and they provide the most actionable guidance for dose adjustment [7]. Third-generation pharmacogenomic panels detect composite genotypes affecting both pharmacokinetics and pharmacodynamics.

Since 2023, meta-analyses and randomized trials indicate that PGx guidance confers small but statistically significant gains in remission/response, most evident in moderate-to-severe or treatment-resistant depression [24]. Patients receiving PGx-guided care were approximately 1.4 times more likely to achieve remission than those receiving treatment-as-usual, and side effects were reduced by avoiding drugs with unfavorable gene–drug interactions. However, across the large trials of GUIDED and PRIME Care, PGx-guided prescribing did not improve primary symptom outcomes and showed at most small, inconsistent advantages on secondary endpoints. Routine implementation remains premature pending genome-wide strategies and validation in diverse populations. *Accordingly, CYP2D6/CYP2C19-based dose adjustment represents the clearest current "actionable" use case, whereas broader panel-based treatment selection should be interpreted more cautiously and remains context-dependent.*

Epigenetic markers—especially DNA methylation signatures that reflect gene–environment interplay—show preliminary utility for predicting nonresponse and treatment resistance, but they require prospective replication, assay harmonization, and clinical calibration [8]. The cost of genomic testing has fallen substantially, and the clinical utility of pharmacogenomics is likely to grow as genomic data are integrated with other omics layers and neuroimaging. For computational and integrative methods, see "Machine learning and multi-omics integration."

14.4 Blood-Based Biomarkers

Inflammatory markers are among the most promising blood-based signatures for depression [9]. Approximately 20–30% of depressed patients have elevated inflammatory biomarkers such as C-reactive protein (CRP) and interleukin-6; this "inflamed depression" subgroup often presents with profound fatigue, anhedonia and psychomotor slowing and responds poorly to conventional antidepressants [25]. Elevated CRP *has been associated with* poorer response to first-line treatments *in group-level studies* and *may* predict better response to anti-inflammatory agents or certain noradrenergic antidepressants. *However, current evidence is insufficient to recommend CRP as a stand-alone treatment-selection biomarker in routine care.* These findings have led experts to propose an inflammatory subtype of major depression and to advocate for adding a "with inflammation" specifier to diagnostic manuals [25].

The neurotrophic hypothesis proposes that depression involves disrupted neuroplasticity and growth-factor signaling. Peripheral brain-derived neurotrophic factor (BDNF) is often lower during acute episodes and tends to rise toward normalization with effective treatment, including antidepressant medication, electroconvulsive therapy, and structured exercise. BDNF levels are frequently reduced in treatment-resistant depression and may help prognosticate treatment response. Because blood assays can index aspects of central neuroplastic change, BDNF remains a promising candidate biomarker for clinical monitoring [10] *but is best regarded as investigational given assay variability and limited prospective calibration for routine use.* Other growth factors, such as vascular endothelial growth factor, are being studied as predictors of treatment response. Future multi-omic strategies will likely integrate inflammatory, neurotrophic and metabolic markers to identify pathophysiologically distinct subtypes.

14.5 Psychosocial Markers

Emotional information-processing biases can serve as markers for mood disorders such as major depression. "Hot" cognition, in which emotion is engaged, is distinguished from "cold" cognition that is relatively affect-independent. Patients with major depressive disorder often show blunted responses to positive stimuli, heightened sensitivity to negative stimuli, and a tendency to interpret ambiguity negatively [11]. These biases map onto biological models of mood disorders and can help predict response to psychopharmacologic treatment, making them candidate predictors of treatment effects. Because these "hot" affective processing disturbances are not reliably remediated by "cold" cognitive training or standard cognitive-restructuring approaches alone, affected patients may benefit more from pharmacotherapy or targeted psychotherapies [12, 13].

To identify patients who require highly specialized care, hierarchical cluster analysis can be applied [14]. This approach has delineated approximately ten clusters that predict the need for tailored interventions, including overall symptom severity, age at onset and course of illness, comorbid psychiatric conditions such as personality and substance use disorders, medical comorbidity, maladaptive coping, childhood trauma, social risk factors, and global psychosocial dysfunction. Comprehensive clinical assessment that integrates clinical and nonclinical factors is, therefore, essential for selecting appropriate treatment.

14.6 Neural Circuit Biomarkers

Advances in neuroimaging have shifted emphasis from isolated brain regions to the dynamics of distributed networks. Depression is increasingly conceptualized as a disorder of network connectivity involving reward, salience, default-mode, and frontoparietal circuits. Resting-state and task-based functional magnetic resonance imaging (fMRI) have shown that depressed patients do not form a monolithic group but instead fall into reproducible "biotypes" distinguished by functional connectivity patterns. A landmark 2024 study examined more than eight hundred individuals with depression or anxiety and derived six biotypes (default mode, salience, frontoparietal attention, negative affect, reward, and cognitive control), each characterized by distinct configurations of neural network activity and correlated with specific symptom constellations and treatment responses [20]. For example, a subtype marked by hyper-activation of cognitive control circuits tended to respond better to serotonin–noradrenaline reuptake inhibitors, whereas a subtype showing excessive coupling of default-mode networks experienced superior outcomes with psychotherapy. Incorporating biotype information into clinical decision-making *within the research sample* improved remission prediction accuracy from roughly one-third with clinical judgement alone to nearly two-thirds when brain data were considered, *but whether this improves real-world outcomes and cost-effectiveness remains unknown.*

The promise of biotype-driven treatment selection has stimulated efforts to translate these findings into practice. Prototype decision-support tools compare an individual's fMRI signatures to reference biotypes and generate ranked treatment suggestions. *At present, these tools should be regarded as research prototypes rather than clinic-ready systems*, and integrating such tools into clinic workflows would require standardized scanning protocols, user-friendly interfaces, and clinician training, but the conceptual shift is clear: rather than treating depression as a unitary syndrome, future clinicians may tailor therapy according to a patient's brain network profile *if prospective validation demonstrates outcome gains over usual care.* Importantly, neural data are one piece of a larger puzzle; combining neuroimaging with clinical, genetic, inflammatory, and psychosocial information will likely yield the most accurate predictions.

Despite the excitement surrounding neuroimaging biomarkers, caution is warranted. Most biotype studies are cross-sectional and conducted in controlled research settings. Larger, prospective studies must confirm that classification improves outcomes in real-world populations and that brain-based algorithms generalize across scanners and demographic groups [28]. Cost and accessibility are additional barriers—fMRI is expensive and not universally available. Nevertheless, as analytic methods advance and scanning costs decline, neural circuit biomarkers are poised to play an increasingly prominent role in personalized psychiatry *if they are prospectively validated and made accessible in routine settings.*

14.7 Digital Biomarkers

Digital phenotyping offers scalable markers for personalization. Passively captured features—especially location variability, device-use time, and communication frequency—are associated with depressive symptom burden, and some screening models report high classification accuracy [23] *in research settings, although external validation and generalizability remain variable.* Smartphone-delivered ecological momentary assessment (EMA) provides active, in situ ground truth for passive digital streams. In clinical settings, EMA shows acceptable reliability and compliance, although adherence declines as sampling burden increases. Prompt timing and task design materially affect completion [32, 33]. When integrated with remote measurement technologies, EMA can support early detection and individualized monitoring of depression in young people. Real-world effectiveness depends on user engagement, context of use, and standardized reporting [26]. Longitudinal, individual-level monitoring can detect early warning signs and help assess whether treatment is working; robust, generalizable prediction of treatment response or relapse remains preliminary. Findings for heart-rate variability are mixed, and sleep variance rather than duration appears more informative. Field-wide standardization of feature engineering and transparent reporting are prerequisites for clinical integration [23].

14.8 Emerging Interventions and Neuromodulation

The burgeoning science of precision psychiatry has coincided with the development of novel interventions that target specific biological mechanisms or utilize digital platforms. Although these treatments remain adjunctive to established pharmacotherapy and psychotherapy, they broaden the therapeutic armamentarium and underscore the trend toward individualized care.

Rapid-acting antidepressants Ketamine and intranasal esketamine produce rapid improvement in many patients with treatment-resistant depression via N-methyl-D-aspartate (NMDA) antagonism with downstream neuroplastic and inflammatory effects. Among pretreatment features, a positive first-degree family history of alcohol use disorder shows the most consistent association with better intravenous ketamine response; analogous associations have not been observed for esketamine. *These associations should be interpreted as exploratory and are not established as selection criteria for routine care.* Post-dose increases in electroencephalogram (EEG) gamma-band power track antidepressant response but are not established pretreatment selection markers; evidence for childhood trauma as a positive predictor is mixed [21].

Personalized psychotherapy Psychotherapies are effective treatments for depression, yet individual responses vary substantially. Attempts to find single predictors of response have been unsuccessful; models integrating multiple predictors are more promising [15]. The personalized advantage index (PAI) uses a combination of baseline characteristics and mediators to recommend whether cognitive-behavioral therapy or interpersonal psychotherapy is more likely to benefit a given patient and provides an estimate of expected advantage [16]. Randomized trials show that matching therapy via the PAI improves long-term outcomes [17]. *Broader clinical adoption of algorithmic matching, however, remains limited.* Future work will need to personalize newer psychotherapies, including mindfulness-based cognitive therapy, acceptance and commitment therapy, and digital interventions. Virtual-reality–assisted behavioral activation is an emerging adjunct that can be tailored to individual cognitive and functional targets [27].

Personalized neuromodulation Transcranial magnetic stimulation is an established treatment for depression, and personalized neuromodulation seeks to reduce nonresponse by tailoring who receives treatment, where the cortex is targeted, and how the course is delivered. Resting-state fMRI can identify individual prefrontal targets with circuit-level relevance [29], yet a large randomized trial found that connectivity-guided targeting did not outperform standard left-dorsolateral prefrontal cortex (DLPFC) approaches [30], so this strategy remains promising but unproven for routine care *and should be considered investigational for routine targeting.* Schedule personalization includes accelerated courses and intermittent theta-burst stimulation that cluster multiple sessions over short intervals and may hasten symptom improvement, though long-term effectiveness and standardized safety monitoring still need confirmation before broad adoption. Biomarker-informed selection and monitoring using EEG features and imaging-derived connectivity show encouraging signals but require independent replication, harmonized pipelines, and evidence of outcome gains over usual selection [31].

Digital therapeutics Prescription digital therapeutics are software-based treatments delivered on mobile platforms that provide structured, evidence-based psychotherapeutic or cognitive-training modules. They adapt content in real time to patient input and support remote monitoring of symptoms and adherence. They may be prescribed alone or as adjuncts to usual care. Early evaluations indicate that these tools can augment standard care and broaden access when face-to-face therapy is limited [22] *with effects best supported as adjunctive rather than replacement treatments*. When integrated with passively collected smartphone and wearable data, they can support just-in-time–style monitoring and prompts, but standardized feature definitions, transparent reporting, and external validation are prerequisites for routine clinical use. Large-scale implementation should foreground privacy, data security, and equitable access.

Machine learning and multi-omics integration Machine-learning techniques are increasingly used to analyze high-dimensional clinical data and build predictive models of antidepressant response. Models based on genomic features alone typically achieve only moderate accuracy; performance improves when clinical, imaging, inflammatory, and digital measures are integrated [19]. Multi-omic approaches combine genomics, epigenomics, transcriptomics, proteomics, metabolomics, and microbiome data to capture the complex biology of depression. Integrating these layers may reveal patient-specific molecular fingerprints—identifying inflammatory, neuroplasticity, or metabolic subtypes that predict treatment response [18]. Although still primarily research tools, AI-driven multi-omic analyses represent a forward-looking strategy for tailoring interventions to each patient's biological profile.

14.9 Challenges and Future Directions

Bridging the Gap Between Research and Practice

Implementing precision-informed personalized care in routine clinical settings requires addressing several technical and methodological challenges. A critical gap often remains between statistical significance in research samples and clinically actionable utility for individual patients. For example, many clinical trials primarily enroll patients with mild-to-moderate depression, which may limit generalizability to more severe or complex presentations. In addition, proposed symptomatic subtypes are frequently inconsistent across studies and may reflect overall severity rather than qualitatively distinct categories. Multi-omic data sets are high-dimensional, and predictive models may not translate readily into clinical decision tools because of heterogeneous data acquisition, limited standardization, and cost and accessibility constraints.

A Pragmatic Approach for Current Clinical Practice

In current practice, personalization is best approached pragmatically and with appropriate caution. Clinicians can individualize care by prioritizing careful clinical profiling such as illness course, prior treatment response, comorbidities, trauma history, adverse-effect vulnerability, patient preferences, and psychosocial context while applying established evidence-based treatments. Where available, clinically mature applications such as CYP2D6 and CYP2C19 based pharmacogenomic dose guidance may be used selectively when supported by evidence and when results are likely to influence prescribing decisions. By contrast, most candidate biomarkers and algorithmic predictions remain investigational and should be interpreted as adjunctive signals rather than determinative criteria. Clear communication with patients is essential to avoid overpromising benefits and to maintain the therapeutic alliance, with technology positioned as supportive of clinical judgment rather than a substitute for it.

Future Aspirations and Ethical Foundations

Over the longer term, the field aims to improve the precision of diagnosis and treatment by refining biotypes, integrating multi-omics and neural circuit measures, and developing interpretable machine-learning models. Translation to practice will require robust infrastructure, including secure computing environments, standardized data pipelines, and large representative data sets that enable continuous external validation. Importantly, future precision strategies should be adopted only when prospective studies demonstrate meaningful improvements in clinical outcomes over usual care, with acceptable harms and favorable cost-effectiveness. Ethical implementation is also central. Precision approaches must protect privacy, avoid discriminatory stratification, and promote equitable access so that advances do not widen existing disparities. Policymakers will need to address reimbursement and regulatory oversight to support safe and equitable deployment. Within these constraints, personalized medicine may progressively evolve from a promising research framework into a practical component of routine depression care.

Declarations

Competing Interests The author(s) has no competing interests to declare that are relevant to the content of this manuscript.

Ethics Approval The author(s) declares that this manuscript does not include primary research with human participants.

The author(s) declares that this manuscript does not include primary studies involving animals.

References

1. American Psychiatric Association, editor. Practice guideline for the treatment of patients with major depressive disorder. 3rd ed. American Psychiatric Association; 2010.
2. Pulciani S, Di Lonardo A, Fagnani C, Taruscio D. P4 medicine versus Hippocrates. Ann Ist Super Sanita. 2017;53(3):185–91. https://doi.org/10.4415/ANN_17_03_02.
3. Češková E, Šilhán P. From personalized medicine to precision psychiatry? Neuropsychiatr Dis Treat. 2021;17:3663–8. https://doi.org/10.2147/NDT.S337814.
4. Trivedi MH, Kahalnik F, Greer TL. Precision medicine for the treatment of depression. In: Trivedi MH, Strakowski SM, editors. Depression. Oxford University Press; 2019. p. 475–86. https://doi.org/10.1093/med/9780190929565.003.0029.
5. Le-Niculescu H, Roseberry K, Gill SS, et al. Precision medicine for mood disorders: objective assessment, risk prediction, pharmacogenomics, and repurposed drugs. Mol Psychiatry. 2021;26(7):2776–804. https://doi.org/10.1038/s41380-021-01061-w.
6. Jukic M, Milosavljević F, Molden E, Ingelman-Sundberg M. Pharmacogenomics in treatment of depression and psychosis: an update. Trends Pharmacol Sci. 2022;43(12):1055–69. https://doi.org/10.1016/j.tips.2022.09.011.
7. Hicks JK, Bishop JR, Sangkuhl K, et al. CPIC guideline for CYP2D6 and CYP2C19 genotypes and dosing of selective serotonin reuptake inhibitors. Clin Pharmacol Ther. 2015;98(2):127–34. https://doi.org/10.1002/cpt.147.
8. Pisoni A, Strawbridge R, Hodsoll J, et al. Growth factor proteins and treatment-resistant depression: a place on the path to precision. Front Psych. 2018;9:386. https://doi.org/10.3389/fpsyt.2018.00386.
9. Drevets WC, Wittenberg GM, Bullmore ET, Manji HK. Immune targets for therapeutic development in depression: towards precision medicine. Nat Rev Drug Discov. 2022;21(3):224–44. https://doi.org/10.1038/s41573-021-00368-1.
10. Suseelan S, Pinna G. Heterogeneity in major depressive disorder: the need for biomarker-based personalized treatments. Adv Clin Chem. 2023;112:1–67. https://doi.org/10.1016/bs.acc.2022.10.001.
11. Elliott R, Zahn R, Deakin JFW, Anderson IM. Affective cognition and its disruption in mood disorders. Neuropsychopharmacology. 2011;36(1):153–82. https://doi.org/10.1038/npp.2010.77.
12. Godlewska BR, Browning M, Norbury R, Cowen PJ, Harmer CJ. Early changes in emotional processing as a marker of clinical response to SSRI treatment

in depression. Transl Psychiatry. 2016;6(11):e957. https://doi.org/10.1038/tp.2016.130.
13. Shiroma PR, Thuras P, Johns B, Lim KO. Emotion recognition processing as early predictor of response to eight-week citalopram treatment in late-life depression. Int J Geriatr Psychiatry. 2014;29(11):1132–9. https://doi.org/10.1002/gps.4107.
14. van Krugten FCW, Goorden M, van Balkom AJLM, Spijker J, Brouwer WBF, Hakkaart-van Roijen L. Indicators to facilitate the early identification of patients with major depressive disorder in need of highly specialized care: a concept mapping study. Depress Anxiety. 2018;35(4):346–52. https://doi.org/10.1002/da.22721.
15. Cuijpers P, Ebert DD, Acarturk C, Andersson G, Cristea IA. Personalized psychotherapy for adult depression: a meta-analytic review. Behav Ther. 2016;47(6):966–80. https://doi.org/10.1016/j.beth.2016.04.007.
16. DeRubeis RJ, Cohen ZD, Forand NR, Fournier JC, Gelfand LA, Lorenzo-Luaces L. The Personalized Advantage Index: translating research on prediction into individualized treatment recommendations. PLoS One. 2014;9(1):e83875. https://doi.org/10.1371/journal.pone.0083875.
17. van Bronswijk SC, DeRubeis RJ, Lemmens LHJM, et al. Precision medicine for long-term depression outcomes using the Personalized Advantage Index approach: cognitive therapy or interpersonal psychotherapy? Psychol Med. 2021;51(2):279–89. https://doi.org/10.1017/S0033291719003179.
18. Stolfi F, Abreu H, Sinella R, et al. Omics approaches open new horizons in major depressive disorder: from biomarkers to precision medicine. Front Psych. 2024;15:1422939. https://doi.org/10.3389/fpsyt.2024.1422939.
19. Comai S, Manchia M, Bosia M, et al. Moving toward precision and personalized treatment strategies in psychiatry. Int J Neuropsychopharmacol. 2025;28(5):pyaf025. https://doi.org/10.1093/ijnp/pyaf025.
20. Tozzi L, Zhang X, Pines A, et al. Personalized brain circuit scores identify clinically distinct biotypes in depression and anxiety. Nat Med. 2024;30(7):2076–87. https://doi.org/10.1038/s41591-024-03057-9.
21. Medeiros GC, Demo I, Goes FS, Zarate CA Jr, Gould TD. Personalized use of ketamine and esketamine for treatment-resistant depression. Transl Psychiatry. 2024;14(1):481. https://doi.org/10.1038/s41398-024-03180-8.
22. Ferrante M, Esposito LE, Stoeckel LE. From palm to practice: prescription digital therapeutics for mental and brain health at the National Institutes of Health. Front Psych. 2024;15:1433438. https://doi.org/10.3389/fpsyt.2024.1433438.
23. Zierer C, Behrendt C, Lepach-Engelhardt AC. Digital biomarkers in depression: a systematic review and call for standardization and harmonization of feature engineering. J Affect Disord. 2024;356:438–49. https://doi.org/10.1016/j.jad.2024.03.163.
24. Barlati S, Minelli A, Nibbio G, et al. The role of pharmacogenetics in the treatment of major depressive disorder: a critical review. Front Psych. 2023;14:1307473. https://doi.org/10.3389/fpsyt.2023.1307473.
25. Miller AH. Advancing an inflammatory subtype of major depression. Am J Psychiatry. 2025;182(6):516–24. https://doi.org/10.1176/appi.ajp.20250289.
26. Song EJ, Tozzi L, Williams LM. Brain circuit–derived biotypes for treatment selection in mood disorders: a critical review and illustration of a functional neuroimaging tool for clinical translation. Biol Psychiatry. 2024;96(7):552–63. https://doi.org/10.1016/j.biopsych.2024.03.016.
27. Jung HW, Jang KW, Nam S, et al. Personalized virtual reality exposure for panic disorder and agoraphobia: a preliminary neurophysiological study. Compr Psychiatry. 2024;129:152447. https://doi.org/10.1016/j.comppsych.2023.152447.
28. Koch E, Pardiñas AF, O'Connell KS, et al. How real-world data can facilitate the development of precision medicine treatment in psychiatry. Biol Psychiatry. 2024;96(7):543–51. https://doi.org/10.1016/j.biopsych.2024.01.001.
29. Cole EJ, Phillips AL, Bentzley BS, et al. Stanford Neuromodulation Therapy (SNT): a double-blind randomized controlled trial. Am J Psychiatry. 2022;179(2):132–41. https://doi.org/10.1176/appi.ajp.2021.20101429.
30. Morriss R, Briley PM, Webster L, et al. Connectivity-guided intermittent theta burst versus repetitive transcranial magnetic stimulation for treatment-resistant depression: a randomized controlled trial. Nat Med. 2024;30:403–13. https://doi.org/10.1038/s41591-023-02764-z.
31. Jin MX, Qin PP, Xia AWL, et al. Neurophysiological and neuroimaging markers of rTMS treatment response in major depressive disorder: a systematic review and meta-analysis of predictive modeling studies. Neurosci Biobehav Rev. 2024;162:105695. https://doi.org/10.1016/j.neubiorev.2024.105695.
32. Stone AA, Schneider S, Smyth JM. Evaluation of pressing issues in ecological momentary assessment. Annu Rev Clin Psychol. 2023;19:107–31. https://doi.org/10.1146/annurev-clinpsy-080921-083128.
33. Tonkin S, Gass J, Wray J, et al. Evaluating declines in compliance with ecological momentary assessment in longitudinal health behavior research: analyses from a clinical trial. J Med Internet Res. 2023;25:e43826. https://doi.org/10.2196/43826.

The Limitations of Antidepressants: Toward Etiology-Based Psychiatry

15

Young-Min Park and Duk-In Jon

15.1 Introduction

Modern individuals are often described as living in an age of widespread depression. Contemporary life is saturated with stress and loneliness, and these conditions have contributed to depression and suicide becoming major social concerns. The World Health Organization has even issued public warnings on the matter [1]. With the growing prevalence of depression, prescriptions for antidepressants have steadily increased. Yet, depression remains a persistent challenge. This chapter seeks to examine the limitations of antidepressants and to consider more appropriate ways of using them.

15.2 Limitations of the Current Diagnostic System

The current dominant psychiatric diagnostic framework, the Diagnostic and Statistical Manual of Mental Disorders (DSM), has been subject to criticism from multiple perspectives [2, 3]. The first concern lies in its symptom-centered structure. Reliance solely on symptom-based diagnosis increases the risk of overdiagnosis or misdiagnosis. The second concern is its limited integration of findings from neurobiological research. For instance, family history has consistently been identified as a strong predictor of bipolar disorder, yet the revised DSM-5 remains largely unchanged from the DSM-IV published in 1994. Although the cautious stance of DSM authors in avoiding premature biological interpretations is understandable, it is nonetheless disappointing that core diagnostic criteria for major disorders such as schizophrenia, bipolar disorder, and major depressive disorder have seen little substantive revision over the past three decades. The third limitation concerns the cross-sectional nature of its diagnostic criteria. Because the DSM defines disorders primarily on the basis of current or recent symptoms, diagnostic errors can easily occur. This complicates differential diagnosis among schizophrenia, bipolar disorder, and major depressive disorder. For example, DSM-5 allows clinicians to diagnose major depressive disorder when five out of nine criteria are fulfilled. Given the combinatorial possibilities, even the minimum threshold of five symptoms can generate 126 distinct diagnostic profiles, reflecting the heterogeneity of this category [4]. Such a symptom-based system likely contributes to overdiagnosis and the inclusion of biologically and psychologically heterogeneous groups, which in turn may reduce the overall effectiveness of antidepressant treatments.

Y.-M. Park (✉)
Brain and Mind Mental Health Clinic, Goyang, Republic of Korea

Brain and Mind Institute, Goyang, Republic of Korea
e-mail: youngminpark007@naver.com

D.-I. Jon
Department of Psychiatry, Dong-A University Hospital, Busan, Republic of Korea

W.-M. Bahk et al. (eds.), *Depressive Disorder*, https://doi.org/10.1007/978-981-92-1331-3_15

15.3 Antidepressants Versus Serotonin Agonists

The term antidepressant may lead psychiatrists or clinicians to mistakenly assume that depressive symptoms should always be treated with these drugs. However, numerous studies have demonstrated that only a subset of depressive disorders respond effectively. In the case of bipolar depression, for example, antidepressant monotherapy has shown no significant advantage over placebo and may even increase the risk of switching to mania or hypomania. Combination therapies for bipolar depression—apart from the U.S. Food and Drug Administration (FDA)-approved olanzapine–fluoxetine combination (OFC)—have likewise produced inconsistent results. Similarly, conditions such as neurotic depression, secondary depression, and persistent depressive disorder lasting more than two years have demonstrated limited responsiveness to antidepressants.

Some researchers have argued that these drugs should instead be renamed according to their mechanisms of action—for example, serotonin agonists—rather than grouped under the broad label of "antidepressants" [5]. One influential meta-analysis demonstrated that in cases of mild-to-moderate depression, antidepressants offered no greater benefit than placebo. In severe depression, the difference reached statistical significance, but the magnitude was small—equivalent to roughly a three-point change on standard symptom rating scales [6]. The STAR*D trial, conducted by the U.S. National Institute of Mental Health, reported a remission rate of only 30% with first-line treatment, and approximately 50% after completion of all four sequential treatment steps [7]. Long-term follow-up of STAR*D participants showed frequent relapses, underscoring the inherent limitations of antidepressant therapy.

15.4 The Shaking Throne of Antidepressants

In 2010, the American psychiatric community entered a period of profound turbulence [8]. Two issues drew major attention: repeated meta-analyses questioning whether antidepressants offered advantages over placebo, and case reports suggesting a possible link to suicidality. The first issue was largely associated with publication bias [9]. When the FDA dataset—including both published and unpublished trials—was examined, results showed almost an even split: just over half indicated some benefit of antidepressants compared to placebo, while nearly half did not. Yet, when only published papers were reviewed, roughly nine out of ten published trials appeared to support antidepressant efficacy, whereas analyses including unpublished data painted a more balanced picture, with results divided almost evenly. This contrast reflected a systemic problem: researchers often hesitated to submit, and journals often avoided studies with negative findings.

A striking example involves lamotrigine in bipolar disorder. Evidence from a meta-analysis [10], indicates that lamotrigine can be considered an effective therapeutic option for bipolar depression. However, a similar pattern was also seen in lamotrigine trials: of nine conducted, two positive studies reached publication, two more emphasized secondary outcomes, while five negative trials remained unpublished, creating a partial and potentially misleading evidence base. Such selective publication may present an incomplete picture of lamotrigine's efficacy and illustrates how non-publication of negative findings can mislead clinicians and overestimate treatment effects.

Clinicians must, therefore, remain mindful of publication bias and actively consider the weight of negative studies. In response, the FDA now mandates prospective registration of clinical trials, and meta-analyses that incorporate unpublished data can provide more balanced perspectives. Even so, meta-analyses remain limited by factors such as selective inclusion of studies. Importantly, one major review found little-to-no difference between antidepressants and placebo in mild-to-moderate depression, but did report greater benefit in severe cases [6]. Thus, treatment decisions should be guided by illness severity.

15.5 The Risk of Suicidality and Aggression

Concerns intensified following reports that some young patients taking antidepressants engaged in aggressive or self-harming behaviors, including suicide attempts and, in rare instances, even acts of violence. These observations prompted a vigorous debate about the safety of antidepressant use in pediatric populations [8, 11, 12]. Current interpretations suggest these risks arise not directly from the drugs themselves, but from unrecognized bipolar vulnerability or medication-induced states such as akathisia. Controlled trials indicate a possible rise in suicidal thoughts or behaviors within certain age groups, though actual completed suicides were not observed [13]. Still, prescribing antidepressants indiscriminately could elevate the risk of harmful outcomes.

15.6 The Collapse of the Serotonin Hypothesis

A comprehensive review by UK researchers revisited the serotonin hypothesis, analyzing data on neurotransmitter levels, receptor activity, transporter function, and experimental tryptophan depletion [14]. The review concluded that current evidence does not provide compelling support for serotonin deficiency as the central mechanism of depression. Critics responded that the analysis underemphasized certain findings and could not establish that serotonin-based treatments are entirely ineffective [15].

Meanwhile, novel treatments such as ketamine—acting through pathways unrelated to serotonin—have shown striking antidepressant effects [16]. Nonetheless, many clinicians observe that patients do improve on serotonin-based medications, often relapsing when these are discontinued. A more nuanced perspective is that only some depressive subtypes involve serotonin dysfunction, and in such cases serotonin-modulating drugs may enhance processes like neurogenesis and functional recovery [17]. For this reason, clinicians should remain receptive both to traditional serotonin-based options and to emerging therapies with alternative mechanisms [18].

15.7 Appropriate Use of Antidepressants

Medicine has historically advanced along two philosophical traditions—Hippocratic and Galenic [19]. The Hippocratic tradition emphasizes a disease-centered approach, with a principle of avoiding unnecessary harm. Diseases were historically classified into three categories: those that remit naturally, those that are amenable to therapeutic intervention, and those resistant to any known treatment. Physicians are urged to intervene only in the second category. By contrast, Galenic practice prioritizes symptom elimination, pursuing aggressive interventions to relieve distress.

Modern psychiatry, in practice, has leaned more toward the Galenic model [19]. Because psychiatric diagnoses often lack precise etiological markers, treatments are typically developed based on observed clinical benefit rather than underlying mechanisms. This fosters a focus on symptoms: antidepressants for low mood, hypnotics for insomnia, antipsychotics for hallucinations.

Clinicians, however, should weigh whether a drug targets root pathology or merely suppresses surface symptoms. Consider a patient with iron-deficiency restless legs syndrome causing profound insomnia. A symptom-oriented approach would use sleeping pills or dopamine agonists. A disease-centered approach, however, would identify and correct iron deficiency. Once the deficiency is corrected, sleep disturbance often subsides, with adjunctive drugs serving only a temporary role. A shift toward etiology-based care could reduce dependence on chronic symptomatic prescriptions.

15.8 Conclusion

Building on these limitations, more concrete clinical guidance is warranted. In routine practice, antidepressant initiation should not be regarded as a default response to depressive symptoms, but rather as a decision informed by illness severity, longitudinal course, and individual risk profiles. Evidence suggests that in mild-to-moderate depression, where antidepressant effects scarcely exceed placebo, first-line strategies may reasonably emphasize psychotherapeutic interventions, psychosocial modification, and watchful waiting, whereas pharmacotherapy should be reserved for cases marked by severe symptom burden, functional impairment, or biological vulnerability.

From an immediate clinical perspective, this implies the need for a structured decision framework that incorporates factors such as prior treatment response, family history of bipolar disorder, age-related suicide risk, and the likelihood of spontaneous remission. Careful screening for bipolar spectrum features and close monitoring during early treatment phases are essential to minimize adverse outcomes.

In contrast, the longer-term implication extends beyond medication choice toward a broader paradigm shift in psychiatric practice. Moving away from symptom-based categorization toward etiology-informed models—integrating neurobiological markers, developmental trajectories, and environmental context—may ultimately improve diagnostic precision and reduce both overtreatment and therapeutic failure. Antidepressants, within this framework, should be viewed not as universal remedies but as selective tools, appropriate only when aligned with an individual patient's underlying pathophysiology and clinical context.

Declarations

Competing Interests The author(s) has no competing interests to declare that are relevant to the content of this manuscript.

Ethics Approval The author(s) declares that this manuscript does not include primary research with human participants.

The author(s) declares that this manuscript does not include primary studies involving animals.

References

1. World Health Organization. Depression: let's talk—says WHO as depression tops list of causes of ill health. Geneva: World Health Organization; 2017.
2. Frances A. Saving normal: an insider's revolt against out-of-control psychiatric diagnosis. New York: HarperCollins; 2013.
3. Wakefield JC. DSM-5, psychiatric epidemiology and the false positives problem. 2015;24(3):188–96. https://doi.org/10.1017/S2045796015000116.
4. Moncrieff J. Are antidepressants overrated? A review of methodological problems in antidepressant trials. J Nerv Ment Dis. 2001;189(5):288–95. https://doi.org/10.1097/00005053-200105000-00003.
5. Kirsch I, Deacon BJ, Huedo-Medina TB, Scoboria A, Moore TJ, Johnson BT. Initial severity and antidepressant benefits: a meta-analysis of data submitted to the FDA. PLoS Med. 2008;5(2):e45. https://doi.org/10.1371/journal.pmed.0050045.
6. Rush AJ, Trivedi MH, Wisniewski SR, et al. Acute and longer-term outcomes in depressed outpatients: STAR*D report. Am J Psychiatry. 2006;163(11):1905–17. https://doi.org/10.1176/ajp.2006.163.11.1905.
7. Whitaker R. Anatomy of an epidemic. New York: Crown Publishing Group; 2010.
8. Turner EH, Matthews AM, Linardatos E, Tell RA, Rosenthal R. Selective publication of antidepressant trials and its influence on apparent efficacy. N Engl J Med. 2008;358(3):252–60. https://doi.org/10.1056/NEJMsa065779.
9. Geddes JR, Calabrese JR, Goodwin GM. Lamotrigine treatment for bipolar depression: a meta-analysis. Br J Psychiatry. 2009;194(1):4–9. https://doi.org/10.1192/bjp.bp.107.048504.
10. Healy D. The antidepressant era. Cambridge, MA: Harvard University Press; 1997.
11. Fergusson D, Doucette S, Glass KC, Shapiro S, Healy D, Hebert P, et al. Association between suicide attempts and SSRIs: a review. BMJ. 2005;330(7488):396. https://doi.org/10.1136/bmj.330.7488.396.
12. Gibbons RD, Brown CH, Hur K, et al. Early evidence on the effects of regulators' suicidality warnings on SSRI prescriptions and suicide in children and adolescents. Am J Psychiatry. 2007;164(9):1356–63. https://doi.org/10.1176/appi.ajp.2007.07030454.
13. Moncrieff J, Cooper RE, Stockmann T, Amendola S, Hengartner MP, Horowitz MA. The serotonin theory

of depression: a systematic umbrella review of the evidence. Mol Psychiatry. 2023;28(8):3243–56. https://doi.org/10.1038/s41380-022-01661-0.
14. Cowen PJ, Browning M. What has serotonin to do with depression? World Psychiatry. 2015;14(2):158–60. https://doi.org/10.1002/wps.20229.
15. Zarate CA Jr, Singh JB, Carlson PJ, Brutsche NE, Ameli R, Luckenbaugh DA, et al. A randomized trial of an N-methyl-D-aspartate antagonist in treatment-resistant major depression. Arch Gen Psychiatry. 2006;63(8):856–64. https://doi.org/10.1001/archpsyc.63.8.856.
16. Malberg JE, Eisch AJ, Nestler EJ, Duman RS. Chronic antidepressant treatment increases neurogenesis in adult rat hippocampus. J Neurosci. 2000;20(24):9104–10. https://doi.org/10.1523/JNEUROSCI.20-24-09104.2000.
17. Duman RS, Aghajanian GK, Sanacora G, Krystal JH. Synaptic plasticity and depression: new insights from stress and rapid-acting antidepressants. Nat Med. 2016;22(3):238–49. https://doi.org/10.1038/nm.4050.
18. von Engelhardt D. Patient vs. disease in medicine: historical perspectives and contemporary concerns. J Nephrol. 2004;17(4):611–8.
19. Ghaemi SN. Clinical psychopharmacology: principles and practice. 2nd ed. New York: Oxford University Press; 2018.

Biological Non-pharmacological Treatments for Depressive Disorder

16

Min-Kyu Song and Jeong Seok Seo

16.1 Introduction

Major depressive disorder (MDD) is among the leading global contributors to disability and disease burden [5, 6]. Even with best-practice pharmacotherapy and psychotherapy, approximately one-third of patients fail to remit or discontinue due to adverse effects, underscoring the need for additional modalities [2, 3]. Biological non-pharmacological treatments modulate brain networks, neuroplasticity, monoaminergic systems, neuroendocrine stress responses, inflammation, and circadian timing. Contemporary guidelines (American psychiatric association (APA) 2023; Canadian network for mood and anxiety treatments (CANMAT) 2023; UK National institute for health and care excellence (NICE) 2022) and KMAP-DD 2025 integrate these modalities within stepped care and treatment-resistance algorithms [4, 7–10] (Table 16.1).

Table 16.1 Roles of major non-pharmacological modalities in depression (guideline snapshot)

Modality	Typical clinical role (summary)
ECT	Highest acute efficacy; severe/psychotic depression, suicidality, catatonia; rapid response needed [3–7]
rTMS	Effective non-invasive option for TRD; iTBS as time-efficient variant; maintenance possible [4, 7–9, 16–18]
tDCS	Modest efficacy; best for non-TRD or as augmentation; portable/home-capable [22–27, 33–36, 43]
VNS	Surgical adjunct for chronic TRD; delayed onset with durable benefit in a subset [28–31, 43]
BLT	First-line for SAD; adjunct for non-seasonal MDD; morning dosing favored [32–36, 44, 47]
Exercise	First-line adjunct across severities; moderate-to-large effects in meta-analyses [51–55]

ECT electroconvulsive therapy; *rTMS* repetitive transcranial magnetic stimulation, *tDCS* transcranial direct current stimulation; *VNS* vagus nerve stimulation; *BLT* bright light therapy; *TRD* treatment-resistant depression; *SAD* seasonal affective disorder.

16.2 Electroconvulsive Therapy (ECT)

Mechanisms and Neurobiological Rationale

ECT induces a controlled generalized seizure under anesthesia, producing widespread modulation of fronto-limbic circuitry, normalization of

M.-K. Song (✉)
Department of Psychiatry, St. Mary's Gong-Gam Mental Health Clinic, Siheung, Republic of Korea
e-mail: somtt0714@gmail.com

J. S. Seo
Department of Psychiatry, College of Medicine, Chung-Ang University, Gwangmyeong Hospital, Gwangmyeong, Republic of Korea

W.-M. Bahk et al. (eds.), *Depressive Disorder*, https://doi.org/10.1007/978-981-92-1331-3_16

subgenual cingulate activity, increased GABAergic tone, monoamine release, and neurotrophic signaling (e.g., brain-derived neurotrophic factor [BDNF]) that promote synaptic remodeling and neurogenesis [7, 9–12].

Efficacy and Comparative Effectiveness

Evidence from randomized controlled trials (RCTs) and meta-analyses consistently demonstrates that ECT remains the most effective acute treatment for severe MDD, including psychotic depression and high-risk states (catatonia, suicidality). Modern series report response rates ≥60–80% and remission ~50–60% [7, 12–14]. Continuation/maintenance strategies (C-ECT ± pharmacotherapy) reduce relapse after successful acute courses [11, 15]. Contemporary network meta-analyses and guideline syntheses consistently rank ECT at the top for acute efficacy [4, 7, 8, 13, 18].

Indications and Protocols

Indications: Severe or psychotic depression; imminent suicide risk; catatonia; medication resistance/intolerance; pregnancy when medications are contraindicated; need for rapid clinical response [3–6].

Protocols: Typically 2–3 sessions/week for 6–12 sessions; electrode placement individualized—bitemporal/bifrontal (maximal efficacy) versus right unilateral (better cognitive profile); ultrabrief pulse (≤0.3 ms) reduces cognitive effects with modest trade-off in speed of response [12, 16, 19]. Maintenance ECT considered in recurrent or highly relapsing courses [11].

Safety and Cognitive Effects

Common adverse effects include headache, myalgia, acute disorientation. Cognitive effects (anterograde/retrograde memory) are dose/placement dependent and usually remit; persistent autobiographical gaps occur in a minority [20]. With appropriate pre-anesthetic screening and monitoring, serious medical risks are rare and comparable to general anesthesia [11, 16, 45].

Box 16.1 ECT Pre-treatment Checklist

- Medical/anesthesia evaluation; electrocardiogram (ECG) and labs as indicated [11, 16]
- Informed consent including discussion of memory effects [20]
- Electrode placement and dosing strategy (threshold titration) [12, 19]
- Relapse prevention plan (C-ECT and/or pharmacotherapy) [11]

16.3 Repetitive Transcranial Magnetic Stimulation (rTMS)

Mechanisms

rTMS modulates cortical excitability and network connectivity via magnetic induction, producing Long-term potentiation (LTP)/ Long-term depression (LTD)-like plasticity in prefrontal-limbic circuits. High-frequency (≥10 Hz) left Dorsolateral prefrontal cortex (DLPFC) increases excitability, whereas low-frequency (≤1 Hz) right DLPFC is inhibitory; neuroimaging shows normalization of DLPFC–subgenual connectivity with response [16, 19–21].

Protocols and Innovations

Standard 10 Hz left DLPFC or 1 Hz right DLPFC deliver ~20–30 sessions over 4–6 weeks. Intermittent theta-burst stimulation (iTBS) is non-inferior to 10 Hz with ~3-minute sessions (THREE-D trial) [17]. Accelerated paradigms (e.g., SAINT; spaced multiple daily sessions) can yield rapid improvement in TRD cohorts [21, 26, 27, 41, 42] (Table 16.2).

Table 16.2 rTMS protocol variants (typical parameters)

Protocol	Target	Frequency	Session time	Notes
10 Hz (HF-L)	Left DLPFC	10 Hz	~37 min	FDA-approved; robust evidence [16, 18, 23–25]
1 Hz (LF-R)	Right DLPFC	1 Hz	~20 min	Alternative/adjunct; lower seizure risk [16]
iTBS	Left DLPFC	50 Hz bursts @ 5 Hz	~3–5 min	Non-inferior to 10 Hz; time-efficient [17]
Accelerated iTBS	Left DLPFC	Multiple/day	1–5 days	Rapid responses in TRD cohorts [21, 26, 27, 41]

Efficacy and Guideline Placement

Meta-analyses and network comparisons confirm superiority to sham with response ~40–55% and remission ~25–35% in TRD, generally below ECT effect sizes [16, 18, 23–26]. CANMAT/NICE/APA endorses rTMS after inadequate antidepressant trials; KMAP-DD 2025 recommends rTMS as a Level-B option when patients prefer non-drug approaches or have intolerance [4, 7–10, 16]. Deep TMS (H-coil) is established for obsessive compulsive disorder (OCD) and is being evaluated in MDD subtypes [46].

Safety and Tolerability

Most common adverse effects: scalp discomfort and transient headache. Seizure risk is <0.1% with protocolized screening/dosing; no consistent cognitive impairment—some studies report modest executive improvements [20, 27–29].

Box 16.2 rTMS Candidacy and Safety Screen

- ≥1–2 adequate antidepressant trials; stable comorbidities [4, 7–10, 16]
- Exclude incompatible cranial ferromagnetic implants/cochlear devices [20]
- Review seizure history, sleep deprivation, and medications lowering threshold [20]

16.4 Transcranial Direct Current Stimulation (tDCS)

Mechanisms

tDCS delivers 1–2 mA constant current via electrodes to shift resting membrane potentials and facilitate N-methyl-D-aspartate (NMDA)-dependent plasticity. Depression protocols typically place the anode over left DLPFC (F3) with cathode over right supraorbital area [31–33].

Efficacy and Combinations

Meta-analyses/IPD syntheses show small-to-moderate antidepressant effects versus sham, strongest in non-TRD and when *combined with selective serotonin reuptake inhibitors (SSRIs)* (e.g., sertraline) [23–26, 32, 34, 35]. Remotely supervised *home-based* tDCS is feasible and may expand access [27, 36]. Parameter and safety consensus continue to evolve [34, 43] (Table 16.3).

Safety, Limitations, and Practical Issues

tDCS is well tolerated (tingling, itch, mild headache/erythema). Serious events are rare with standard protocols [34, 35]. Effects are modest and heterogeneous; sham blinding and inter-individual anatomical variability (skull thickness, gyrifica-

Table 16.3 Typical tDCS parameters in depression

Montage	Current	Duration	Frequency	Notes
Anode L-DLPFC / cathode Relative sleep onset advance (R-SOA)	1–2 mA	20–30 min	5×/week × 2–6 weeks	Standard protocol [22–26, 31–33]
+ SSRI augmentation	2 mA	30 min	5×/week × 4–6 weeks	Additive effects versus either alone [24]
Remote-supervised home tDCS	1–2 mA	20–30 min	Programmed	Feasibility shown [27, 36]

tion) complicate signal detection [37, 40, 41]. Good practice includes skin inspection, consistent electrode prep, and adherence monitoring [34, 43].

Box 16.3 Selecting Patients for tDCS

- Mild–moderate MDD; limited access/tolerance to rTMS/ECT [23–26]
- Preference for low-cost, portable option; ability for frequent sessions [27, 36]
- Avoid in patients with implanted electronics or active scalp disease [34, 35, 43]

16.5 Vagus Nerve Stimulation (VNS)

Mechanisms and Clinical Profile

Implanted left cervical VNS projects to nucleus tractus solitarius and onward to locus coeruleus and dorsal raphe, modulating NE/5-HT systems and limbic-prefrontal circuits [31]. Acute RCTs showed limited short-term separation versus sham, but long-term observational/registry data indicate sustained benefits over months–years in subsets of chronic TRD, particularly with concomitant pharmacotherapy [28–31, 40–42].

Indications, Safety, and Expectations

VNS is considered after multiple adequate trials (often including ECT/rTMS). Common stimulation-related effects: hoarseness, throat discomfort, cough/dyspnea; surgical complications are uncommon (infection, lead issues). Onset is delayed—set expectations for gradual improvement over several months [28–31, 40–43].

16.6 Bright Light Therapy (BLT) and Chronotherapy

Mechanisms and Protocols

BLT entrains circadian rhythms via intrinsically photosensitive retinal ganglion cells projecting to the Suprachiasmatic nucleus (SCN), normalizing melatonin secretion and interacting with monoaminergic systems [46].

Protocol: 10,000 lux at eye level for ~30 minutes each morning over several weeks; lower lux requires longer duration [32–34, 46, 50].

Efficacy and Safety

BLT is first-line for *seasonal affective disorder* and effective as an adjunct in non-seasonal MDD, with some RCTs showing faster improvement when combined with SSRIs [32, 34–36, 44, 47–49]. Side effects are usually mild (eye strain, headache, agitation/insomnia if late). Use caution with retinal disease and photosensitizing medications; consider midday timing in bipolar depression to mitigate switch risk [34–36, 50].

Box 16.4 Practical Tips for BLT/Chronotherapy

- Consistent *morning* use; avoid late-day sessions [32–36, 44, 47]
- Combine with sleep phase advance/Cognitive behavioral therapy for insomnia (CBT-I) when circadian misalignment is prominent [36, 46, 48]
- Educate on distance (~50 cm), angle, and open-eye exposure (no direct stare into LEDs) [50]

16.7 Exercise

Mechanisms and Clinical Effects

Exercise increases BDNF and hippocampal neurogenesis, modulates monoamines, improves sleep, and reduces systemic inflammation, translating into antidepressant effects across severities [51–53].

Efficacy and Prescription

RCTs and umbrella/meta-analyses confirm moderate-to-large effect sizes; aerobic exercise (e.g., brisk walking/cycling) is particularly effective, with resistance training also beneficial [51–55]. APA/CANMAT endorse structured exercise as first-line adjunctive care [4, 7–9] (Table 16.4).

Table 16.4 Recommended exercise prescription in depression

Component	Recommendation
Frequency	≥3 sessions/week
Duration	30–60 min/session
Intensity	Moderate (≈50–70% HRmax; Retinal pigment epithelium (RPE) 12–14)
Type	Aerobic ± resistance; mind–body (yoga/tai-chi) as adjunct

16.8 Nutraceuticals

Overview

Nutritional agents with evidence include *omega-3 polyunsaturated fatty acids (PUFAs)*, *S-adenosyl methionine (SAMe)*, *folate/L-methylfolate*, and *vitamin D*. They are generally safe and can be considered in partial responders or phenotype-guided contexts (e.g., inflammation, folate deficiency) [56–61, 64–67].

Specific Agents

- *Omega-3 PUFAs:* Multiple meta-analyses show antidepressant benefits, especially with European Psychiatric Association *(EPA)-dominant* formulations (≥60% EPA), typically *1–2 g/day* as augmentation [57–59, 61–63].
- *SAMe:* Effective as mono/adjunctive therapy in RCTs (e.g., 800–1600 mg/day); favorable tolerability [62, 63, 65].
- *Folate/L-methylfolate:* Augmentation is beneficial, particularly in folate deficiency or Methylenetetrahydrofolate reductase (MTHFR) polymorphisms; *L-methylfolate 15 mg/day* is commonly studied [60, 64, 65].
- *Vitamin D:* Evidence mixed; meta-analyses suggest modest benefit in deficient populations—supplement to sufficiency [66, 67].

Box 16.5 Practical Guide to Nutraceuticals in Depression

- *Omega-3 (EPA-dominant)*: 1–2 g/day EPA; consider in partial responders/inflammatory phenotype [57–59, 61–63]
- *SAMe*: 800–1600 mg/day; monitor for activation/GI upset [62, 63]
- *L-methylfolate*: 15 mg/day augmentation; check folate/B12 status [64, 65]
- *Vitamin D*: Replete deficiency to 25(OH)D sufficiency; monitor levels [66, 67]

16.9 Brief Note on DBS and Other Emerging Approaches

Deep brain stimulation (DBS) of subcallosal cingulate, ventral capsule/ventral striatum, or medial forebrain bundle shows promising long-term outcomes in selected TRD but remains investigational; closed-loop neuromodulation illustrates personalized, biomarker-guided stimulation with early case-level success [37–40]. These approaches are restricted to specialized centers/clinical trials.

16.10 Conclusion

Among biological non-pharmacological treatments, electroconvulsive therapy (ECT) provides the most rapid and robust efficacy for severe or psychotic depression. Repetitive transcranial magnetic stimulation (rTMS) is an effective, well-tolerated non-invasive option, with intermittent theta burst stimulation (iTBS) offering a more time-efficient protocol. Transcranial direct current stimulation (tDCS) confers modest benefits with excellent portability and safety, making it best suited as an augmentative strategy or for non–treatment-resistant depression. Vagus nerve stimulation (VNS) yields delayed but durable benefits in chronic, treatment-resistant depression. Bright light therapy (BLT) is established as a first-line treatment for seasonal affective disorder and serves as an evidence-based adjunct for non-seasonal major depression. Exercise and nutraceuticals remain accessible and generally safe adjunctive options that can produce clinically meaningful effects.

Contemporary guideline consensus (APA, CANMAT, NICE, with alignment to KMAP-DD 2025) endorses their integration into stepped-care frameworks, tailored to illness severity, comorbidities, patient preferences, and resource availability [4, 7–10]. Future directions include the development of biomarker-guided treatment selection, refinement of stimulation protocols (e.g., accelerated TMS), and exploration of multimodal combinations to enhance and sustain long-term remission.

Declarations

Competing Interests The author(s) has no competing interests to declare that are relevant to the content of this manuscript.

Ethics Approval The author(s) declares that this manuscript does not include primary research with human participants.

The author(s) declares that this manuscript does not include primary studies involving animals.

References

1. Rush AJ, Trivedi MH, Wisniewski SR, et al. Acute and longer-term outcomes in depressed outpatients requiring one or several treatment steps: a STAR*D report. Am J Psychiatry. 2006;163(11):1905–17.
2. Gaynes BN, Lux L, Gartlehner G, et al. Defining treatment-resistant depression. Depress Anxiety. 2020;37(2):134–45.
3. Fava M. Diagnosis and definition of treatment-resistant depression. Biol Psychiatry. 2003;53(8):649–59.
4. Kennedy SH, Lam RW, McIntyre RS, et al. CANMAT 2023 clinical guidelines for the management of adults with major depressive disorder. Can J Psychiatr. 2023;68(2):80–134.
5. Bromet E, Andrade LH, Hwang I, et al. Cross-national epidemiology of DSM-IV major depressive episode. BMC Med. 2011;9:90.
6. Kessler RC, Bromet EJ. The epidemiology of depression across cultures. Annu Rev Public Health. 2013;34:119–38.
7. American Psychiatric Association. Practice guideline for the treatment of patients with major depressive disorder. 4th ed. Washington, DC: APA Publishing; 2023.
8. Lam RW, Kennedy SH, Parikh SV, et al. Canadian network for mood and anxiety treatments (CANMAT) guidelines. J Affect Disord. 2023;336:12–27.
9. European Psychiatric Association. EPA guidance on treatment of depression. Eur Psychiatry. 2022;65(1):e39.
10. Korean Medication Algorithm Project for Depressive Disorder (KMAP-DD 2025). Seoul: Korean Society for Affective Disorders; 2025.
11. Kellner CH, Obbels J, Sienaert P. When to consider electroconvulsive therapy (ECT). Acta Psychiatr Scand. 2020;141(4):304–15.
12. UK ECT Review Group. Efficacy and safety of electroconvulsive therapy in depressive disorders: a systematic review and meta-analysis. Lancet. 2003;361(9360):799–808.
13. Heijnen WT, Birkenhäger TK, Wierdsma AI, van den Broek WW. Antidepressant pharmacotherapy failure and response to subsequent electroconvulsive therapy. J Clin Psychopharmacol. 2010;30(5):616–9.

14. Kellner CH, Greenberg RM, Murrough JW, et al. Electroconvulsive therapy in treatment-resistant depression. Am J Psychiatry. 2012;169(12):1238–44.
15. Andrade C. Maintenance ECT for treatment-resistant depression: clinical considerations. J Clin Psychiatry. 2014;75(10):e1223–6.
16. O'Connor DW, Knapp R, Husain MM, et al. The efficacy and safety of right unilateral ECT. Br J Psychiatry. 2010;196(3):226–34.
17. Bahji A, Hawken ER, Sepehry AA, et al. ECT beyond unipolar major depression: systematic review and meta-analysis. J ECT. 2019;35(1):4–15.
18. Milev RV, Giacobbe P, Kennedy SH, et al. CANMAT 2016 guidelines: ECT and neurostimulation treatments. Can J Psychiatr. 2016;61(9):561–75.
19. Fink M. What was learned: studies by the Consortium for Research in ECT (CORE). Acta Psychiatr Scand. 2014;129(6):417–26.
20. Semkovska M, McLoughlin DM. Objective cognitive performance associated with ECT: meta-analysis. Br J Psychiatry. 2010;197(3):197–208.
21. Lefaucheur JP, Aleman A, Baeken C, et al. Evidence-based guidelines on the therapeutic use of rTMS. Clin Neurophysiol. 2020;131(2):474–528.
22. Blumberger DM, Vila-Rodriguez F, Thorpe KE, et al. Effectiveness of theta burst vs high-frequency rTMS in depression. JAMA Psychiatry. 2018;75(11):1192–200.
23. Mutz J, Vipulananthan V, Carter B, et al. Comparative efficacy and acceptability of non-surgical brain stimulation for depression: network meta-analysis. BMJ. 2019;364:l1079.
24. Berlim MT, van den Eynde F, Daskalakis ZJ. High-frequency rTMS for major depression: meta-analysis. Psychol Med. 2013;43(11):2245–54.
25. George MS, Post RM. Daily left prefrontal rTMS for acute treatment of depression. CNS Spectr. 2011;16(5):56–62.
26. Fitzgerald PB, Hoy KE, Elliot D, et al. Accelerated rTMS for depression: randomized controlled trial. Am J Psychiatry. 2018;175(5):427–33.
27. Trevizol AP, Downar J, Vila-Rodriguez F, et al. Efficacy of accelerated intermittent theta burst stimulation in TRD. J Affect Disord. 2020;278:542–8.
28. Berlim MT, McGirr A, Rodrigues Dos Santos N, et al. Efficacy of bilateral rTMS in depression: meta-analysis. Psychol Med. 2014;44(12):2255–66.
29. Health Canada. Non-invasive brain stimulation in depression: evidence and recommendations. Ottawa; 2021.
30. Kito S, Hasegawa T, Koga Y. rTMS as a therapeutic tool for MDD. Curr Psychiatry Rep. 2020;22(8):41.
31. Nitsche MA, Paulus W. Excitability changes induced in the human motor cortex by weak tDCS. J Physiol. 2000;527(3):633–9.
32. Brunoni AR, Moffa AH, Fregni F, et al. tDCS for acute major depressive episodes: meta-analysis. Br J Psychiatry. 2016;208(6):522–31.
33. Mutz J, Edgcumbe DR, Brunoni AR, Fu CH. Efficacy and acceptability of non-invasive brain stimulation for depression: updated systematic review and meta-analysis. JAMA Psychiatry. 2022;79(5):424–34.
34. Palm U, Hasan A, Strube W, Padberg F. tDCS for depression: state of the art 2022. Brain Stimul. 2022;15(4):918–26.
35. Razza LB, Palumbo P, Moffa AH, et al. tDCS for depression: individual patient data meta-analysis. Br J Psychiatry. 2020;216(4):186–91.
36. Valiengo L, Goerigk S, Gordon PC, et al. Efficacy of home-based tDCS for depression. J Affect Disord. 2022;303:289–97.
37. Brunoni AR, Boggio PS, De Raedt R, et al. Clinical research with tDCS in major depression: challenges and future directions. Brain Stimul. 2012;5(3):175–95.
38. Nemeroff CB, Mayberg HS, Krahl SE, et al. Vagus nerve stimulation for treatment-resistant depression: randomized controlled trial. Neuropsychopharmacology. 2006;31(11):2325–35.
39. Rush AJ, Marangell LB, Sackeim HA, et al. VNS for treatment-resistant depression: outcomes in a naturalistic study. Biol Psychiatry. 2005;58(5):347–54.
40. Aaronson ST, Sears P, Ruvuna F, et al. Five-year observational outcomes with VNS vs treatment as usual in TRD. Am J Psychiatry. 2017;174(7):640–8.
41. Conway CR, Xiong W, Rosenthal SZ, et al. Long-term VNS outcomes in depression. Brain Stimul. 2018;11(3):600–8.
42. Berry SM, Broglio K, Bunker M, et al. VNS for depression: updated evidence. CNS Drugs. 2013;27(4):287–98.
43. Müller H, Moeller S, Neumaier B, et al. Clinical guidelines for invasive neuromodulation in TRD. World J Biol Psychiatry. 2020;21(6):424–49.
44. Golden RN, Gaynes BN, Ekstrom RD, et al. Bright light therapy for nonseasonal depression: meta-analysis. Am J Psychiatry. 2005;162(4):656–62.
45. Lam RW, Levitt AJ, Levitan RD, et al. Efficacy of BLT in seasonal affective disorder. Am J Psychiatry. 2006;163(4):805–12.
46. Wirz-Justice A, Benedetti F, Terman M. Chronotherapeutics for affective disorders: a clinician's manual for light and wake therapy. 2nd ed. Basel: Karger; 2013.
47. Al-Karawi D, Jubair L. BLT in nonseasonal depression: updated meta-analysis. J Affect Disord. 2016;198:64–71.
48. Geoffroy PA, Schroder CM, Bourgin P. Chronobiology and depression: therapeutic perspectives. Dialogues Clin Neurosci. 2019;21(1):63–72.
49. Zhou X, Teng T, Zhang Y, et al. Comparative efficacy of psychotherapies, BLT, and exercise for depression: network meta-analysis. Psychol Med. 2019;49(6):773–83.
50. Terman M, Terman JS. Light therapy for mood disorders: safety considerations. CNS Spectr. 2005;10(8):647–63.
51. Schuch FB, Vancampfort D, Firth J, et al. Physical activity and incident depression: meta-

analysis of prospective cohorts. Am J Psychiatry. 2018;175(7):631–48.
52. Kandola A, Ashdown-Franks G, Hendrikse J, et al. Physical activity in MDD: meta-analysis. J Affect Disord. 2020;274:85–96.
53. Cooney GM, Dwan K, Greig CA, et al. Exercise for depression. Cochrane Database Syst Rev. 2013;(9):CD004366.
54. Stubbs B, Vancampfort D, Rosenbaum S, et al. An evidence synthesis of exercise as treatment for depression. Curr Psychiatry Rep. 2016;18(6):45.
55. Morres ID, Hatzigeorgiadis A, Stathi A, et al. Aerobic exercise for major depressive disorder: RCT evidence. Depress Anxiety. 2019;36(1):39–53.
56. Sarris J, Logan AC, Akbaraly TN, et al. Nutritional medicine in psychiatric practice: a consensus position. Lancet Psychiatry. 2015;2(3):271–4.
57. Mocking RJT, Harmsen I, Assies J, et al. Omega-3 fatty acids in depression: meta-analysis and meta-regression. Transl Psychiatry. 2016;6(3):e756.
58. Grosso G, Pajak A, Marventano S, et al. Omega-3 PUFAs and depression: systematic review and meta-analysis. Crit Rev Food Sci Nutr. 2014;54(4):443–50.
59. Mischoulon D, Freeman MP. Omega-3 fatty acids in psychiatry: a review. Psychiatr Clin North Am. 2013;36(1):15–23.
60. Taylor MJ, Carney SM, Goodwin GM, Geddes JR. Folate for depressive disorders: systematic review & meta-analysis. J Psychopharmacol. 2004;18(2):251–6.
61. Freeman MP, Rapaport MH. Omega-3 fatty acids and depression: clinical update. Curr Opin Psychiatry. 2011;24(1):12–7.
62. Papakostas GI, Mischoulon D, Shyu I, et al. S-adenosyl-L-methionine (SAMe) augmentation and monotherapy for MDD: randomized controlled trials. Am J Psychiatry. 2010;167(8):942–8.
63. Sharma A, Gerbarg PL, Bottiglieri T, et al. SAMe for depression: review of antidepressant efficacy. J Clin Psychiatry. 2017;78(6):e656–71.
64. Coppen A, Bailey J. Enhancement of the antidepressant action of fluoxetine by folic acid. Lancet. 2000;356(9237):79–85.
65. Papakostas GI, Shelton RC, Zajecka JM, et al. L-methylfolate as adjunctive therapy for SSRI-resistant MDD: randomized double-blind trial. Am J Psychiatry. 2012;169(12):1267–74.
66. Spedding S. Vitamin D and depression: systematic review and meta-analysis. Br J Psychiatry. 2014;205(2):100–7.
67. Shaffer JA, Edmondson D, Wasson LT, et al. Vitamin D supplementation for depression: meta-analysis of randomized controlled trials. Psychosom Med. 2014;76(3):190–6.

Part IV

Miscellaneous

17 Suicide and Depression

Tae Hui Kim and Beomwoo Nam

17.1 Global Epidemiology of Suicide

In 2021, more than 720,000 people worldwide died by suicide, accounting for approximately 1.1% of all deaths [1]. Suicide ranked as the third leading cause of death among individuals aged 15–29 years, and approximately 73% of all suicides occurred in low- and middle-income countries [1]. Among older adults aged 65 years and above, the suicide mortality rate was 15.99 per 100,000, higher than in other age groups. The rate was markedly higher in men, and firearm-related suicide deaths in older adults were nearly twice as frequent as those observed in all age groups combined [2]. From 2000 to 2019, the global age-standardized suicide mortality rate decreased by about 23%, from 12.97 to 9.93 per 100,000 population. In Europe, the reduction was even greater, declining from 16.26 to 10.22, a decrease of 37% [3] These global patterns vary across countries. In the United States, more than 49,000 suicide deaths were recorded in 2023, the highest number on record, with about 55% involving firearms [4]. In South Korea, the suicide rate reached 27.3 in 2023, an increase from the previous year, and continued to rise in 2024 [5]. Within the Organisation for Economic Co-operation and Development (OECD), the average suicide rate in 2020 was 11.0, while South Korea reported 24.1, the highest among member states [6].

Since the establishment of the Korea Psychological Autopsy Center in 2015, South Korea has strengthened its national suicide prevention infrastructure with the launch of the Korea Foundation for Suicide Prevention (KFSP) in 2021 [7]. The KFSP coordinates national policies and implements annual initiatives to reinforce prevention and mental health promotion. Nevertheless, the national suicide rate remains more than twice the OECD average. At the global level, the International Association for Suicide Prevention (IASP) [8], founded in 1960, works in close collaboration with the World Health Organization (WHO) to guide global suicide prevention strategies, and South Korea's policies broadly reflect the WHO recommendations and align with the IASP priorities.

17.2 Suicide Risk in Major Depressive Disorder and Bipolar Disorder

Suicide risk is closely associated with mental disorders, and a large proportion of suicide deaths involve psychiatric disorders, most com-

T. H. Kim (✉)
Department of Psychiatry, Yonsei University Wonju College of Medicine, Wonju, Republic of Korea

Department of Psychiatry, Yonsei University Wonju Severance Christian Hospital, Wonju, Republic of Korea
e-mail: gooddr@yonsei.ac.kr

B. Nam
Nam Psychiatric Clinic, Chungju, Republic of Korea

W.-M. Bahk et al. (eds.), *Depressive Disorder*, https://doi.org/10.1007/978-981-92-1331-3_17

monly mood disorders [9]. Recent evidence suggests that increased use of digital media and reduced sleep duration may be associated with the rising prevalence of mood disorders and suicidality [10].

Recent meta-analyses demonstrate that the risk of suicide mortality is similarly elevated in major depressive disorder (MDD) and bipolar disorder (BD), at approximately 8.6–8.7 times higher than in the general population [11]. Suicide risk is highest in the early phase after diagnosis and rises markedly during the first year of hospitalization or the initial months following discharge, emphasizing the necessity of close monitoring during these critical phases. Across depressive disorder, consistent predictors of suicide behavior include the severity of hopelessness, prior suicidal ideation (SI) or attempts, severe depressive symptoms, psychotic features, delayed remission, and sleep disturbance [12]. These factors represent shared targets for suicide prevention across mood disorders, while important disorder-specific patterns also exist (Table 17.1).

Table 17.1 Comparison of suicide risk characteristics in major depressive disorder (MDD) and bipolar disorder (BD)

Domain	MDD	BD
High-risk clinical phases	Time-anchored risk: early post-diagnosis; first year after diagnosis or post-hospitalization	State-dependent risk: depressive and mixed episodes across the illness course
Core shared predictors	Hopelessness, prior SI/SA, severe depression, psychotic symptoms, sleep disturbance	Hopelessness, prior SI/SA, depressive polarity, mixed features, impulsivity
Disorder-specific high-risk features	Depressive mixed state; anxious depression	Mixed episodes; polarity of first episode
Lifetime suicide attempt rate	Approximately 30%	30–50%
Conceptual framework	Subtype-and symptoms-oriented risk	Progressive accumulation of depressive and mixed episodes

MDD is strongly associated with suicide, with up to 87% of suicide decedents carrying this diagnosis [13]. Among individuals with MDD, suicidal ideation (SI) occurs in 37.7%, suicide attempts (SA) in 31%, and suicide planning (SP) in 15.1% [14, 15]. Compared with borderline personality disorder, substance use disorder, and delusional disorder, patients with MDD show 2.9 times higher risk of SI, 9.5 times higher risk of SP, and 3.5 times higher risk of SA, while suicide mortality rates are broadly comparable across diagnosis [16]. Recent large-scale research found that approximately 1.4% of patients with MDD exhibit suicidal behavior. This figure reflects a realistic estimate by including data from diverse healthcare settings. These findings confirm suicidal behavior as a prognostic marker associated with excess mortality, healthcare utilization, and socioeconomic burden over time. It was observed that the period between MDD diagnosis and suicide death averaged 4.5 years, and a significant number of deaths occurred in the first year after diagnosis. This underscores the urgent need for systematic management and tailored interventions to reduce suicide risk in this high-risk group [17]. Beyond classical depressive presentations, specific MDD subtypes are closely associated with suicide risk. Depressive mixed states (DMX), characterized by depressive episodes with subthreshold manic or hypomanic symptoms, and anxious depression (AD), defined by prominent anxiety during depressive episodes, both independently predict suicidal behavior. Patients exhibiting co-occurring DMX and AD represent the highest-risk group, highlighting the need for early identification, vigilant monitoring, and intensive treatment strategies [18]. In *Diagnostic and Statistical Manual of Mental Disorders*, Fifth Edition (DSM-5), AD corresponds largely to the "with anxious distress" specifier, while DMX resemble the "with mixed features" specifier. However, DSM-5 criteria may underdetect subthreshold mixed presentations that still carry elevated suicide risk [18].

BD is also strongly linked to suicide. Suicidal behavior occurs predominantly during depressive and mixed episodes, with the elevated risk in mixed states largely attributable to their depressive features rather than to mixed polarity itself [19]. By contrast, suicidal behavior is comparatively uncommon during euphoric mania, hypomania, or euthymic periods. Overall, patients with BD have about a 30 times higher risk of SA than the general population [20], with 30–50% reporting a lifetime history of SA and 15–20% eventually die by suicide [21]. The combination of a BD diagnosis and a prior history of SA is regarded as one of the strongest predictors of suicide [22].

The polarity of the first episode also influences long-term suicide risk. Patients presenting with an initial mixed episode show the highest rates of suicide attempts over 40%, followed by those with an initial depressive episode around 30%, while those with an initial manic episode exhibit comparatively lower risk [23]. Findings from the FondaMental Advanced Center of Expertise-Bipolar Disorders (FACE-BD) cohort support conceptualizing suicidality in BD as a staged process, progressing from ideation to planning and attempts, with depressive and mixed episodes acting as critical drivers at each stage. This staging approach underscores the need for phase-specific preventive strategies and vigilant monitoring throughout the course of illness [24]. A recent systematic review and meta-analysis further demonstrated that bipolar II disorder (BD-II) patients carry suicide completion rates comparable to those with bipolar I disorder (BD-I), challenging the traditional view of BD-II as a "milder" form and underscoring its clinical severity [25]. Despite current suicide prevention guidelines being primarily focused on BD-I, the comparable mortality risk in BD-II highlights the urgent need for systematic and tailored treatment recommendations for this population [26].

17.3 The Complexity of Suicide Risk Prediction and Prevention

Suicide risk is associated not only with mental disorders but also with a wide range of social, economic, and cultural contexts, including unemployment, bankruptcy, indebtedness, medical illness, family and interpersonal conflict, and cultural factors [27, 28]. To date, no established biological marker has been identified that can reliably predict suicidal behavior. However, recent studies employing precision medicine approaches have reported that blood-based gene expression biomarkers can predict suicidality states and subsequent psychiatric hospitalizations, suggesting new possibilities for biological prediction [29]. Nevertheless, genetic predisposition appears to be polygenic, partially diagnosis-specific, and varies according to subphenotypes as well as between single and repeated suicide attempts [30, 31]. This complexity renders suicide risk prediction inherently difficult, indicating that while risk factors may be useful for identifying high-risk groups, they have limited value in accurately predicting imminent suicide at the individual level [28, 32].

The development of quantitative prediction models to complement clinical decision-making has progressed rapidly in recent years. For example, machine learning models based on electronic health records (EHR) have predicted suicide attempts or deaths within 90 days with higher accuracy than traditional clinical screening [33]. In addition, models analyzing voice signals using machine learning have demonstrated the potential of voice as a non-invasive biomarker for suicidal behavior [34]. Plasma folate and homocysteine levels have also been reported to show age-specific patterns associated with suicide risk, suggesting their potential utility in risk assessment [35]. The Oxford Mental Illness and Suicide Tool (OxMIS) and the Oxford Suicide Attempt Tool (OxSATS), developed in the United Kingdom and trained on Swedish national registry and clinical data, are structured prediction tools that generate probabilistic estimates of suicide mortality and attempts. Although evidence has suggested their feasibility in clinical practice, further research is needed to establish their robustness and applicability [36–38]. Moreover, recent advances in technology have introduced approaches using large language models to automatically extract suicide-related social determinants of health from unstructured text data, indicating new possibilities for risk assessment [39].

Suicide risk assessment inevitably entails uncertainty in prediction, yet it remains the critical entry point for clinical intervention and the bridge between evaluation and prevention [40]. Because suicide is shaped by overlapping biological, psychological, and social determinants, it cannot be prevented through a single factor or a single strategy [41]. Effective prevention, therefore, requires a multilevel, evidence-based combination of strategies, integrating advances in digital and biological approaches with the clinician's qualitative judgment. Ultimately, such integrative efforts hold promises for enhancing the real-world effectiveness of suicide prevention and for bridging the gap between clinical practice and public health.

17.4 Concept and Clinical Implication of Suicidality

Suicidality refers to the overall risk or potential for suicide. It is conceptually distinct from completed suicide but is regarded as a clinically significant warning signal [16, 42]. Epidemiological data further illustrates its prevalence. For example, a European population-based study reported a point prevalence of 3.6%, a 12-month prevalence of 2.9%, and a lifetime prevalence of 5.55%; notably, approximately 21% of individuals reported having wished to be dead at some point during their lifetime [43]. Among adolescents and young people, considerably higher rates have been observed, with SI ranging from 14% to 23%, SP from 4% to 24%, and SA from 5% to 16%, underscoring important age-related differences [44].

Evidence indicates that SI, SP, and SA are not aligned with a simple linear continuum. Some individuals attempt suicide without prior planning, while the severity of SI does not necessarily predict subsequent behavior. This discrepancy between ideation and action has been consistently demonstrated across clinical settings. For instance, only 22% of patients who eventually died by suicide reported suicidal ideation at their last outpatient visit [45], and an analysis of data from more than 300,000 individuals demonstrated that the relationship between suicidal intent and actual suicide events cannot be explained by a simple linear prediction [46]. Likewise, among 76 inpatients who died by suicide, 78% had denied SI prior to the act, and a "no-suicide contract" was not protective [47]. Nevertheless, individuals with SI, SP, or SA consistently demonstrate a markedly higher risk of future suicide compared with those without such experiences, highlighting the clinical importance of evaluating trajectories [16, 42].

In contrast to these non-linear patterns, large-scale cohort data suggest that suicidality can also be conceptualized dimensionally through staging. The FACE-BD cohort study classified patients into four stages: no suicidality, SI only, single attempt (non-violent/non-serious vs. violent/serious), and repeated attempts [24]. Each stage was characterized by distinct clinical correlations and risk factors. For instance, repeated attempts had longer illness duration, higher rates of alcohol use disorder, and depressive episodes, while serious single attempts were strongly associated with childhood trauma and alcohol misuse. Importantly, the staging framework showed significant predictive validity, with higher stages strongly associated with suicide attempts during one-year follow-up. These findings suggest that while suicidality is heterogeneous and often discontinuous, a staging approach can offer a clinically useful framework for risk stratification and intervention planning in certain subgroups.

Beyond staging, another critical issue is its relationship with psychiatric diagnoses. Although suicidality is strongly associated with mood and other psychiatric disorders, approximately 10–37% of individuals with suicidality do not meet diagnostic criteria for any psychiatric condition [42, 48]. Moreover, suicidality may arise even among well-treated patients or within the general population, and no pharmacological intervention has been shown to eliminate suicidality per se. These observations argue that suicidality should be considered not only as a symptom within psychiatric disorders but also as a potential independent diagnostic and therapeutic target.

Assessment and intervention for suicidality are directly linked to preventive outcomes. School-based awareness programs have reduced SI and SA among adolescents, while antidepressant treatment in late life has been associated with reductions in SA and suicide mortality [16, 41]. Taken together, these findings underscore that systematic assessment of suicidality is essential, serving as the foundation for timely and effective preventive strategies.

17.5 Clinical Assessment of Suicidality

Clinical assessment aims to rapidly identify the patient's current state and short-term risk, and it also represents a critical moment for establishing trust between patient and clinician that may lead to therapeutic engagement. Suicide risk can be classified into acute high-risk, chronic high-risk, moderate urgent-risk, and low-risk groups. Acute high-risk patients are those with a high likelihood of attempting suicide within hours to several months, requiring immediate and proactive intervention. Chronic high-risk patients, by contrast, remain vulnerable over years and therefore need long-term management and treatment. In patients with depressive disorders, suicide risk often fluctuates between acute and chronic states depending on the course of illness and environmental factors, highlighting the necessity of repeated assessments in the same individual [49].

While a history of SA or family history offers important clues for long-term vulnerability, evaluation of the patient's current symptoms and subjective distress is crucial in determining immediate risk [50]. Anxiety, insomnia, hopelessness, anhedonia, and impulsivity are closely associated with suicide risk. Clinicians should work with patients to identify their most distressing "target symptoms" and assess their intensity and tolerability, as perceiving suicide as the "only escape" may occur regardless of the explicit presence of suicidal ideation [49, 50].

Clinical assessment of suicidality must be able to detect risk even when patients do not explicitly report suicidal ideation. In this context, the recently proposed Narrative Crisis Model of Suicide (NCM) provides a multi-stage dynamic framework that integrates long-term vulnerability factors with short-term crisis variables [51]. Whereas many traditional models have treated the expression of SI as a pivotal transition point, the NCM is clinically valuable in that it explains suicidal crises regardless of whether SI is overtly reported.

The central concepts of this model are the individual's suicidal narrative and the suicide crisis syndrome (SCS). The suicidal narrative refers to the progressive development of distorted self-perceptions such as "I am worthless, isolated, and a burden to others." As this narrative intensifies, hopelessness and suicide risk escalate, eventually culminating in the acute psychological state of SCS. SCS is characterized by profound psychological pain, a sense of entrapment with no escape, and extreme urgency, and it is regarded as a clinical marker of imminent risk even when suicidal ideation is not explicitly reported [52].

The model also identifies trait vulnerabilities and stressors as key background factors that precipitate crisis states. Vulnerabilities such as childhood trauma, impulsivity, and chronic hopelessness do not predict suicide in isolation but increase risk through interaction with current psychological states. Stressful events, including job loss or interpersonal difficulties, may further amplify this risk depending on the individual's subjective interpretation and attribution of meaning [51].

Therefore, the NCM conceptualizes suicide risk not as a fixed trait but as the interaction of four stages: vulnerabilities, stressors, suicidal narrative, and acute crisis. This perspective emphasizes that suicide risk assessment must go beyond the mere reporting of suicidal ideation, highlighting the importance of detecting underlying psychological narratives and acute warning signs as the core of preventive intervention.

17.6 Systematic Assessment of Suicidality

Clinical assessment of suicidality focuses on detecting both acute and chronic risk, but more systematic and reproducible evaluation requires the use of structured interviews, standardized scales, and biological markers. Such approaches complement assessments that rely solely on clinical intuition and contribute to long-term monitoring as well as research applications.

Clinical Interview-Based Assessment

Systematic suicide risk assessment should be based on structured clinical interviews that evaluate risk across multiple domains, regardless of whether patients explicitly report suicidal ideation [49].

First, suicide risk assessment should integrate sociodemographic context, developmental history, medical comorbidity, recent life stressors, and the circumstances leading to clinical contact, as these factors may function as either risk or protective variables. Particular attention should be paid to high-risk exposure such as domestic violence, substance misuse, childhood abuse or neglect, bullying experiences, and sexual minority status. Recent major life changes and overall health status, including relevant medical history, should also be considered as part of a comprehensive assessment.

Second, the history of identified problems and symptoms is central to suicide risk assessment and builds upon the sociodemographic context. This encompasses the patient's main symptoms and difficulties, the presence or absence of psychiatric diagnoses, the age of onset and course of illness, the persistence or episodic nature of symptoms, and factors that exacerbate or relieve them. Equally important is the functional impact of these symptoms and the patient's own explanatory model of distress. Treatment history, including prior interventions, adherence, response, and hospitalization outcomes, further informs illness insight, coping capacity, and current vulnerability.

Third, the assessment of current suicidality should address suicidal thoughts, intent, specific planning and rehearsal, feasibility, lethality, temporal proximity, impulsivity, aggression, and hopelessness, as these dimensions determine the likelihood that suicidal thoughts may transition into action.

Fourth, a careful evaluation of suicide history is required, including the number, methods, lethality, and circumstances of past attempts, as well as post-attempt medical, psychological, and interpersonal consequences.

Fifth, the history of suicide among family members or close friends is another critical consideration, as exposure to attempts or deaths in one's social network significantly increases individual vulnerability.

Sixth, social, environmental, psychiatric, and personal risk factors should be evaluated in an integrated manner, as their interaction can give rise to maladaptive suicidal narratives and precipitate acute crises. Social risks include instability in family structure, loss of significant relationships, persistent interpersonal conflict, and social isolation. Environmental risks encompass limited access to health and mental healthcare, housing instability, unemployment, legal difficulties, and easy access to lethal means. Personal vulnerabilities, including maladaptive coping styles, difficulties in problem-solving, low self-esteem, hopelessness, impulsivity, and aggression, may further amplify suicide risk, particularly during periods of acute stress or clinical deterioration.

Seventh, protective factors serve to buffer against these risks. Strong family and social support networks, stable and trusting relationships, religious or spiritual beliefs, effective coping strategies, engagement with treatment, and a sense of purpose or meaning in life all act to reduce suicide risk and should be systematically explored in clinical assessment.

Suicide Risk Assessment Instruments

Instruments for the assessment of suicide risk and suicidality can supplement clinical evaluation [53]. Nevertheless, no single instrument demonstrates sufficient sensitivity or specificity for predicting suicide outcomes [54]. Therefore, suicide risk assessment tools should not replace a thorough clinical assessment, and none have been specifically validated for bipolar disorder [55]. An overview of commonly used instruments, organized by assessment format and primary clinical purpose, is provided in Table 17.2.

For adults, interview-based instruments used to assess and stratify the risk of suicide attempts or deaths include the Scale for Suicide Ideation (SSI), the Scale for Suicide Ideation–Worst (SSI-W), the Suicide Intent Scale (SIS), the Risk–Rescue Rating (RRR), the SAD PERSONS scale, the Columbia–Suicide Severity Rating Scale (C-SSRS), and the Ask Suicide-Screening Questions (ASQ). Suggested clinical cutoffs are generally greater than or equal to 3 for the SSI, greater than or equal to 2 for the SSI-W, and 19 or above for an elevated SIS risk category. These thresholds have low positive predictive value ranging from 1.4% to 9.7%) but high negative predictive value over 95% for suicide death. The SAD PERSONS scale uses a simple mnemonic to represent ten major suicide risk factors with each letter standing for Sex (male), Age (less than 19 or greater than 45), Depression, Previous suicide attempt, Excess alcohol or substance use, Rational thinking loss, Separated divorced or widowed, Organized suicide plan, No social support, and Sickness which refers to poor physical health. Although its sensitivity and specificity are low, especially in psychiatric populations, it helps clinicians quickly assess initial risk but should be used with caution as a standalone tool [56]. The C-SSRS is an internationally standardized tool for quantifying the severity of suicidal thoughts and behaviors, widely used in clinical and research settings, and is currently one of the most widely used instruments worldwide [57]. The ASQ, developed by the National Institute of Mental Health (NIMH), is a brief four-item screening tool that can be administered in less than 20 s in emergency departments or primary care settings, with versions used across age groups, including adolescents [58].

Self-report instruments include the Adult Suicidal Ideation Questionnaire (ASIQ), the Beck Hopelessness Scale (BHS), the Suicide Probability Scale (SPS), the Psychache Scale (PS), the Columbia Suicide Screen (CSS), and the Reasons for Living Inventory (RFL). Depression rating scales also contain items related to suicide risk, such as the Hamilton Rating Scale for Depression (HAM-D, interview-based), the Beck Depression Inventory (BDI), and the Center for Epidemiological Studies Depression Scale (CES-D), which include four suicide-related items [56].

For older adults, interview-based scales are limited, but a SIS total score ≥19 in individuals aged 55 years and older demonstrated a sensitivity of 90%, specificity of 60.3%, and positive predictive value of 22.5% for suicide mortality [59]. The Geriatric Suicide Ideation Scale (GSIS) is a multidimensional self-report instrument specifically developed for older adults, assessing suicid-

Table 17.2 Overview of suicide risk assessment instruments

Assessment format	Primary clinical purpose	Representative instruments
Interview-based	Acute risk screening	Ask Suicide-Screening Questions (ASQ); Columbia–Suicide Severity Rating Scale (C-SSRS, screening version); SAD PERSONS scale
	Severity and intent assessment	Scale for Suicide Ideation (SSI); Scale for Suicide Ideation–Worst (SSI-W); Suicide Intent Scale (SIS); Risk–Rescue Rating (RRR)
	Longitudinal assessment	Columbia–Suicide Severity Rating Scale (C-SSRS, full version)
Self-report	Suicidal ideation and cognitive risk factors	Beck Hopelessness Scale (BHS); Adult Suicidal Ideation Questionnaire (ASIQ); Suicide Probability Scale (SPS); Psychache Scale (PS)
	Protective factors	Reasons for Living Inventory (RFL)
	Age-specific assessment	Geriatric Suicide Ideation Scale (GSIS) Suicidal Ideation Questionnaire (SIQ)
	Repeated monitoring	Computerized Adaptive Test for Suicide Risk (CAT-SS)

ality, hopelessness, and loss of life purpose, with confirmed reliability and validity [60].

For children and adolescents, interview-based instruments include the Diagnostic Interview for Children and Adolescents (DICA), the Interview Schedule for Children and Adolescents (ISCA), and the Schedule for Affective Disorders and Schizophrenia, School-Age Epidemiologic Version (K-SADS-E), while self-report instruments include the Suicidal Ideation Questionnaire (SIQ) [56].

More recently, the Computerized Adaptive Test for Suicide Risk (CAT-SS), based on item response theory (IRT), has been introduced as a transdiagnostic and age-spanning self-report instrument applicable across adolescent and adult populations. It minimizes the number of items while maintaining measurement precision, can be completed in about 2 min, and demonstrates strong predictive validity in clinical populations [61].

Biological Assessment

Ongoing research continues to explore blood-based, genetic, and proteomic biomarkers for suicide risk. Classical findings have suggested several biological alterations in suicide decedents, including increased subtypes of serotonin receptors, reduced serotonin metabolites (e.g., 5-hydroxyindoleacetic acid), elevated platelet 5-HT_2A receptors, abnormal results in the dexamethasone suppression test (DST), decreased serum brain-derived neurotrophic factor (BDNF) as an indicator of hypothalamic–pituitary–adrenal (HPA) axis dysfunction, and abnormalities in receptor-linked signaling mechanisms such as phosphoinositide and adenylyl cyclase [62]. Despite these observations, no single biological marker has demonstrated sufficient accuracy for clinical prediction or diagnostic use.

In more recent studies, elevated neutrophil-to-lymphocyte ratio (NLR) and monocyte-to-lymphocyte ratio (MLR) have been observed among suicide attempters. Importantly, these measures are not significantly influenced by antidepressant treatment and thus may reflect both short- and long-term vulnerability to suicidality [63, 64]. Similarly, inflammatory and serotonergic markers, including increased plasma thrombospondin-2 and C-reactive protein (CRP) and decreased peripheral serotonin levels, have been associated with recent SI and SA, although their predictive utility remains limited [65].

A large population-based cohort study using the UK Biobank demonstrated that phenotypic age acceleration (PhenoAge) was significantly associated with both SI and SA. Individuals in the highest quartile had 22% increased risk of SA and 13% increased risk of SI, suggesting that suicide risk may be linked not only to psychiatric pathology but also to processes of biological aging [66].

Molecular research has further clarified biological mechanisms related to suicidality. Among patients with MDD, differential gene expression in both brain and blood has been reported between those who died by suicide and those who died by other causes [67]. In BD, a large cohort study identified three candidate proteins (SCGB1A1, ANXA10, and CETN2) that were significantly associated with future suicide attempts, although their standalone predictive power remains limited [68]. Postmortem studies have also identified alterations in proteins related to the endocannabinoid system and cell death pathways in the dorsolateral prefrontal cortex of suicide decedents, including GSTT1 proposed as a potential biomarker [68, 69].

From a neuroimaging perspective, white matter hyperintensities (WMH) have been reported to be more frequent among patients with BD who attempt suicide. However, it remains uncertain whether these findings reflect suicide risk per se or are attributable to the underlying diagnosis and vascular risk factors [55].

Taken together, no single hematological, genetic, or neuroimaging biomarker is currently established as a clinically reliable tool for suicide risk assessment [28]. Nonetheless, multi-modal approaches integrating biological, clinical, and psychological markers may offer a more promising direction for improving the precision of suicide risk prediction in the future.

17.7 Suicide Prevention and Intervention

Integrated Suicide Preventive Strategies: Policy-Level and Digital Interventions

Suicide prevention strategies are commonly divided into three categories: universal, selective, and indicated interventions [70]. Among these, environmental regulatory measures, such as restricting access to toxic substances and securing jumping sites, have shown the strongest preventive effects. Early detection and treatment of psychiatric disorders, particularly depression, and school-based mental health education also contributed to suicide reductions. In contrast, strategies such as primary care screening, gatekeeper training, and telephone- or Internet-based interventions show variable effectiveness, particularly in real-world implementation [41]. These findings highlight the limitations of single interventions and suggest that preventive effects are context-dependent, varying across intervention type and setting [71, 72].

Digital interventions, including safety planning mobile applications, crisis text lines, and automated short message service (SMS), have emerged as adjunctive tool that may reduce suicidal ideation and improve linkage to follow-up care after emergency department visits [73, 74]. While these approaches provide anonymity and accessibility, their effectiveness remains heterogeneous, with challenges related to user engagement, appropriateness, clinical integration, and data protection [72].

Overall, suicide prevention requires an integrated and multilayered approach in which environmental regulation, mental health treatment, school-based education, and digital strategies operate in a complementary ways, supported by cross-sector collaboration and broad societal engagement [70–73].

Pharmacological Treatment for Suicide Risk

Antidepressant treatment plays a central role in the management of suicide risk, yet concerns have long been raised that these medications may themselves increase suicide risk in certain age groups and patient populations. In 2004, U.S. Food and Drug Administration (FDA) issued a black-box warning based on evidence that selective serotonin reuptake inhibitors (SSRIs) and other antidepressants were associated with increased suicidal thoughts and behaviors among children and adolescents [75]. This warning has been repeatedly examined in subsequent clinical studies and meta-analyses, and its relevance has been reaffirmed in a recent analysis of the FDA Adverse Event Reporting System (FAERS, 2017–2023). Findings indicated that suicide risk reports were approximately 7.4 times higher in children (ages 8–17) and 3.5 times higher in young adults (ages 18–24), whereas no statistically significant increase was observed in adults aged 65 years and older [76]. These results suggest that the FDA's original warning remains valid, but primarily for children and young adults.

Differences in suicide risk have also been reported across antidepressants. When compared with fluoxetine as the reference drug, desvenlafaxine and vilazodone were associated with lower reported suicide risk, likely related to their cytochrome P450 3A4 (CYP3A4) metabolic pathways. In contrast, trazodone was linked to an increased risk, while levomilnacipran showed a risk level comparable to fluoxetine [76]. These findings suggest that not only metabolic pathways but also broader pharmacological properties of antidepressants may influence suicide risk.

Lithium has been consistently associated with reduced suicide risk across studies from multiple regions and remains the most well-established pharmacological agent with anti-suicidal properties [77]. It is considered a preventive rather than an acute intervention and carries the potential for lethality in overdose [55]. Its effect is not clearly distinguishable from mood stabilization or reductions in impulsivity and aggression, and recent meta-analyses have reported somewhat smaller preventive effects than previously recognized [78]. Lithium's role is, therefore, centered on long-term prevention rather than acute crisis management. Protective effects have been demonstrated in children and adolescents, whereas no significant differences compared with fluoxetine were observed in young adults or older adults [76]. Other mood stabilizers, such as valproate, carbamazepine, and lamotrigine, also show some degree of anti-suicidal effect, though to a lesser extent than lithium [77].

Ketamine, including its S-enantiomer esketamine, has emerged as a rapid-acting treatment for reducing suicidal ideation. Evidence from randomized and observational studies demonstrates short-term reductions in suicidal ideation, with the most consistent effects observed following intravenous administration [79]. Esketamine exhibits greater affinity for N-methyl-D-aspartate (NMDA) receptors and has been suggested to be more effective for treatment-resistant depression (TRD) [80]. In 2019, the FDA approved intranasal esketamine for the treatment of TRD, allowing for greater convenience compared with intravenous administration and facilitating broader clinical use [81]. However, evidence supporting intranasal esketamine remains limited, particularly regarding durability of effect and relapse prevention. Safety concerns, including dissociation, dizziness, nausea, and somnolence, require careful monitoring, and potential risk related to misuse with long-term repeated administration underscore the need for ongoing evaluation [82, 83].

Among atypical antipsychotics, clozapine is the only agent approved by the FDA for reducing suicide risk, but this indication is limited to patients with schizophrenia [84]. Other agents such as quetiapine, lurasidone, and the olanzapine/fluoxetine combination are used in the treatment of bipolar depression and carry a lower risk of manic switch, yet the evidence supporting their anti-suicidal effects remains limited [55, 77]. Moreover, some atypical antipsychotics can induce akathisia or agitation, which may paradoxically increase suicide risk. Electroconvulsive therapy (ECT) is considered a crucial intervention in emergency situations for patients at high risk of suicide, with studies demonstrating superior anti-suicidal effects compared to pharmacological treatment in both unipolar and bipolar depression [85, 86]. However, its long-term impact on reducing suicide risk in bipolar depression has not been firmly established [42].

Despite their central role in treating depression, pharmacological interventions alone are insufficient for comprehensive suicide risk management, given delayed onset of efficacy, age-dependent risk profiles, and the potential for mood switching [77, 87]. Accordingly, pharmacotherapy should be integrated with evidence-base psychological interventions, such as interpersonal therapy and dialectical behavioral therapy, to effectively reduce suicide ideation and behavior [88, 89].

Management of Patients in Acute Suicidal Crisis

The optimal management for patients in an acute suicidal crisis is psychiatric hospitalization, although admission is often limited by the patient's autonomy and by institutional or legal constraints. As a result, clinicians are frequently required to manage even high-risk patients in outpatient settings.

To bridge this gap, Safety Planning Intervention (SPI) has emerged as a standardized and practical approach. Through collaborative planning between patients and clinicians, SPI identifies warning signs, personal coping strategies, sources of social support, and professional resources, which are organized into a structured plan [90]. In a randomized trial of emergency department patients, SPI combined with brief follow-up phone contacts reduced suicide attempts by 45% and significantly improved treatment engagement [91]. Consistent with these findings, a systematic review demonstrated associations between SPI and reduced suicidal ideation and behavior across diverse clinical settings [92]. Although digital and mobile adaptations have broadened implementation, challenges related to privacy, emotional burden, cultural and linguistic adaptation, and application during periods of acute distress remain [93].

Clinicians should incorporate SPI within a problem-solving framework to collaboratively address seemingly uncontrollable suicidal urges [42]. Clinical management during acute crises should integrate SPI with simultaneous suicide risk assessment and symptom-oriented medical stabilization. Pharmacologic strategies may include antidepressants, mood stabilizers, or antipsychotics, tailored to the patient's comorbid psychiatric conditions. For acute anxiety, insomnia, or alcohol-related crises, sedating atypical antipsychotics, benzodiazepines with lower disinhibition potential, or short-term hypnotics may be considered. However, such interventions primarily serve to stabilize acute symptoms and should be understood as adjunctive rather than definitive strategies for long-term suicide prevention [77].

Equally crucial is the establishment of short-term goals that validate the patient's emotional pain while fostering emotional connectedness and a sense of support. Engaging significant others can be particularly protective for high-risk patients. Clinical intervention should also focus on problem-solving approaches that replace maladaptive coping with constructive alternatives. For adolescents, the stability of family resources must be assessed, whereas in older adults, losses associated with aging and related psychosocial difficulties should be carefully evaluated. Based on these assessments, integration of social support networks and community resources represents a key component of effective suicide crisis management [42].

Declarations

Competing Interests The author(s) has no competing interests to declare that are relevant to the content of this manuscript.

Ethics Approval The author(s) declares that this manuscript does not include primary research with human participants.

The author(s) declares that this manuscript does not include primary studies involving animals.

References

1. World Health Organization. Suicide worldwide in 2021: global health estimates. Geneva: World Health Organization; 2025.
2. Cho H, Kim S, Son Y, Jang W, Kim HJ, Lee H, et al. Method-specific suicide mortality rates among older adults in 47 countries and territories, 1996-2021, with projections to 2050: a global time series and modelling study. Lancet Healthy Longev. 2025;6(7):100719.
3. Rotejanaprasert C, Thanutchapat P, Phoncharoenwirot C, Mekchaiporn O, Chienwichai P, Maude RJ. Global spatiotemporal analysis of suicide epidemiology and risk factor associations from 2000 to 2019 using Bayesian space time hierarchical modeling. Sci Rep. 2025;15(1):12785.
4. Centers for Disease Control and Prevention. Suicide data and statistics [Internet] 2025 [cited 2025 Aug 24]. Available from: https://www.cdc.gov/suicide/facts/data.html.
5. SW RSBSJMKHLJKJK. Changes in suicide rate trend after implementation of suicide prevention policy: an interrupted time series study on the fifth master plan for suicide prevention. J Korean Neuropsychiatr Assoc. 2024;63(4):237–45.
6. Organisation for Economic Co-operation and Development. Society at a Glance 2024: OECD social indicators. Paris: OECD Publishing; 2024.
7. Korea Foundation for Suicide Prevention. Korea Foundation for Suicide Prevention official website. [Internet]. [cited 2025 Aug 30]. Available from: https://www.kfsp.or.kr/web.
8. International Association for Suicide Prevention. International Association for Suicide Prevention official website [cited 2025 Aug 30]. Available from: https://www.iasp.info/.
9. Sutar R, Kumar A, Yadav V. Suicide and prevalence of mental disorders: a systematic review and meta-analysis of world data on case-control psychological autopsy studies. Psychiatry Res. 2023;329:115492.
10. Twenge JM, Cooper AB, Joiner TE, Duffy ME, Binau SG. Age, period, and cohort trends in mood disorder indicators and suicide-related outcomes in a nationally representative dataset, 2005–2017. J Abnorm Psychol. 2019;128(3):185.
11. Arnone D, Karmegam SR, Ostlundh L, Alkhyeli F, Alhammadi L, Alhammadi S, et al. Risk of suicidal behavior in patients with major depression and bipolar disorder – a systematic review and meta-analysis of registry-based studies. Neurosci Biobehav Rev. 2024;159:105594.
12. Riera-Serra P, Navarra-Ventura G, Castro A, Gili M, Salazar-Cedillo A, Ricci-Cabello I, et al. Clinical predictors of suicidal ideation, suicide attempts and suicide death in depressive disorder: a systematic review and meta-analysis. Eur Arch Psychiatry Clin Neurosci. 2024;274(7):1543–63.
13. Nordentoft M, Mortensen PB, Pedersen CB. Absolute risk of suicide after first hospital contact in mental disorder. Arch Gen Psychiatry. 2011;68(10):1058–64.
14. Cai H, Jin Y, Liu S, Zhang Q, Zhang L, Cheung T, et al. Prevalence of suicidal ideation and planning in patients with major depressive disorder: a meta-analysis of observation studies. J Affect Disord. 2021;293:148–58.
15. Dong M, Zeng L-N, Lu L, Li X-H, Ungvari GS, Ng CH, et al. Prevalence of suicide attempt in indi-

viduals with major depressive disorder: a meta-analysis of observational surveys. Psychol Med. 2019;49(10):1691–704.
16. Cai H, Xie X-M, Zhang Q, Cui X, Lin J-X, Sim K, et al. Prevalence of suicidality in major depressive disorder: a systematic review and meta-analysis of comparative studies. Front Psych. 2021;12:690130.
17. Lundberg J, Cars T, Lampa E, Ekholm Selling K, Leval A, Gannedahl A, et al. Determinants and outcomes of suicidal behavior among patients with major depressive disorder. JAMA Psychiatry. 2023;80(12):1218–25.
18. Ota K, Shinzato H, Otsuka N, Zamami Y, Kurihara K, Futenma K, et al. Depressive mixed state and anxious distress as risk factors for suicidal behavior during major depressive episodes. Sci Rep. 2025;15(1):11918.
19. Dome P, Rihmer Z, Gonda X. Suicide Risk in Bipolar Disorder: A Brief Review. Medicina (Kaunas). 2019;55(8):403.
20. Goodwin FK, Jamison KR. Manic-depressive illness: bipolar disorders and recurrent depression. Oxford University Press; 2007.
21. Oliva V, Fico G, De Prisco M, Gonda X, Rosa AR, Vieta E. Bipolar disorders: an update on critical aspects. Lancet Reg Health Eur. 2025;48:101135.
22. Antypa N, Antonioli M, Serretti A. Clinical, psychological and environmental predictors of prospective suicide events in patients with bipolar disorder. J Psychiatr Res. 2013;47(11):1800–8.
23. Eroglu MZ, Karakus G, Tamam L. Bipolar disorder and suicide. Dusunen Adam. 2013;26(2):139.
24. Auxilia AM, Olie E, Dubois J, Capuzzi E, Aubin V, Aouizerate B, et al. staging of suicidality in bipolar disorder: findings from the FACE-Bd cohort (FondaMental Advanced centre of Expertise for Bipolar Disorders). Eur Psychiatry. 2025;68:1–50.
25. Dev DA, Le GH, Kwan ATH, Wong S, Arulmozhi A, Ceban F, et al. Comparing suicide completion rates in bipolar I versus bipolar II disorder: a systematic review and meta-analysis. J Affect Disord. 2024;361:480–8.
26. Berk M, Corrales A, Trisno R, Dodd S, Yatham LN, Vieta E, et al. Bipolar II disorder: a state-of-the-art review. World Psychiatry. 2025;24(2):175–89.
27. Baldessarini RJ, Tondo L, Pinna M, Nuñez N, Vázquez GH. Suicidal risk factors in major affective disorders. Br J Psychiatry. 2019;215(4):621–6.
28. Turecki G, Brent DA, Gunnell D, O'Connor RC, Oquendo MA, Pirkis J, et al. Suicide and suicide risk. Nat Rev Dis Primers. 2019;5(1):74.
29. Bhagar R, Gill SS, Le-Niculescu H, Yin C, Roseberry K, Mullen J, et al. Next-generation precision medicine for suicidality prevention. Transl Psychiatry. 2024;14(1):362.
30. Lee D, Baek JH, Ha K, Cho E-Y, Choi Y, Yang S-Y, et al. Dissecting the genetic architecture of suicide attempt and repeated attempts in Korean patients with bipolar disorder using polygenic risk scores. Int J Bipolar Disord. 2022;10(1):3.
31. Mullins N, Bigdeli TB, Børglum AD, Coleman JR, Demontis D, Mehta D, et al. GWAS of suicide attempt in psychiatric disorders and association with major depression polygenic risk scores. Am J Psychiatry. 2019;176(8):651–60.
32. Franklin JC, Ribeiro JD, Fox KR, Bentley KH, Kleiman EM, Huang X, et al. Risk factors for suicidal thoughts and behaviors: a meta-analysis of 50 years of research. Psychol Bull. 2017;143(2):187.
33. Adams R, Haroz EE, Rebman P, Suttle R, Grosvenor L, Bajaj M, et al. Developing a suicide risk model for use in the Indian Health Service. Npj Ment Health Res. 2024;3(1):47.
34. Krautz AE, Volkening J, Raue J, Otte C, Eickhoff SB, Ahlers E, et al. Prediction of suicide using web based voice recordings analyzed by artificial intelligence. Sci Rep. 2025;15(1):23855.
35. Zhang A, Qin Y, Wang H, Lyu N, Zhao Q, Zhang L, et al. Serum folate and homocysteine as biomarkers for suicide risk in major depressive disorder: insights in males and younger patients. BMC Psychiatry. 2025;25(1):745.
36. Senior M, Burghart M, Yu R, Kormilitzin A, Liu Q, Vaci N, et al. Identifying predictors of suicide in severe mental illness: a feasibility study of a clinical prediction rule (Oxford Mental Illness and Suicide Tool or OxMIS). Front Psych. 2020;11:268.
37. Sariaslan A, Fanshawe T, Pitkanen J, Cipriani A, Martikainen P, Fazel S. Predicting suicide risk in 137,112 people with severe mental illness in Finland: external validation of the Oxford Mental Illness and Suicide tool (OxMIS). Transl Psychiatry. 2023;13(1):126.
38. Torino G, Moltrasio C, Callari A, Delvecchio G. Validity and feasibility of the oxford mental illness suicide tool (OxMIS): a mini-review and meta-analysis. J Affect Disord. 2025;381:321–8.
39. Haebom, Lee HJ, Oh S, Song Y-K, Cavanagh L, Pollard JT. A multi-stage large language model framework for extracting suicide-related social determinants of health. Commun Med (Lond). 2025; https://doi.org/10.1038/s43856-025-01114-z.
40. Hawgood J, De Leo D. Suicide prediction–a shift in paradigm is needed. Hogrefe Publishing; 2016.
41. Zalsman G, Hawton K, Wasserman D, van Heeringen K, Arensman E, Sarchiapone M, et al. Suicide prevention strategies revisited: 10-year systematic review. Lancet Psychiatry. 2016;3(7):646–59.
42. Chiles JA, Roberts LW. Clinical manual for assessment and treatment of suicidal patients. American Psychiatric Pub; 2018.
43. Castillejos MC, Huertas P, Martin P, Moreno KB. Prevalence of suicidality in the European general population: a systematic review and meta-analysis. Arch Suicide Res. 2021;25(4):810–28.
44. Van Meter AR, Knowles EA, Mintz EH. Systematic review and meta-analysis: international prevalence of suicidal ideation and attempt in youth. J Am Acad Child Adolesc Psychiatry. 2023;62(9):973–86.

45. Klonsky ED, Dixon-Luinenburg T, May AM. The critical distinction between suicidal ideation and suicide attempts. World Psychiatry. 2021;20(3):439–41.
46. Xiao Y, Bi K, Yip PS, Cerel J, Brown TT, Peng Y, et al. Decoding suicide decedent profiles and signs of suicidal intent using latent class analysis. JAMA Psychiatry. 2024;81(6):595–605.
47. Busch KA, Fawcett J, Jacobs DG. Clinical correlates of inpatient suicide. J Clin Psychiatry. 2003;64(1):14–9.
48. Oquendo MA, Baca-Garcia E. Suicidal behavior disorder as a diagnostic entity in the DSM-5 classification system: advantages outweigh limitations. World Psychiatry. 2014;13(2):128.
49. Association AP. Practice guideline for the assessment and treatment of patients with suicidal behaviors. Arlington: American Psychiatric Association; 2023.
50. Hendin H. The American Psychiatric Publishing textbook of suicide assessment and management. Am J Psychiatry. 2006;163(2):331.
51. Menon V. The narrative-crisis model of suicide as an emerging framework for suicide risk stratification, management, and prevention. Indian J Psychol Med. 2024;46(4):285–8.
52. Galynker I, Bloch-Elkouby S, Cohen LJ. Suicide crisis syndrome: a specific diagnosis to aid suicide prevention. World Psychiatry. 2024;23(3):362–3.
53. Bernert RA, Hom MA, Roberts LW. A review of multidisciplinary clinical practice guidelines in suicide prevention: toward an emerging standard in suicide risk assessment and management, training and practice. Acad Psychiatry. 2014;38:585–92.
54. Runeson B, Odeberg J, Pettersson A, Edbom T, Jildevik Adamsson I, Waern M. Instruments for the assessment of suicide risk: a systematic review evaluating the certainty of the evidence. PLoS One. 2017;12(7):e0180292.
55. Miller JN, Black DW. Bipolar disorder and suicide: a review. Curr Psychiatry Rep. 2020;22:1–10.
56. Park S-J, Lim A, Park S, Na R, Hong JP. A review on predictive validity of suicide assessment measures. Anxiety Mood. 2013;9(1):10–8.
57. Giddens JM, Sheehan KH, Sheehan DV. The Columbia-suicide severity rating scale (C-SSRS): has the "gold standard" become a liability? Innov Clin Neurosci. 2014;11(9–10):66–80.
58. Horowitz LM, Bridge JA, Teach SJ, Ballard E, Klima J, Rosenstein DL, et al. Ask Suicide-Screening Questions (ASQ): a brief instrument for the pediatric emergency department. Arch Pediatr Adolesc Med. 2012;166(12):1170–6.
59. Niméus A, én M, Träskman-Bendz L. High suicidal intent scores indicate future suicide. Arch Suicide Res. 2002;6(3):211–9.
60. Heisel MJ, Flett GL. Investigating the psychometric properties of the Geriatric Suicide Ideation Scale (GSIS) among community-residing older adults. Aging Ment Health. 2016;20(2):208–21.
61. Gibbons RD, Kupfer D, Frank E, Moore T, Beiser DG, Boudreaux ED. Development of a computerized adaptive test suicide scale-the CAT-SS. J Clin Psychiatry. 2017;78(9):1376–82.
62. Pandey GN. Biological basis of suicide and suicidal behavior. Bipolar Disord. 2013;15(5):524–41.
63. Ninla-Aesong P, Kietdumrongwong P, Neupane SP, Puangsri P, Jongkrijak H, Chotipong P, et al. Relative value of novel systemic immune-inflammatory indices and classical hematological parameters in predicting depression, suicide attempts and treatment response. Sci Rep. 2024;14(1):19018.
64. Velasco A, Lengvenyte A, Rodriguez-Revuelta J, Jimenez-Trevino L, Courtet P, Garcia-Portilla MP, et al. Neutrophil-to-lymphocyte ratio, platelet-to-lymphocyte ratio, and monocyte-to-lymphocyte ratio in depressed patients with suicidal behavior: a systematic review. Eur Psychiatry. 2023;67(1):1–25.
65. Lengvenyte A, Belzeaux R, Olie E, Hamzeh-Cognasse H, Seneque M, Strumila R, et al. Associations of potential plasma biomarkers with suicide attempt history, current suicidal ideation and subsequent suicidal events in patients with depression: a discovery study. Brain Behav Immun. 2023;114:242–54.
66. Hu W, Shen Z, Tian G, Liu B, Jia C. Associations of clinical biomarker-based biological aging with suicide attempts and suicidal ideation: evidence from 124,529 UK Biobank participants. Transl Psychiatry. 2025;15(1):204.
67. Sandberg JV, Hansson C, Göteson A, Joas E, Jakobsson J, Pålsson E, et al. Proteins associated with future suicide attempts in bipolar disorder: a large-scale biomarker discovery study. Mol Psychiatry. 2022;27:1–7.
68. Kim MJ, Do M, Han D, Son M, Shin D, Yeo I, et al. Proteomic profiling of postmortem prefrontal cortex tissue of suicide completers. Transl Psychiatry. 2022;12(1):142.
69. Pinna G. Endocannabinoids and precision medicine for mood disorders and suicide. Front Psych. 2021;12:658433.
70. Pirkis J, Gunnell D, Hawton K, Hetrick S, Niederkrotenthaler T, Sinyor M, et al. A public health, whole-of-government approach to national suicide prevention strategies. Hogrefe Publishing; 2023.
71. Sakashita T, Oyama H. Suicide prevention interventions and their linkages in multilayered approaches for older adults: a review and comparison. Front Public Health. 2022;10:842193.
72. Yosep I, Hikmat R, Mardhiyah A, Hernawaty T. A scoping review of digital-based intervention for reducing risk of suicide among adults. J Multidiscip Healthc. 2024;17:3545–56.
73. Burr SK, Yu M, Clark D, Alonzo D, Gearing RE. Digital interventions for suicide prevention. Crisis. 2025;46(3):176–86.
74. Cullen SW, Olfson M, Xie M, Marcus SC. Impact of emergency department safety planning on 30-day mental health service use. Psychiatr Serv. 2024;75(6):528–33.

75. Friedman RA. Antidepressants' black-box warning—10 years later. N Engl J Med. 2014;371(18):1666–8.
76. Eugene AR. Country-specific psychopharmacological risk of reporting suicidality comparing 38 antidepressants and lithium from the FDA Adverse Event Reporting System, 2017–2023. Front Psych. 2024;15:1442490.
77. Tondo L, Baldessarini RJ. Suicidal behavior in mood disorders: response to pharmacological treatment. Curr Psychiatry Rep. 2016;18:1–11.
78. Nabi Z, Stansfeld J, Plöderl M, Wood L, Moncrieff J. Effects of lithium on suicide and suicidal behaviour: a systematic review and meta-analysis of randomised trials. Epidemiol Psychiatr Sci. 2022;31:e65.
79. Shen Z, Gao D, Lv X, Wang H, Yue W. A meta-analysis of the effects of ketamine on suicidal ideation in depression patients. Transl Psychiatry. 2024;14(1):248.
80. Zeilhofer HU, Swandulla D, Geisslinger G, Brune K. Differential effects of ketamine enantiomers on NMDA receptor currents in cultured neurons. Eur J Pharmacol. 1992;213(1):155–8.
81. Kim J, Farchione T, Potter A, Chen Q, Temple R. Esketamine for treatment-resistant depression – first FDA-approved antidepressant in a new class. N Engl J Med. 2019;381(1):1–4.
82. Wilkinson ST, Ballard ED, Bloch MH, Mathew SJ, Murrough JW, Feder A, et al. The effect of a single dose of intravenous ketamine on suicidal ideation: a systematic review and individual participant data meta-analysis. Am J Psychiatry. 2018;175(2):150–8.
83. Voort JLV, Morgan RJ, Kung S, Rasmussen KG, Rico J, Palmer BA, et al. Continuation phase intravenous ketamine in adults with treatment-resistant depression. J Affect Disord. 2016;206:300–4.
84. Meltzer HY, Alphs L, Green AI, Altamura AC, Anand R, Bertoldi A, et al. Clozapine treatment for suicidality in schizophrenia: International Suicide Prevention Trial (InterSePT). Arch Gen Psychiatry. 2003;60(1):82–91.
85. Association AP. The practice of electroconvulsive therapy: recommendations for treatment, training, and privileging (A task force report of the American Psychiatric Association). American Psychiatric Pub; 2008.
86. Liang CS, Chung CH, Ho PS, Tsai CK, Chien WC. Superior anti-suicidal effects of electroconvulsive therapy in unipolar disorder and bipolar depression. Bipolar Disord. 2018;20(6):539–46.
87. Machado-Vieira R, Baumann J, Wheeler-Castillo C, Latov D, Henter ID, Salvadore G, et al. The timing of antidepressant effects: a comparison of diverse pharmacological and somatic treatments. Pharmaceuticals. 2010;3(1):19–41.
88. Weitz E, Hollon SD, Kerkhof A, Cuijpers P. Do depression treatments reduce suicidal ideation? The effects of CBT, IPT, pharmacotherapy, and placebo on suicidality. J Affect Disord. 2014;167:98–103.
89. DeCou CR, Comtois KA, Landes SJ. Dialectical behavior therapy is effective for the treatment of suicidal behavior: a meta-analysis. Behav Ther. 2019;50(1):60–72.
90. Stanley B, Brown GK. Safety planning intervention: a brief intervention to mitigate suicide risk. Cogn Behav Pract. 2012;19(2):256–64.
91. Stanley B, Brown GK, Brenner LA, Galfalvy HC, Currier GW, Knox KL, et al. Comparison of the safety planning intervention with follow-up vs usual care of suicidal patients treated in the emergency department. JAMA Psychiatry. 2018;75(9):894–900.
92. Ferguson M, Rhodes K, Loughhead M, McIntyre H, Procter N. The effectiveness of the safety planning intervention for adults experiencing suicide-related distress: a systematic review. Arch Suicide Res. 2022;26(3):1022–45.
93. O'Connor E, Rhodes K, Procter N, Loughhead M, Procter A, Reilly J-A, et al. The experiences of consumers, clinicians and support persons involved in the safety planning intervention for suicide prevention: a qualitative systematic review and meta-synthesis. Front Psych. 2024;15:1482924.

18 Effects of Parental Depression on Child Development

Chan-Mo Yang and Hyung-Mo Sung

Major depressive disorder is one of the most common mental illnesses, with a one-year prevalence rate of about 7% in adults. It is most frequently diagnosed before the age of 30, and the prevalence in women is known to be 1.5 to 3 times higher than in men [1]. Approximately 10–16% of women experience major depressive disorder during pregnancy or postpartum [2]. Like general depression, maternal depression not only increases the risk of self-harm through suicidal ideation but depression during pregnancy is also known to increase fetal and childbirth-related complications. Moreover, postpartum depression can negatively affect child-rearing and also have a detrimental impact on the next generation by causing various problems related to childhood development. For these reasons, maternal depression is considered a sufficiently important issue that the World Health Organization (WHO) has prioritized it as one of the most urgent global health problems [3].

The role of the mother in providing the foundational environment for child development is universally recognized as crucial. A healthy nurturing environment provided by a healthy mother is essential for normal and healthy child development. This nurturing process creates a dynamic interaction between mother and child, bringing emotional regulation and stability to each other through mutual feedback like facial expressions and speech. Globally, there is a rapid increase in interest in the mental health of children and adolescents, which has led to a rise in academic and policy discussions aimed at promoting the mental health of people throughout their lives. In fact, a substantial body of research suggests that healthy childhood development is a crucial foundation for reducing lifelong health disparities and social inequality, and therefore should be treated as a key component of national policy [4].

Maternal depression is known to not only increase perinatal complications such as low birth weight and preterm birth but also to be directly related to problems in children's emotional, cognitive, and interpersonal skills, and to affect neuroendocrine and brain function [5]. From a mental health perspective, it is already well-known that maternal depression is associated with increased insecure attachment, a lack of social skills, academic problems, and internalizing and externalizing issues in children, as well as a rise in mental illness [6, 7]. Specifically regarding childhood mental illness, the prevalence of depression is particularly high in children of mothers with depression, showing a prevalence rate of depressive disorder about three times higher than in normal control groups. What's even more interesting is that more than half of the children with depressive

C.-M. Yang (✉)
Department of Psychiatry, Wonkwang University Hospital, School of Medicine, Wonkwang University, Iksan, Republic of Korea
e-mail: ychanmo@wku.ac.kr

H.-M. Sung
Department of Psychiatry, Soonchunhyang University Hospital Gumi, Gumi, Republic of Korea

W.-M. Bahk et al. (eds.), *Depressive Disorder*, https://doi.org/10.1007/978-981-92-1331-3_18

disorders experience an early onset before adulthood [8]. Children born to mothers with depression who subsequently develop depression generally have a worse prognosis than children with typical adolescent depression, with earlier onset, a longer duration of the illness, greater functional impairment, and a higher relapse rate [5]. It is known that postpartum depression and maternal mental health problems affect a child's psychological development, and the severity is even greater when both postpartum depression and other mental health problems are present [9]. The more severe and chronic the symptoms of maternal depression, the more harmful the outcome for the child. Therefore, the severity and chronicity of maternal depression symptoms can be a potential predictor for the prognosis of depression that may appear in the child [10]. Thus, the early detection and appropriate treatment of maternal depression should be handled with great importance when considering the prevention and treatment of adolescent depression.

Most of the research on the effects of parental depression on child development has focused exclusively on its association with maternal depression. However, paternal depression is also reported to influence the occurrence of depression in children. Statistically, it is common for fathers to have depression when mothers do, which is likely influenced by assortative mating or living with a spouse who has a mental illness [11]. For this reason, the need for systematic research on paternal depression has been raised, but studies focusing solely on paternal depression's effect on childhood depression account for only about 1% of the total research, and its prevalence and the extent of its impact on child development appear to be less than those of maternal depression. The reason for the lack of research on paternal depression seems to be the societal perception that fathers, as providers, spend most of their time away from home and thus have little influence on a child's development [12]. However, this perception is changing due to the recent increase in women's participation in the workforce and fathers' greater interest and involvement in childcare. As a result, the need for research on the impact of paternal depression on children is growing [13]. In fact, the mean effect size of recent studies on the impact of paternal depression on children's internalizing problems is similar to that of maternal depression, suggesting that paternal depression can have a significant impact on child development, just as maternal depression does. Of course, studies on the effects of paternal depression have methodological limitations, such as small sample sizes and the absence of structured psychopathological diagnostic criteria. Therefore, systematic and longitudinal studies on paternal depression and child development and psychopathology are needed. The impact of paternal depression on children is known to cause a decrease in prosocial behavior and more problems in peer relationships in children [14]. It is also known to influence anger disorders, substance use disorders, and physical health. Furthermore, paternal depression has been reported to affect development during adolescence, being associated with lower academic achievement, reduced social competence, and an increase in suicide attempts [15]. The mechanisms by which paternal depression affects child development include impaired parental role performance due to the father's depression and the impact on the mother's psychological state [16]. However, research on paternal depression and child development and psychopathology is relatively limited and shows mixed results for internalizing behaviors [17]. In this chapter, we aim to examine the effects of parental depression on child development, including not only maternal depression but also paternal depression, which has been relatively under-researched.

There are many factors besides maternal depression that influence child development. These include parent-related factors such as parental psychopathology and parenting styles, child-related factors such as the child's temperament or congenital diseases, and socioenvironmental factors such as community involvement. Maternal psychological stress, including depression, is commonly observed during pregnancy, with over 30% of mothers known to experience stress. For most women, stress experienced during pregnancy persists after childbirth and has a significant impact on their child's development.

These research findings can be very helpful in establishing policies for prevention and early intervention to reduce the risks to childhood development [18]. The WHO Commission on Social Determinants of Health, in its final report, also argued that a more comprehensive approach to early life should include comprehensive support and care for mothers before, during, and after pregnancy, and this should include interventions to help address perinatal maternal mental health issues [19].

Large-scale cohort studies have shown that maternal depression, including prenatal depression, as well as premature birth, low community participation, and low parent-child interaction, is known to have a negative impact on childhood development. Conversely, parental well-being, self-efficacy in child-rearing, community participation, a strong social support system, and daily repeated interactions between caregiver and child act as factors that protect against developmental problems [20]. The experience of stress by the primary caregiver mother during childhood has been found to affect not only childhood development but also anxiety, depression, and low self-efficacy in adulthood, which demonstrates the importance of early detection and treatment of maternal stress and depression [21].

This chapter aims to investigate the influence of maternal depression on major areas of child development, including language, cognitive, and emotional development. Within each developmental domain, key findings are described according to the child's developmental stage. While many studies have been reported on the relationship between maternal depression and child development, including large-scale community-based cohort studies, it is still difficult to draw definitive conclusions. This is partly due to the inability to make clear, objective evaluations because of the characteristics of the research and its participants, as well as the failure to fully control for other factors that could affect a child's development. This chapter reviews recent research to explore the effects of maternal and paternal depression—specifically within the context of maternal stress related to pregnancy and childbirth—on childhood development. Through this, it aims to confirm the importance of appropriate intervention for parental depression to ensure a child's normal and healthy development.

18.1 Impact on the Development of Language and Communication Skills

The development of language is crucial not only for its intrinsic importance but also because it serves as a foundation for the development of a child's cognitive functions and communication abilities. Around five months of age, infants begin to vocalize by imitating the sounds of their caregivers. Subsequently, their language gradually develops as they imitate and repeat their caregivers' speech. The stimuli and feedback provided by the caregiver during this period of language and communication skill development play a vital role. Consequently, depression in the primary caregiver—the mother—inevitably affects the child's language and communication skill development.

A closer examination of the relationship between maternal depression and a child's language development more clearly reveals its negative effects. Depressive symptoms can cause problems in mother–child interactions, such as caring for and responding appropriately to the child, which in turn degrades the quality of the dynamic interactions between them. Mothers with depression tend to have less physical contact and conversation with their children, show appropriate facial expressions less frequently, and may even display more negative facial expressions. As with other areas of childhood development, interaction with the caregiver, especially face-to-face interaction, is critical for language development. Maternal depression affects the quantity and quality of these crucial interactions, increasing the likelihood of negative consequences for the child's development of language and many other cognitive functions [22]. In fact, studies have shown that mothers with depression differ significantly from non-depressed mothers in their tone of voice, the content of their speech, the feedback they provide, and the degree of focus they give the child when speaking [23]. In other words, there is a potential lack of maternal responses and behaviors that are essential for a child's language development, which will have a highly negative impact on the development of their language and communication skills. Indeed, several related studies confirm that maternal depression affects the development of language and communication skills. Maternal depression has an impact from the earliest stages of language and communication skill development. A study on postpartum depression and the development of communication skills up to age two found that postpartum depressive symptoms were associated with lower communication skills in children under two by delaying not only non-verbal communication abilities but also language development. This highlights that postpartum depression is a very important issue in the development of a child's early communication skills [20, 24].

The relationship between maternal depression and delays in language and communication skills remains a topic of debate. In particular, there are likely many opinions on the mechanisms by which maternal depression hinders this development. It has not been definitively concluded whether this is due to an actual neurodevelopmental delay caused by genetic or epigenetic factors, or if it is a secondary effect resulting from problems in mother–infant interaction, as mentioned earlier. The current literature suggests that maternal depression negatively affects language development, and the more severe and prolonged the depressive symptoms, the worse the outcome for the child's language and communication skill development [25].

18.2 Impact on Cognitive Development

As previously mentioned, maternal depression affects a child's language development, which in turn impacts the development of cognitive functions that are based on language. Furthermore, maternal depression directly influences the development of cognitive functions, including intelligence (hereafter IQ), supported by numerous studies.

Some studies investigating the relationship between maternal depression and cognitive development from the neonatal to infancy period have reported that postpartum depression affects the development of cognitive functions in infancy [26]. However, there have been no studies that directly assess or systematically investigate the effects of maternal depression on development before the age of one. This seems to be largely due to the difficulty of adequately assessing cognitive functions in such a young age group. A domestic study in Korea, which used the Korean Bayley Scales of Infant and Toddler Development to examine six-month-old infants, also found that maternal depressive symptoms and stress were associated with delays in cognitive development during infancy. Cohort studies on the relationship between maternal depression and cognitive development during the toddler years [27] (under 3 years old) generally report that both prenatal and postpartum depression are associated with delays in cognitive development, and the effect of maternal depression on cognitive development during this period is reported to have a moderate effect size [28].

Similarly, studies on the relationship between cognitive development and maternal depression in preschool children, though few in number like those for earlier periods, have generally reported that prenatal or postpartum stress and depression are associated with deficits in cognitive development, such as lower intelligence [29]. In contrast, there is a relatively larger body of research on cognitive development and maternal stress in school-aged children, likely because standardized intelligence tests and other cognitive function assessments become feasible at this age. A review of these studies indicates that maternal stress, including depression, is clearly associated with delays in cognitive development. Furthermore, the cognitive delays observed in studies of school-aged children appear to be more clearly influenced by prenatal stress and changes in cortisol levels during pregnancy rather than by postpartum stress [30].

Although the principles or factors behind this phenomenon are not yet clear, it is evident that maternal depression has a negative impact on the development of cognitive functions. Children of mothers with depression show more problems in the development of cognition, language, and IQ. These problems, similar to other developmental aspects, are influenced by the stage of brain development at the time of exposure to maternal depression and the duration of the depression. The risk becomes significantly greater with longer periods of maternal depression [31]. Because chronicity is a crucial factor, the importance of early detection and treatment of maternal depression must be emphasized.

18.3 Impact on Emotional Development

As previously discussed, maternal depression has a significantly negative impact on a child's negative emotions, mental disorders, and emotional development, such as by increasing the prevalence of depression in childhood and adolescence. Among perinatal maternal stresses, maternal depression and anxiety have long been known as significant factors that induce internalizing behaviors during a child's development. Furthermore, the child's response to the mother's prolonged pathological mental health condition has been shown to depend on the instability of maternal attachment. For this reason, interventions focused on mother–child interaction, attachment, and the mother's mental health—including depression and anxiety—are emphasized [32].

Regarding emotional development in infancy, some studies have reported that postpartum stress, in connection with mental disorders like postpartum depression or generalized anxiety disorder, affects the emotional and social development of infants. However, it is difficult to draw clear conclusions considering the characteristics of the study subjects and methodologies [18]. Research on the relationship between maternal depression and emotional development in toddlers is also limited, though many reports suggest that maternal depression negatively affects it. Yet, there may be considerable disagreement as to whether these outcomes are due to genetic, biological, or psychosocial factors. Based on a review of related studies, the most crucial factor through which maternal depression negatively impacts a child's emotional development appears to be the chronicity of the symptoms [33].

A recent study on preschool children, a large-scale mother–child cohort study in Norway, confirmed that parental depressive symptoms are associated with children's internalizing and externalizing problems, with maternal depression showing a particularly strong correlation. Maternal depression was found to especially affect children's emotional and behavioral problems when it occurred in early childhood or persisted into this period. The association with internalizing problems was also found to increase as the child's age increased, confirming the significant impact of maternal depression on the development of preschool-aged children [34].

There is a relatively large body of research on the relationship between school-aged children's emotions and maternal stress, including cohort studies with several thousand participants. A synthesis of these studies shows that maternal stress during pregnancy and the first year after childbirth, including depression, negatively affects the emotional development of school-aged children. This stress includes accumulated prenatal stress, anxiety in the third trimester, postpartum depression and anxiety, and parenting stress. Several studies have reported that anxiety may have a greater impact than postpartum depression [30]. Synthesizing various studies, it can be inferred that maternal anxiety is more highly associated with preschool children, while maternal depression is more associated with adolescent children [35]. Additionally, a review of research on the impact of paternal depression on adolescent depression and anxiety has reported effects similar to those of maternal depression [36].

18.4 Impact on Psychomotor Development

Numerous studies on the effects of maternal depression on children's psychomotor development have been published, but they show conflicting results. Furthermore, most studies only suggest a correlation between maternal depression and the prevalence of psychomotor developmental delays. More systematic research is needed, considering that most studies may not have adequately controlled for other factors besides maternal depression or stress that could affect psychomotor development. According to research on infants under one year of age, high prenatal anxiety shows a strong association with delays in psychomotor development. There are also reports that maternal stress, particularly high stress and anxiety related to parenting, may be associated with overall developmental delays in infancy, but a link to maternal depression has not been established [18, 37–39]. Studies on the impact of maternal depression on psychomotor development during the toddler years also show contradictory findings. However, among the studies that do report a connection, the prevalence of psychomotor developmental delays was higher in children whose mothers had postpartum depression, especially when it was chronic [40].

18.5 Impact on Behavioral Development

Although substantial evidence suggests that maternal depression affects a child's behavioral development, there is currently insufficient research to draw specific conclusions. Research on the relationship between maternal stress and behavioral development in infancy is also lacking, making it difficult to form any conclusions. However, two community-based studies suggest that stress during the third trimester of pregnancy, in particular, affects the behavioral development of infants under one year of age, with chronic and persistent anxiety appearing to have a greater impact than acute anxiety [18]. Studies on the relationship between problem behaviors during the toddler years and maternal depression also show mixed results. Although some studies have reported an association, they were either small-scale or, even when statistical significance was reported, the effect size was too small to conclude whether prenatal or postpartum depression independently affects the behavior of toddlers.

Research on the relationship between behavioral problems in preschool children and maternal depression appears to be extremely limited. A longitudinal study from Sweden seems to be the only large-scale research on the topic. This study reported that postpartum depression is related to behavioral problems in children of this age. It found that chronic maternal depression, where a mother caring for a preschooler has ongoing depressive symptoms, is more dangerous than a past history of postpartum depression. The study also emphasized the importance of early detection and treatment, as postpartum depression has a recurrence rate more than six times higher than that of general depression [41]. Related studies on school-aged children (including seven community-based studies conducted in five countries, including the United States) show that prenatal and postnatal maternal stress, especially maternal depression, has a significant correlation with behavioral problems that appear during the school years. Among these behavioral problems, attention-deficit/hyperactivity disorder (ADHD) was the most common, with the highest odds ratio at 9.30. These studies also confirmed that the child's gender acts as an important mediating factor, with a stronger association observed in boys [30].

18.6 Impact on Neurobiological Development

With the recent development of diagnostic tools, including various neuroimaging devices, many studies have been reported on the effects of maternal depression on a child's brain development [42]. The relatively consistent findings from brain imaging studies of children born to mothers with prenatal depression include observations such as decreased cortical thickness in the prefrontal cortex and other various regions, increased amygdala size, and changes in functional connectivity. Furthermore, persistent microstructural changes, such as decreased anisotropy and increased diffusion, were observed in the cingulum. Maternal depressive symptoms also affected the functional connectivity of the limbic structure with the mesocortical and mesolimbic networks. A decrease in cortical thickness is a part of the normal brain maturation process during childhood, which suggests that children exposed to maternal depression may experience premature brain maturation. While it has been suggested that paternal stress could affect offspring through genetic changes by causing alterations in mRNA [43], the morphological differences in the amygdala and cerebrum have shown no association with paternal depression during pregnancy. This indicates that these neurodevelopmental abnormalities are related to maternal depression, particularly prenatal depression during the period of fetal brain development [44]. Studies using functional neuroimaging have shown that adolescents of depressed mothers have decreased activity in the anterior prefrontal cortex and anterior cingulate cortex, as well as impaired executive function, which is fundamental for coping skills under stress [45]. Although it is not yet clear whether maternal depression is a direct cause or through which mechanisms it affects brain development, it seems certain that it does have an impact on the child's brain development. Interestingly, the effects of maternal depression on brain structure show a similar pattern to those of maternal anxiety. While changes in hippocampal size were associated only with maternal anxiety, changes in the amygdala, frontal lobe, and temporal lobe were similar in both conditions, suggesting that these areas are more generally associated with pathological levels of stress during pregnancy. A synthesis of recent studies using functional magnetic resonance imaging (fMRI) and DTI suggests that prenatal stress affects the development of the connectome through hypothalamic–pituitary–adrenal (HPA) axis activation and epigenetic changes. Consequently, not only the structural but also the functional connectivity of the brain differs from that of a normal brain, and this abnormal connectivity is presumed to have an overall impact on a child's neurocognitive development [46].

The changes in the amygdala, which have garnered attention in relation to depression, are presumed to be the result of altered cortisol and hormone levels due to maternal stress and depression. Considering that the amygdala is directly related to mood reactivity and mood disorders, this could serve as a scientific basis for the transmission of vulnerability to depression from mother to child. These structural changes in the brain are thought to mediate the relationship between stress during pregnancy, such as depression, and the cognitive, behavioral, and emotional problems that cause mental health issues in children, with genetic differences, environmental factors, and epigenetic changes also appearing to play a role. For example, when exposed to perinatal maternal stress, the reduction in functional connectivity of the amygdala, thalamus, hypothalamus, brainstem, and insular cortex was amplified when combined with the condition of being born prematurely [47]. These facts suggest that early intervention in mental health, starting from early pregnancy, is critically important [48, 49].

Since maternal depression can affect the emotions and behavior of children with normal neurocognitive functions, continuous research on its impact on neurocognitive development is necessary for the prevention and intervention of emotional and behavioral problems in children. Regarding its effect on neonatal sleep, children of mothers with depression have been observed to have not only a reduction in total sleep time but also more frequent awakenings and changes in sleep architecture, such as decreased non-rapid eye movement (NREM) and REM sleep. This may suggest that the prenatal fetal environment (especially maternal depression) can increase a child's future vulnerability to developing depression and may reduce neuroplasticity [50]. The UK Millennium Cohort Study, involving over 17,000 participants, reported that maternal depression affects externalizing symptoms like conduct problems and hyperactivity, as well as internalizing symptoms related to emotions and peer relationships. This is said to occur because maternal depression impacts the development of a child's working memory and decision-making functions [51]. According to a recent genetic study from an epigenetic perspective on one-year-old infants born to mothers with major depressive disorder, maternal depression also negatively affects children genetically. It was found to particularly influence the development and function of the central nervous system, providing clues to the neurobiological mechanisms of maternal depression's impact on child development [52].

18.7 Summary

Maternal depression is hypothesized to affect a child's development through several mechanisms. First, when a mother experiences depression, biological changes such as increased cortisol due to alterations in the HPA axis can affect the fetal brain, leading to changes in brain development during the fetal period and beyond. Second, genetic factors can be considered. Genetic factors that cause parental psychopathology or are epigenetically altered can lead to abnormalities in the child's development and psychopathology. Third, interactional problems arising from maternal depression can cause secondary developmental issues. When a mother caring for a child is depressed, an inadequate nurturing environment, reduced responsiveness to the child's speech and actions, and decreased physical and emotional exchange can have a significant impact on childhood development after birth. Fourth, various parenting problems, such as increased family discord secondary to maternal depression and abuse resulting from that discord, can also affect a child's development. Paternal depression, in particular, is likely to have a significant direct and indirect influence on interactions and secondary family discord through impaired parenting and its effects on the mother's psychological state. In addition, many other biological or environmental factors can be seen as directly or indirectly mediating the relationship between maternal depression and abnormal child development. As these many elements interact in a highly complex manner, it is impossible to distinguish each individual effect; the impact will also vary depending on the stage of child development at which maternal depression occurred, and the chronicity and severity of the symptoms.

A synthesis of studies on the relationship between maternal depression and child development shows that maternal depression negatively affects not only a child's emotional development but also various other domains, including language, cognition, and behavioral development. Paternal depression, being associated with maternal depression, can also directly and indirectly affect child development. Recent studies using neuroimaging provide a scientific basis for this, suggesting that maternal depression causes neurobiological changes, including changes in the brain parenchyma, thereby affecting the child's development. Despite extensive research, it is difficult to clearly distinguish whether the negative effects of maternal depression on child development are direct or indirect, or to specify the exact mechanisms or mediating factors involved. However, many researchers agree that the severity and chronicity of depressive symptoms are important prognostic factors for these negative effects. Therefore, from the perspective of child development and mental health, the early detection of and intervention for maternal depression should be treated as a crucial issue not only in individual psychiatric care but also in the formulation and implementation of relevant national policies. Interventions should not target the mother's depression alone but should be carried out with an interest in the psychopathology and interactions of all family members. Further research is needed, based on the understanding that a child is raised by both mother and father, and that their development can be affected not only by direct factors like parental mental illness and stress exposure but also by indirect methods such as all stress related to psychopathology [53].

Declarations

Competing Interests The author(s) has no competing interests to declare that are relevant to the content of this manuscript.

Ethics Approval The author(s) declares that this manuscript does not include primary research with human participants.

The author(s) declares that this manuscript does not include primary studies involving animals.

References

1. American Psychiatric Association. Diagnostic and statistical manual of mental disorders. 5th ed. Washington, DC: American Psychiatric Association; 2013.
2. Kessler R. Epidemiology of women and depression. J Affect Disord. 2003;74(1):5–13.
3. Surkan PJ, Patel SA, Rahman A. Preventing infant and child morbidity and mortality due to maternal depression. Best Pract Res Clin Obstet Gynaecol. 2016;36:156–68.
4. Hertzman C. The state of child development in Canada: are we moving toward, or away from, equity from the start? Paediatr Child Health. 2009;14(10):673–6.
5. Goodman SH. Depression in mothers. Annu Rev Clin Psychol. 2007;3:107–35.
6. Beardslee WR, Versage EM, Gladstone TR. Children of affectively ill parents: a review of the past 10 years. J Am Acad Child Adolesc Psychiatry. 1998;37(11):1134–41.
7. Downey G, Coyne JC. Children of depressed parents: an integrative review. Psychol Bull. 1990;108(1):50–76.
8. Hammen C, Brennan P. Severity, chronicity, and timing of maternal depression and risk for adolescent offspring diagnoses in a community sample. Arch Gen Psychiatry. 2003;60(3):253–8.
9. Closa-Monasterolo R, Gispert-Llauradó M, Canals J, Luque V, Zaragoza-Jordana M, Koletzko B, et al. The effect of postpartum depression and current mental health problems of the mother on child behaviour at eight years. Matern Child Health J. 2017;21(8):1563–72.
10. Ashman SB, Dawson G, Panagiotides H. Trajectories of maternal depression over 7 years: relations with child psychophysiology and behavior and role of contextual risks. Dev Psychopathol. 2008;20(1):55–77.
11. Mathews CA, Reus VI. Assortative mating in the affective disorders: a systematic review and meta-analysis. Compr Psychiatry. 2001;42(4):257–62.
12. Cabrera N, Tamis-LeMonda CS, Bradley RH, Hofferth S, Lamb ME. Fatherhood in the twenty-first century. Child Dev. 2000;71(1):127–36.
13. Cabrera NJ, Volling BL, Barr R. Fathers are parents, too! Widening the lens on parenting for children's development. Child Dev Perspect. 2018;12(3):152–7.
14. Davé S, Sherr L, Senior R, Nazareth I. Associations between paternal depression and behaviour problems in children of 4-6 years. Eur Child Adolesc Psychiatry. 2008;17(5):306–15.
15. Lewinsohn PM, Olino TM, Klein DN. Psychosocial impairment in offspring of depressed parents. Psychol Med. 2005;35(10):1493–503.
16. Ramchandani P, Psychogiou L. Paternal psychiatric disorders and children's psychosocial development. Lancet. 2009;374(9690):646–53.
17. Tichovolsky MH, Griffith SF, Rolon-Arroyo B, Arnold DH, Harvey EA. A longitudinal study of fathers' and young children's depressive symptoms. J Clin Child Adolesc Psychol. 2016;45(6):1–15.
18. Kingston D, Tough S, Whitfield H. Prenatal and postpartum maternal psychological distress and infant development: a systematic review. Child Psychiatry Hum Dev. 2012;43(5):683–714.
19. World Health Organization. Closing the gap in a generation: health equity through action on the social determinants of health. Final report of the Commission on Social Determinants of Health. Geneva: WHO; 2008.
20. McDonald S, Kehler H, Bayrampour H, Fraser-Lee N, Tough S. Risk and protective factors in early child development: results from the All Our Babies (AOB) pregnancy cohort. Res Dev Disabil. 2016;58:20–30.
21. Nilsen W, Dion J, Karevold EB, Skipstein A. Maternal psychological distress and offspring psychological adjustment in emerging adulthood: findings from over 18 years. J Dev Behav Pediatr. 2016;37(9):746–52.
22. Valla L, Wentzel-Larsen T, Smith L, Birkeland MS, Slinning K. Association between maternal postnatal depressive symptoms and infants' communication skills: a longitudinal study. Infant Behav Dev. 2016;45:83–90.
23. Porritt LL, Zinser MC, Bachorowski JA, Kaplan PS. Depression diagnoses and fundamental frequency-based acoustic cues in maternal infant-directed speech. Lang Learn Dev. 2014;10(1):51–67.
24. Kawai E, Takagai S, Takei N, Itoh H, Kanayama N, Tsuchiya KJ. Maternal postpartum depressive symptoms predict delay in non-verbal communication in 14-month-old infants. Infant Behav Dev. 2017;46:33–45.
25. Sohr-Preston SL, Scaramella LV. Implications of timing of maternal depressive symptoms for early cognitive and language development. Clin Child Fam Psychol Rev. 2006;9(1):65–83.
26. Murray L. The impact of postnatal depression on infant development. J Child Psychol Psychiatry. 1992;33(3):543–61.
27. Bhang SY, Ha E, Park H, Ha M, Hong YC, Kim BN, et al. Maternal stress and depressive symptoms and infant development at six months: the Mothers and Children's Environmental Health (MOCEH) prospective study. J Korean Med Sci. 2016;31(6):843–51.

28. Kingston D, McDonald S, Austin MP, Tough S. Association between prenatal and postnatal psychological distress and toddler cognitive development: a systematic review. PLoS One. 2015;10(4):e0126929.
29. Slykerman RF, Thompson JM, Pryor JE, Becroft DM, Robinson E, Clark PM, et al. Maternal stress, social support and preschool children's intelligence. Early Hum Dev. 2005;81(10):815–21.
30. Kingston D, Tough S. Prenatal and postnatal maternal mental health and school-age child development: a systematic review. Matern Child Health J. 2014;18(7):1728–41.
31. van der Waerden J, Bernard JY, De Agostini M, Saurel-Cubizolles MJ, Peyre H, Heude B, et al. Persistent maternal depressive symptoms trajectories influence children's IQ: the EDEN mother-child cohort. Depress Anxiety. 2017;34(2):105–17.
32. Reck C, Nonnenmacher N, Zietlow AL. Intergenerational transmission of internalizing behavior: the role of maternal psychopathology, child responsiveness and maternal attachment style insecurity. Psychopathology. 2016;49(4):277–84.
33. Prenoveau JM, Craske MG, West V, Giannakis A, Zioga M, Lehtonen A, et al. Maternal postnatal depression and anxiety and their association with child emotional negativity and behavior problems at two years. Dev Psychol. 2017;53(1):50–62.
34. Gjerde LC, Eilertsen EM, Reichborn-Kjennerud T, McAdams TA, Zachrisson HD, Zambrana IM, et al. Maternal perinatal and concurrent depressive symptoms and child behavior problems: a sibling comparison study. J Child Psychol Psychiatry. 2017;58(7):779–86.
35. Ma X, Biaggi A, Sacchi C, Lawrence AJ, Chen PJ, Pollard R, et al. Mediators and moderators in the relationship between maternal childhood adversity and children's emotional and behavioural development: a systematic review and meta-analysis. Psychol Med. 2022;52(10):1817–37.
36. Wickersham A, Leightley D, Archer M, Fear NT. The association between paternal psychopathology and adolescent depression and anxiety: a systematic review. J Adolesc. 2020;79:232–46.
37. Buitelaar JK, Huizink AC, Mulder EJ, de Medina PG, Visser GH. Prenatal stress and cognitive development and temperament in infants. Neurobiol Aging. 2003;24(Suppl 1):S53–60.
38. Punamäki RL, Repokari L, Vilska S, Poikkeus P, Tiitinen A, Sinkkonen J, et al. Maternal mental health and medical predictors of infant developmental and health problems from pregnancy to one year: does former infertility matter? Infant Behav Dev. 2006;29(2):230–42.
39. Slykerman RF, Thompson JM, Clark PM, Becroft DM, Robinson E, Pryor JE, et al. Determinants of developmental delay in infants aged 12 months. Paediatr Perinat Epidemiol. 2007;21(2):121–8.
40. Cornish AM, McMahon CA, Ungerer JA, Barnett B, Kowalenko N, Tennant C. Postnatal depression and infant cognitive and motor development in the second postnatal year: the impact of depression chronicity and infant gender. Infant Behav Dev. 2005;28(4):407–17.
41. Josefsson A, Sydsjö G. A follow-up study of postpartum depressed women: recurrent maternal depressive symptoms and child behavior after four years. Arch Womens Ment Health. 2007;10(3):141–5.
42. Cattarinussi G, Aarabi MH, Sanjari Moghaddam H, Homayoun M, Ashrafi M, Soltanian-Zadeh H, et al. Effect of parental depressive symptoms on offspring's brain structure and function: a systematic review of neuroimaging studies. Neurosci Biobehav Rev. 2021;131:451–65.
43. Bowers ME, Yehuda R. Intergenerational transmission of stress in humans. Neuropsychopharmacology. 2016;41(1):232–44.
44. El Marroun H, Tiemeier H, Muetzel RL, Thijssen S, van der Knaap NJ, Jaddoe VW, et al. Prenatal exposure to maternal and paternal depressive symptoms and brain morphology: a population-based prospective neuroimaging study in young children. Depress Anxiety. 2016;33(7):658–66.
45. Reising MM, Bettis AH, Dunbar JP, Watson KH, Gruhn M, Hoskinson KR, et al. Stress, coping, executive function, and brain activation in adolescent offspring of depressed and nondepressed mothers. Child Neuropsychol. 2017;23(2):147–64.
46. Scheinost D, Sinha R, Cross SN, Kwon SH, Sze G, Constable RT, et al. Does prenatal stress alter the developing connectome? Pediatr Res. 2017;81(1–2):214–26.
47. Scheinost D, Kwon SH, Lacadie C, Sze G, Sinha R, Constable RT, et al. Prenatal stress alters amygdala functional connectivity in preterm neonates. Neuroimage Clin. 2016;12:381–8.
48. Rifkin-Graboi A, Bai J, Chen H, Hameed WB, Sim LW, Tint MT, et al. Prenatal maternal depression associates with microstructure of right amygdala in neonates at birth. Biol Psychiatry. 2013;74(11):837–44.
49. Rifkin-Graboi A, Meaney MJ, Chen H, Bai J, Hameed WB, Tint MT, et al. Antenatal maternal anxiety predicts variations in neural structures implicated in anxiety disorders in newborns. J Am Acad Child Adolesc Psychiatry. 2015;54(4):313–21.
50. Bat-Pitault F, Sesso G, Deruelle C, Flori S, Porcher-Guinet V, Stagnara C, et al. Altered sleep architecture during the first months of life in infants born to depressed mothers. Sleep Med. 2017;30:195–203.
51. Flouri E, Ruddy A, Midouhas E. Maternal depression and trajectories of child internalizing and externalizing problems: the roles of child decision making and working memory. Psychol Med. 2017;47(6):1138–48.
52. Cicchetti D, Hetzel S, Rogosch FA, Handley ED, Toth SL. Genome-wide DNA methylation in 1-year-old infants of mothers with major depressive disorder. Dev Psychopathol. 2016;28(5):1413–29.
53. Aktar E, Qu J, Lawrence PJ, Tollenaar MS, Elzinga BM, Bögels SM. Fetal and infant outcomes in the offspring of parents with perinatal mental disorders: earliest influences. Front Psych. 2019;10:391.

Trauma and Depression

19

Sun Mi Kim and Kyoung Joon Min

19.1 Introduction

Trauma and depression are closely interconnected phenomena from both clinical and public health perspectives. Exposure to trauma in childhood or adulthood has been consistently linked to an elevated risk of major depressive disorder (MDD). This association is shaped by a complex interplay of neurobiological mechanisms, psychological vulnerabilities, and sociocultural contexts. This chapter provides an overview of the association between trauma and depression. We first review epidemiological evidence linking different types of trauma to depressive outcomes. We then discuss proposed explanations for the comorbidity of posttraumatic stress disorder (PTSD) and depression, risk and protective factors for depression after traumatic events, trauma exposure in children and adolescents, and childhood trauma as a risk factor for adult depression. Key neurobiological mechanisms—such as stress system dysregulation, immune and inflammatory pathways, and altered neuroplasticity—are also summarized, along with recent advances in the field. Together, these perspectives clarify how trauma contributes to depression and highlight opportunities for prevention and intervention.

S. M. Kim (✉) · K. J. Min
Department of Psychiatry, Chung-Ang University Hospital, Seoul, Republic of Korea
e-mail: sunmikim706@cauhs.or.kr

19.2 Types of Traumatic Events and the Prevalence of MDD Following Trauma

Traumatic events can be classified into several categories, including interpersonal trauma, accident-related trauma, disaster-related trauma, trauma associated with life-threatening illness, and war-related trauma [1]. Exposure to traumatic events is highly common; population-based self-report surveys indicate that approximately 70.4% of individuals worldwide have experienced at least one traumatic event [1]. Encountering multiple traumatic events across the lifespan is not the exception but rather the norm [2]. Globally, the number of individuals affected by trauma continues to rise and may further increase due to factors such as climate change–related natural disasters, religious extremism, terrorism, and political violence [3]. In recent years, unprecedented large-scale natural disasters have occurred worldwide, leading to substantial mortality and leaving overwhelming numbers of survivors vulnerable to a wide range of psychiatric difficulties. While it is well recognized that posttraumatic stress disorder (PTSD) frequently develops after exposure to trauma, depression also constitutes a major mental health consequence—and one that has often been underrecognized relative to PTSD.

Among survivors with severe exposure to community disasters, up to one-third have been reported to develop PTSD, and up to one-quarter

W.-M. Bahk et al. (eds.), *Depressive Disorder*, https://doi.org/10.1007/978-981-92-1331-3_19

meet criteria for MDD [4]. From a longer-term perspective, however, depression may represent an even more common sequela of disasters than PTSD, given its generally higher prevalence in the population [5]. The prevalence of MDD following disasters varies widely, influenced by factors such as the baseline prevalence of depression in the affected population, the method of symptom assessment, sampling design, severity of disaster exposure, and the availability of social support post-disaster [5]. For example, approximately 5% of the Texas population affected by Hurricane Ike met criteria for MDD one month after the disaster [6], whereas about one in ten adult residents of New York met criteria for MDD one month after the September 11 World Trade Center attacks [7]. Among disaster-exposed children and adolescents, depression emerged as the second most common psychiatric outcome after PTSD [8]. Prevalence estimates were highly variable, ranging from 1.6 to 81% in the first year and 5.4 to 76% at one year post-disaster. Comorbidity was also frequent, with depression occurring in 8 to 88.6% of those presenting with PTSD symptoms [8].

19.3 Comorbidity of PTSD and Depression

Comorbidity of PTSD with Other Psychiatric Disorders

Psychiatric disorders that develop in the aftermath of trauma are commonly characterized by comorbidity [9]. In the U.S. National Comorbidity Survey, 88% of men and 79% of women with chronic PTSD met criteria for at least one additional psychiatric disorder [10]. Similarly, in a national survey conducted in Australia, 85% of men and 80% of women diagnosed with PTSD within the past 12 months had at least one comorbid psychiatric disorder [11]. Another study reported that 83% of individuals with PTSD had at least one comorbid disorder, compared with 44% among those with other psychiatric disorders, demonstrating a marked difference [12]. Across these studies, MDD consistently emerged as one of the most common comorbid conditions with PTSD.

The Relationship Between PTSD and MDD

Several causal hypotheses have been proposed to explain the relationship between PTSD and MDD [13]. The first is the shared vulnerability model, which posits that each disorder increases susceptibility to the other. In other words, a preexisting diagnosis of MDD may heighten vulnerability to developing PTSD after a traumatic event, while preexisting PTSD may increase the risk of subsequent MDD [10, 14]. Supporting this hypothesis is the observation that many risk factors—such as a history of depression, exposure to severe trauma, childhood abuse, and female gender—are common to both disorders [15, 16]. Taken together, these findings suggest that comorbid PTSD and MDD following trauma are best explained within a unified traumatic stress etiology model.

A second hypothesis suggests that PTSD and MDD represent distinct outcomes of trauma exposure. For instance, one study analyzing diverse posttraumatic symptoms found that a two-factor model of PTSD and depression provided the best fit for the data, rather than a one-factor model, which would have supported a shared response to trauma [17].

More recent research has examined predictors of PTSD and MDD at multiple time points—at discharge, and at 3 and 12 months posttrauma—to further clarify their relationship [9]. The findings indicated that most posttraumatic psychopathology is better explained by a shared traumatic stress etiology model, supporting the notion that PTSD and MDD share substantial overlapping pathophysiology. Specifically, factors such as trauma characteristics (severity, hospital ward type), individual characteristics (prior psychiatric disorders and trauma history), negative appraisals of injury and its potential consequences, PTSD symptom severity, initial depressive affect, and dissociation in the first week were identified as common predictors for both conditions. However, at the three-month mark, MDD exhibited some distinct predictors not observed in PTSD, and at 12 months, MDD showed a more favorable prognosis than PTSD [9]. These findings suggest that while PTSD and MDD may present with relative distinctions during the acute posttrauma phase, their differentiation becomes less clear as psychopathology becomes chronic. At the same time, MDD may demonstrate relatively greater potential for recovery compared with PTSD.

19.4 Risk Factors for MDD Following Traumatic Events

The development of MDD after traumatic exposure is best understood as a multifactorial process. Rather than arising from a single cause, posttraumatic depression emerges through the interaction of three broad domains: pre-existing vulnerabilities, the characteristics of the traumatic event itself, and the post-event context.

Adults

In adults, several risk factors have been identified in the aftermath of natural disasters. Pre-existing vulnerabilities include a history of traumatic exposure, low educational attainment, religious beliefs, and female gender [18]. The effect of trauma history is consistent with previous findings that cumulative lifetime exposure to violent events increases the risk of depression. Education plays an indirect role by shaping access to economic resources, social networks, and coping strategies; individuals with higher education may, therefore, show greater resilience [19]. Interestingly, religious belief has also been linked to increased vulnerability, possibly due to interpretations of disasters as divine punishment, which may intensify feelings of guilt and sadness [20]. Event-related characteristics such as fear, injury, bereavement, unemployment, property loss, and housing damage further increase risk [18]. Additional studies highlight that preexisting psychopathology, the severity of the event, and the presence of concurrent stressors also elevate risk [4].

Adolescents

Among adolescents, individual-level factors appear to play a stronger role than event-related characteristics in predicting posttraumatic depression [3]. Important personal risk factors include female gender, low socioeconomic status, early depressive symptoms, comorbid PTSD symptoms, exaggerated fear responses to non-threatening stimuli, limited family and social support, introverted temperament, psychotic features, and low tolerance for distress. However, event- and trauma-related characteristics may also contribute to the risk of depression, including violent assault, kidnapping, However, event- and trauma-related characteristics may also contribute to the risk of depression, including violent assault, kidnapping, witnessing severe injury, trauma severity, prior exposure to trauma or interpersonal violence, negative life events, resource loss, housing damage, and disaster-related displacement.

19.5 Protective Factors for the Development of MDD Following Trauma

The onset and course of MDD following trauma are not determined solely by the accumulation of risk factors. Rather, they should be understood within a framework in which protective factors at the individual, family, and community levels interact to buffer symptom expression and promote recovery.

Adults

In adults, the most consistently reported protective factor is social support. Prospective cohort studies have shown that emotional and instrumental support networks established prior to a disaster are associated with a reduced incidence of depression following natural disasters [21]. Perceived social support after a disaster has repeatedly been reported to buffer the association between stress and depressive symptoms [22, 23]. Among individual psychological resources, coping self-efficacy has been observed to play a protective role. High levels of self-efficacy are thought to reduce vulnerability to depression by enhancing a sense of control and promoting problem-solving strategies, thereby facilitating resilience in the face of adversity [24]. From a behavioral and lifestyle perspective, physical activities such as group exercise and daily walking, as well as social participation, have been associated with decreased depressive symptoms among older adult disaster survivors, suggesting that the combination of behavioral activation and social connectedness may enhance protective effects [25].

Adolescents

In adolescents, family functioning has consistently been identified as a protective factor. Higher levels of family cohesion, communication, and problem-solving have been associated with reduced exacerbation of internalizing symptoms such as depression and anxiety following natural disasters [26]. Furthermore, low family resilience—the ability of the family to respond positively to adverse situations—has been linked to post-disaster emotional problems in children, including feelings of unhappiness, worry, fear, nervousness, and somatic complaints [27].

19.6 Trauma Exposure and Depression in Children and Adolescents

Children and adolescents are particularly vulnerable to traumatic events because they are in a developmental stage during which the brain is still maturing [3]. At this stage, psychological strengths and coping capacities are not yet firmly established, limiting their ability to employ effective coping strategies. Moreover, the absence of socioeconomic stability can exacerbate the impact of trauma. In this context, depression arising from severe traumatic events may negatively affect one's sense of life purpose and contribute to existential anxiety.

Moreover, community-level disasters can disrupt family functioning and precipitate parental psychopathology, thereby heightening the risk of mental disorders among child and adolescent survivors [8]. This is because children's sense of security and resilience is strongly influenced by the adaptive capacities of parents and caregivers. In addition, children are particularly susceptible to secondary stressors associated with disasters, such as separation from family members or pets, scarcity of food and water, destruction of the home, and interruption of schooling [28]. Consequently, there is growing attention to the psychiatric sequelae experienced by child and adolescent survivors of community disasters, as well as to the need for welfare services and psychosocial support for this vulnerable population.

19.7 Childhood Trauma and Adult Depression

There is growing recognition that childhood traumas such as abuse, neglect, separation from parents, and parental psychopathology constitute significant risk factors for the development of depressive disorders in adulthood [29]. Some studies have reported that childhood trauma may increase the risk of an earlier onset of depression [30]. In general, individuals with depression report having experienced more severe adversity during childhood compared to those without depression [29]. Childhood trauma exerts detrimental effects on the development of children and adolescents and may leave long-lasting consequences that persist into adulthood. Accumulating evidence further suggests that individuals exposed to trauma early in life may be more sensitive to the adverse effects of subsequent stressors, thereby showing increased vulnerability to stress-related disorders and depression.

Childhood Abuse and Adult Psychopathology

Research on the relationship between childhood abuse and adult psychopathology provides substantial evidence for the impact of early trauma on the development of depressive disorders in adulthood. Childhood abuse is generally categorized into four types: sexual abuse, physical abuse, psychological-emotional abuse, and neglect. Among these, considerable research has focused on the association between childhood sexual abuse and the onset of psychiatric disorders in adulthood. There is extensive evidence that childhood sexual abuse increases the likelihood of a wide range of symptoms, including depression, anxiety, low self-esteem, guilt, fear, sexual difficulties, suicidal ideation, and self-harming behaviors [31]. Moreover, sexual abuse in childhood has been shown to be strongly associated with the onset of depression in adulthood and to significantly increase the risk of chronic depression, suicidal behavior, and impulsivity [31]. The negative consequences of sexual abuse are further exacerbated when accompanied by other adverse experiences, such as parental neglect, psychological or physical abuse, or poor parental care [32].

As sexual abuse is often accompanied by physical abuse, childhood physical abuse—frequently co-occurring with other forms of maltreatment—is relatively common and significantly associated with adult depression, anxiety, and anger [33]. Psychological–emotional abuse has likewise been linked to an increased lifetime risk of depressive disorders and appears to elevate the risk of comorbidity and chronicity in adult depression [34]. Psychological trauma can profoundly impair a child's social, emotional, neurological, physical, and sensory development, with particularly severe consequences when psychological-emotional abuse is repeated or chronic [35]. Unlike physical abuse, the effects of psychological-emotional abuse are more difficult to detect, as the scars are internal rather than external.

Another form of maltreatment, neglect, also exerts widespread negative effects on lifelong mental health functioning. Adults with MDD report significantly higher rates of childhood neglect compared with healthy controls, and neglect has been associated with earlier onset of depression [36] as well as with more frequent depressive episodes [37]. Recent meta-analytic evidence further indicates that among the various forms of childhood abuse, psychological–emotional abuse and neglect show particularly strong associations with depression [29]. However, in clinical reality, exposure to one type of childhood abuse often coincides with exposure to other types, and cumulative experiences of multiple forms of abuse appear to be linked to more complex psychopathology in adulthood [38].

Pathophysiology of Childhood Trauma and Adult Depression

In the pathophysiology of MDD, genetic factors are estimated to account for approximately 30–40% of the risk, while the remaining 60–70% is influenced by environmental factors [39]. These environmental influences largely consist of adverse childhood experiences, abuse, other traumatic events, low social support, marital difficulties, and various interpersonal stressors occurring either in childhood or later in life [39]. Among these, childhood traumatic experiences appear to play a particularly central role in the onset of depression. Traumatic events during critical developmental periods can alter both the structure and function of brain systems, and such alterations may persist into adulthood.

This interplay between environment and biology has also been conceptualized within the framework of epigenetic mechanisms, whereby external environmental conditions can modify gene expression [29]. From a biological perspective, childhood trauma may interact with genetic vulnerability and the hypothalamic–pituitary–adrenal (HPA) axis, thereby increasing susceptibility to depression. In addition, maladaptive response patterns to stress contribute to vulnerability through psychological pathways. For instance, withdrawal in the face of stress may be highly adaptive in the context of childhood abuse, yet in adulthood the same behavioral response becomes maladaptive and may generate additional stress. Ultimately, the accumulation of such adverse factors increases the risk for depression.

19.8 Neurobiology of Posttraumatic Depression

The interactions among genetic, environmental, and neurobiological factors in the relationship between trauma and depression are highly complex, and research in this field remains at a relatively early stage.

Polymorphic Variants of the Serotonin Transporter

Research has explored potential interactions between polymorphic variants of the serotonin transporter gene (5-HTT), exposure to environmental stressors across the lifespan, and vulnerability to depression. This body of work has largely adopted a gene–environment interaction framework, focusing on whether genetic variation moderates the association between traumatic experiences and depressive outcomes rather than establishing direct causal pathways [40, 41]. Among polymorphisms in the promoter region of the 5-HTT gene (5-HTTLPR), the short (s) allele has been most extensively studied as a potential moderator of stress-related depression risk. Early studies reported that, in individuals without childhood abuse, no significant association was observed between genotype and depression, whereas among those exposed to childhood trauma, depression risk appeared to differ by genotype, with short–short (ss) homozygotes showing higher risk than long–short (ls) or long–long (ll) genotypes. These findings were interpreted as suggesting both stress-dose and gene-dose patterns [40, 41]. Similar genotype-dependent associations were initially reported for stressful life events in adulthood. For example, major stressors occurring between ages 21 and 26 were more strongly associated with depression among carriers of the allele, whereas no such association was observed in individuals reporting low levels of stress [40]. Together, these early findings contributed to the hypothesis that variation in the serotonin transporter gene may influence individual sensitivity to environmental stressors. However, subsequent replication studies and large-scale meta-analyses have yielded mixed and sometimes inconsistent findings regarding the 5-HTTLPR × stress interaction [42, 43]. In particular, evidence from a large meta-analysis including more than 38,000 individuals did not demonstrate consistent support for this interaction in predicting depression [42]. These findings underscore ongoing debates regarding the robustness and clinical relevance of this gene–environment interaction. Accordingly, while 5-HTTLPR research has contributed to theoretical models of stress vulnerability, these findings should be interpreted as preliminary rather than definitive.

Hypothalamic-Pituitary-Adrenal (HPA) Axis Dysregulation

In a subset of patients with depression, activation of the stress response system is accompanied by elevated peripheral cortisol levels, a finding commonly interpreted as reflecting altered regulation of the HPA axis. Although abnormalities of HPA axis function have been widely reported in the depression literature, evidence of HPA dysregulation is not uniformly observed across all individuals with depressive disorders and appears to characterize only specific clinical subgroups [44]. Notably, depression occurring in the context of childhood trauma has been consistently associated with markers of altered HPA axis function. Observational studies indicate that exposure to severe and persistent traumatic events beginning in childhood is associated with a higher prevalence of subsequent depressive and anxiety disorders, as well as indices suggestive of HPA axis dysregulation [44]. Traumatic experiences during sensitive developmental periods—

such as physical or sexual abuse, or parental loss—have been linked to long-lasting changes in stress responsivity at the level of the central nervous system [45]. However, these findings are primarily based on correlational data, and causal inferences regarding the direct effects of early trauma on enduring HPA axis alterations remain limited. From a theoretical or teleological perspective, sustained activation of the stress response system under conditions of chronic or severe stress has been hypothesized to confer short-term adaptive advantages by maintaining a heightened state of physiological vigilance in the face of perceived threat. At the same time, prolonged elevations in cortisol levels have been associated with adverse long-term health outcomes in individuals with MDD, including increased risk of coronary heart disease, type 2 diabetes mellitus, and osteoporosis [39]. Importantly, these associations do not establish a direct causal pathway but rather suggest that chronic HPA axis activation may represent one of several interrelated biological processes linking depression, stress exposure, and physical health outcomes.

Other Neurobiological Mechanisms

In addition, trauma-, stress-, and depression-related cellular and structural alterations may arise through multiple mechanisms involving the proliferation, growth, survival, and functional changes of neurons and glial cells. These mechanisms include altered neurotrophic and growth factors, glutamatergic excitotoxicity, inflammatory cytokines, metabolic and vascular changes, viral infections, and brain injury caused by physical trauma [46]. The interaction between genetic factors and exposure to life stressors contributes to an individual's vulnerability or resilience to psychopathology [46]. The psychopathological consequences of such interactions may occur acutely following a single major traumatic event or may gradually develop over time as one or more traumatic experiences accumulate. Research in neurobiology holds immense potential and promise for clarifying the pathophysiology of mental disorders and for serving as a foundation for the development of novel treatments.

19.9 Recent Trends

In the context of recent global disasters caused by the pandemic and climate change, the association between trauma and depression has garnered increasing attention. During coronavirus disease 2019 (COVID-19), the prevalence of depressive symptoms was more than three times higher compared with pre-pandemic estimates, and individuals with lower social resources, limited economic means, or greater exposure to stressors such as job loss reported a substantially greater burden of depressive symptoms [47]. Furthermore, natural disasters driven by climate change have been reported to exert long-term negative effects on community mental health, markedly increasing the risk of depression [48]. Meanwhile, International Classification of Diseases, 11th revision (ICD-11) has introduced the expanded diagnostic category of complex PTSD, emphasizing that difficulties in emotion regulation, interpersonal problems, and chronic depressive symptoms may be included [49]. These developments suggest that trauma should be understood not merely as a single syndrome but along a close continuum with depression.

19.10 Summary

Trauma serves as a critical precipitating factor not only for PTSD but also for major depressive disorder (MDD), with adverse childhood experiences, abuse, and other traumatic events acting as major environmental risk factors. In particular, trauma experienced during developmental periods induces structural and functional alterations in brain systems that can persist into adulthood, while maladaptive stress response patterns further exacerbate psychological vulnerability to depression. PTSD and MDD show high comorbidity, and although distinct predictors may appear in the early stages, over time the two disorders increasingly converge on shared traumatic stress–related etiologies. Mechanistically, childhood trauma heightens vulnerability to adult depression, with gene–environment interactions (e.g., 5-HTTLPR) and dysregulation of the HPA axis identified as key biological pathways. Clinically, early intervention following trauma, strengthening of family and social support, psychoeducation, and systematic assessment of childhood trauma history are essential. Taken together, these findings highlight the necessity of comprehensive strategies that encompass biological, psychological, and social dimensions in both research and clinical practice. Future studies should further clarify the mechanisms linking trauma and depression to guide the development of more effective preventive and therapeutic interventions.

Declarations

Competing Interests The author(s) has no competing interests to declare that are relevant to the content of this manuscript.

Ethics Approval The author(s) declares that this manuscript does not include primary research with human participants.

The author(s) declares that this manuscript does not include primary studies involving animals.

References

1. Geoffrion S, Goncalves J, Robichaud I, Sader J, Giguère C, Fortin M, et al. Systematic review and meta-analysis on acute stress disorder: rates following different types of traumatic events. Trauma Violence Abuse. 2022;23(1):213–23. https://doi.org/10.1177/1524838020933844.
2. Kilpatrick DG, Resnick HS, Milanak ME, Miller MW, Keyes KM, Friedman MJ. National estimates of exposure to traumatic events and PTSD prevalence using DSM-IV and DSM-5 criteria. J Trauma Stress. 2013;26(5):537–47. https://doi.org/10.1002/jts.21848.
3. Kar N. Depression in youth exposed to disasters, terrorism and political violence. Curr Psychiatry Rep. 2019;21(8):73. https://doi.org/10.1007/s11920-019-1061-9.
4. North CS, Pfefferbaum B. Mental health response to community disasters: a systematic review. JAMA. 2013;310(5):507–18. https://doi.org/10.1001/jama.2013.107799.
5. Goldmann E, Galea S. Mental health consequences of disasters. Annu Rev Public Health. 2014;35:169–83. https://doi.org/10.1146/annurev-publhealth-032013-182435.
6. Tracy M, Norris FH, Galea S. Differences in the determinants of posttraumatic stress disorder and depression after a mass traumatic event. Depress Anxiety. 2011;28(8):666–75. https://doi.org/10.1002/da.20838.
7. Galea S, Ahern J, Resnick H, Kilpatrick D, Bucuvalas M, Gold J, et al. Psychological sequelae of the September 11 terrorist attacks in New York City. N Engl J Med. 2002;346(13):982–7. https://doi.org/10.1056/NEJMsa013404.
8. Wang CW, Chan CL, Ho RT. Prevalence and trajectory of psychopathology among child and adolescent survivors of disasters: a systematic review of epidemiological studies across 1987-2011. Soc Psychiatry Psychiatr Epidemiol. 2013;48(11):1697–720. https://doi.org/10.1007/s00127-013-0731-x.
9. O'Donnell ML, Creamer M, Pattison P. Posttraumatic stress disorder and depression following trauma: understanding comorbidity. Am J Psychiatry. 2004;161(8):1390–6. https://doi.org/10.1176/appi.ajp.161.8.1390.
10. Kessler RC, Sonnega A, Bromet E, Hughes M, Nelson CB. Posttraumatic stress disorder in the National Comorbidity Survey. Arch Gen Psychiatry. 1995;52(12):1048–60. https://doi.org/10.1001/archpsyc.1995.03950240066012.
11. Creamer M, Burgess P, McFarlane AC. Posttraumatic stress disorder: findings from the Australian National Survey of Mental Health and Well-being. Psychol Med. 2001;31(7):1237–47. https://doi.org/10.1017/s0033291701004287.
12. Breslau N, Davis GC, Andreski P, Peterson E. Traumatic events and posttraumatic stress disorder in an urban population of young adults. Arch Gen Psychiatry. 1991;48(3):216–22. https://doi.org/10.1001/archpsyc.1991.01810270028003.
13. Breslau N, Davis GC, Peterson EL, Schultz LR. A second look at comorbidity in victims of trauma: the posttraumatic stress disorder-major depression connection. Biol Psychiatry. 2000;48(9):902–9. https://doi.org/10.1016/s0006-3223(00)00933-1.
14. Breslau N, Davis GC, Peterson EL, Schultz L. Psychiatric sequelae of posttraumatic stress disorder in women. Arch Gen Psychiatry. 1997;54(1):81–7. https://doi.org/10.1001/archpsyc.1997.01830130087016.
15. Carlson EB, Rosser-Hogan R. Trauma experiences, posttraumatic stress, dissociation, and depression in Cambodian refugees. Am J Psychiatry. 1991;148(11):1548–51. https://doi.org/10.1176/ajp.148.11.1548.
16. Kendler KS, Gardner CO, Prescott CA. Toward a comprehensive developmental model for major depression

in women. Am J Psychiatry. 2002;159(7):1133–45. https://doi.org/10.1176/appi.ajp.159.7.1133.
17. Blanchard EB, Buckley TC, Hickling EJ, Taylor AE. Posttraumatic stress disorder and comorbid major depression: is the correlation an illusion? J Anxiety Disord. 1998;12(1):21–37. https://doi.org/10.1016/s0887-6185(97)00047-9.
18. Tang B, Liu X, Liu Y, Xue C, Zhang L. A meta-analysis of risk factors for depression in adults and children after natural disasters. BMC Public Health. 2014;14:623. https://doi.org/10.1186/1471-2458-14-623.
19. Lee J. Pathways from education to depression. J Cross Cult Gerontol. 2011;26(2):121–35. https://doi.org/10.1007/s10823-011-9142-1.
20. Chen YY, Koenig HG. Traumatic stress and religion: Is there a relationship? A review of empirical findings. J Rel Health. 2006;45:371–81.
21. Sasaki Y, Aida J, Tsuji T, Koyama S, Tsuboya T, Saito T, et al. Pre-disaster social support is protective for onset of post-disaster depression: prospective study from the Great East Japan Earthquake & Tsunami. Sci Rep. 2019;9(1):19427. https://doi.org/10.1038/s41598-019-55953-7.
22. Rung AL, Gaston S, Robinson WT, Trapido EJ, Peters ES. Untangling the disaster-depression knot: the role of social ties after Deepwater Horizon. Soc Sci Med. 2017;177:19–26. https://doi.org/10.1016/j.socscimed.2017.01.041.
23. McGuire AP, Gauthier JM, Anderson LM, Hollingsworth DW, Tracy M, Galea S, et al. Social support moderates effects of natural disaster exposure on depression and posttraumatic stress disorder symptoms: effects for displaced and nondisplaced residents. J Trauma Stress. 2018;31(2):223–33. https://doi.org/10.1002/jts.22270.
24. Benight CC, Bandura A. Social cognitive theory of posttraumatic recovery: the role of perceived self-efficacy. Behav Res Ther. 2004;42(10):1129–48. https://doi.org/10.1016/j.brat.2003.08.008.
25. Tsuji T, Sasaki Y, Matsuyama Y, Sato Y, Aida J, Kondo K, et al. Reducing depressive symptoms after the Great East Japan earthquake in older survivors through group exercise participation and regular walking: a prospective observational study. BMJ Open. 2017;7(3):e013706. https://doi.org/10.1136/bmjopen-2016-013706.
26. McDermott BM, Cobham VE. Family functioning in the aftermath of a natural disaster. BMC Psychiatry. 2012;12:55. https://doi.org/10.1186/1471-244x-12-55.
27. McDermott BM, Cobham VE, Berry H, Stallman HM. Vulnerability factors for disaster-induced child post-traumatic stress disorder: the case for low family resilience and previous mental illness. Aust N Z J Psychiatry. 2010;44(4):384–9. https://doi.org/10.3109/00048670903489916.
28. Belfer ML. Caring for children and adolescents in the aftermath of natural disasters. Int Rev Psychiatry. 2006;18(6):523–8. https://doi.org/10.1080/09540260601048877.
29. Mandelli L, Petrelli C, Serretti A. The role of specific early trauma in adult depression: a meta-analysis of published literature. Childhood trauma and adult depression. Eur Psychiatry. 2015;30(6):665–80. https://doi.org/10.1016/j.eurpsy.2015.04.007.
30. Dunn EC, McLaughlin KA, Slopen N, Rosand J, Smoller JW. Developmental timing of child maltreatment and symptoms of depression and suicidal ideation in young adulthood: results from the National Longitudinal Study of Adolescent Health. Depress Anxiety. 2013;30(10):955–64. https://doi.org/10.1002/da.22102.
31. Gladstone G, Parker G, Wilhelm K, Mitchell P, Austin MP. Characteristics of depressed patients who report childhood sexual abuse. Am J Psychiatry. 1999;156(3):431–7. https://doi.org/10.1176/ajp.156.3.431.
32. Hill J, Pickles A, Burnside E, Byatt M, Rollinson L, Davis R, et al. Child sexual abuse, poor parental care and adult depression: evidence for different mechanisms. Br J Psychiatry. 2001;179:104–9. https://doi.org/10.1192/bjp.179.2.104.
33. Springer KW, Sheridan J, Kuo D, Carnes M. Long-term physical and mental health consequences of childhood physical abuse: results from a large population-based sample of men and women. Child Abuse Negl. 2007;31(5):517–30. https://doi.org/10.1016/j.chiabu.2007.01.003.
34. Hovens JG, Giltay EJ, Wiersma JE, Spinhoven P, Penninx BW, Zitman FG. Impact of childhood life events and trauma on the course of depressive and anxiety disorders. Acta Psychiatr Scand. 2012;126(3):198–207. https://doi.org/10.1111/j.1600-0447.2011.01828.x.
35. Garbarino J, Garbarino A. Emotional maltreatment of children. 2nd ed. Chicago: National Committee to Prevent Child Abuse; 1994.
36. Bifulco A, Moran PM, Baines R, Bunn A, Stanford K. Exploring psychological abuse in childhood: II. Association with other abuse and adult clinical depression. Bull Menn Clin. 2002;66(3):241–58. https://doi.org/10.1521/bumc.66.3.241.23366.
37. Bernet CZ, Stein MB. Relationship of childhood maltreatment to the onset and course of major depression in adulthood. Depress Anxiety. 1999;9(4):169–74.
38. Putnam KT, Harris WW, Putnam FW. Synergistic childhood adversities and complex adult psychopathology. J Trauma Stress. 2013;26(4):435–42. https://doi.org/10.1002/jts.21833.
39. Hasler G. Pathophysiology of depression: do we have any solid evidence of interest to clinicians? World Psychiatry. 2010;9(3):155–61. https://doi.org/10.1002/j.2051-5545.2010.tb00298.x.
40. Caspi A, Sugden K, Moffitt TE, Taylor A, Craig IW, Harrington H, et al. Influence of life stress on depression: moderation by a

polymorphism in the 5-HTT gene. Science (New York, NY). 2003;301(5631):386–9. https://doi.org/10.1126/science.1083968.
41. Kendler KS, Kuhn JW, Vittum J, Prescott CA, Riley B. The interaction of stressful life events and a serotonin transporter polymorphism in the prediction of episodes of major depression: a replication. Arch Gen Psychiatry. 2005;62(5):529–35. https://doi.org/10.1001/archpsyc.62.5.529.
42. Culverhouse RC, Saccone NL, Horton AC, Ma Y, Anstey KJ, Banaschewski T, et al. Collaborative meta-analysis finds no evidence of a strong interaction between stress and 5-HTTLPR genotype contributing to the development of depression. Mol Psychiatry. 2018;23(1):133–42. https://doi.org/10.1038/mp.2017.44.
43. Risch N, Herrell R, Lehner T, Liang KY, Eaves L, Hoh J, et al. Interaction between the serotonin transporter gene (5-HTTLPR), stressful life events, and risk of depression: a meta-analysis. JAMA. 2009;301(23):2462–71. https://doi.org/10.1001/jama.2009.878.
44. Heim C, Plotsky PM, Nemeroff CB. Importance of studying the contributions of early adverse experience to neurobiological findings in depression. Neuropsychopharmacology. 2004;29(4):641–8. https://doi.org/10.1038/sj.npp.1300397.
45. Shelton RC. The molecular neurobiology of depression. Psychiatr Clin North Am. 2007;30(1):1–11. https://doi.org/10.1016/j.psc.2006.12.005.
46. Duman RS. Neuronal damage and protection in the pathophysiology and treatment of psychiatric illness: stress and depression. Dialogues Clin Neurosci. 2009;11(3):239–55. https://doi.org/10.31887/DCNS.2009.11.3/rsduman.
47. Ettman CK, Abdalla SM, Cohen GH, Sampson L, Vivier PM, Galea S. Prevalence of depression symptoms in US adults before and during the COVID-19 pandemic. JAMA Netw Open. 2020;3(9):e2019686. https://doi.org/10.1001/jamanetworkopen.2020.19686.
48. Thompson R, Lawrance EL, Roberts LF, Grailey K, Ashrafian H, Maheswaran H, et al. Ambient temperature and mental health: a systematic review and meta-analysis. Lancet Planet Health. 2023;7(7):e580–e9. https://doi.org/10.1016/s2542-5196(23)00104-3.
49. Organization WH. The ICD-11 for mortality and morbidity statistics. https://icd.who.int/browse11/l-m/en (2018). Accessed 26 Aug 2025.

GPSR Compliance

The European Union's (EU) General Product Safety Regulation (GPSR) is a set of rules that requires consumer products to be safe and our obligations to ensure this.

If you have any concerns about our products, you can contact us on ProductSafety@springernature.com

In case Publisher is established outside the EU, the EU authorized representative is:

Springer Nature Customer Service Center GmbH
Europaplatz 3
69115 Heidelberg, Germany

Batch number: 10731395

Printed by Printforce, the Netherlands